'A valuable and creative stimulus to our knowledge of the human chaos that occurs when individuals and communities are exposed to horrific and life threatening situations. This work makes a unique contribution in its integration of disaster, war and other studies.'

From the Foreword by Professor Raphael

The aims of this book are twofold – to improve understanding of the human experience of trauma at the individual and community levels, and to help the victims of trauma. The range of issues covered is impressive, from the psychosocial development of the experience of terror through the biological basis of posttraumatic stress reactions to practical strategies for prevention and treatment. The editors have sought to impart understanding, order, and predictability to the experience of trauma and disasters in the belief that the way to recovery is through the mastery and structuring of chaotic events.

The contributors, among them the leading clinicians and research workers in this field, present observational reports and empirical studies which range from responses to individual acts of violence to the effects of well-known disasters affecting hundreds or thousands of people. Distinctions are drawn between responses to manmade and natural disasters, and the particular needs of rescue and disaster workers are considered.

The emphasis throughout this book is on preparedness, prevention and care through psychiatric and other interventions in both civilian and military settings. This is a book which will inform clinicians, administrators and research workers who recognize that, if disaster plans do not consider the psychological effects of trauma, the consequences will overwhelm all available services and resources, exhausting rescue workers as well as victims.

INDIVIDUAL AND COMMUNITY
RESPONSES TO TRAUMA AND DISASTER:
THE STRUCTURE OF HUMAN CHAOS

INDIVIDUAL AND COMMUNITY RESPONSES TO TRAUMA AND DISASTER: THE STRUCTURE OF HUMAN CHAOS

Edited by

ROBERT J. URSANO

BRIAN G. McCAUGHEY

CAROL S. FULLERTON

Foreword by

BEVERLEY RAPHAEL

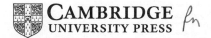

Published by the Press Syndicate of the University of Cambridge
The Pitt Building, Trumpington Street, Cambridge CB2 1RP
40 West 20th Street, New York, NY 10011-4211, USA
10 Stamford Road, Oakleigh, Melbourne 3166, Australia

© Cambridge University Press 1994

First published 1994

Printed in Great Britain at the University Press, Cambridge

A catalogue record for this book is available from the British Library

Library of Congress cataloguing in publication data

Individual and community responses to trauma and disaster: the
  structure of human chaos / edited by Robert J. Ursano, Brian G.
  McCaughey, Carol S. Fullerton; foreword by Beverley Raphael.
    p.   cm.
    Includes index.
    ISBN 0-521-41633-7 (hardback)
    1. Disasters – Psychological aspects. 2. Post-traumatic stress
  disorder. I. Ursano, Robert J., 1947– . II. McCaughey, Brian G. III. Fullerton, Carol S.
  [DNLM: 1. Stress Disorders, Post-Traumatic. 2. Disasters.
  3. Survival. WM 170 I39 1994]
  BF789.D5I63   1994
  155.9'35 – dc20
  DNLM/DLC
  for Library of Congress   93-13036   CIP

ISBN 0 521 41633 7   hardback

Contents

Contributors

Paul T. Bartone, PhD
Research Psychologist, Department of Military Psychiatry, Walter Reed Army Institute of Research, Washington, DC

Andrew Baum, PhD
Professor, Departments of Medical Psychology, Psychiatry, and Neuroscience, Uniformed Services University of the Health Sciences, F. Edward Hebert School of Medicine, Bethesda, Maryland

Laura M. Davidson, PhD
Research Assistant Professor, Departments of Medical Psychology, and Psychiatry, Uniformed Services University of the Health Sciences, F. Edward Hebert School of Medicine, Bethesda, Maryland; Consultant, Departments of Psychiatry and Neurology, Dwight D. Eisenhower Army Medical Center, Fort Gordon, Georgia

Michael P. Dinneen, MD, PhD
Director, Residency Training, Department of Psychiatry, National Naval Medical Center, Bethesda, Maryland

Alan Fontana, PhD
Director, PTSD Evaluations, VA Northeast Program Evaluation Center, Evaluation Division of the National Center for PTSD, Westhaven, Connecticut; Senior Research Scientist, Department of Psychiatry, Yale University School of Medicine, New Haven, Connecticut

Carol S. Fullerton, PhD
Assistant Professor (Research), Department of Psychiatry, Uniformed Services University of the Health Sciences, F. Edward Hebert School of Medicine, Bethesda, Maryland

Ellen T. Gerrity, PhD
Chief, Emergency Research Program, Violence and Traumatic Research Branch, National Institute of Mental Health, Rockville, Maryland

Mary C. Grace, MEd, MS
Senior Research Associate, Traumatic Stress Study Center, Department of Psychiatry, University of Cincinnati College of Medicine, Cincinnati, Ohio

Bonnie L. Green, PhD
Professor of Psychiatry, Georgetown University, Washington, DC

Jesse J. Harris, DSW
Dean, School of Social Work, University of Maryland, Baltimore, Maryland

Pal Herlofsen, MD
Military Psychiatrist, Joint Norwegian Armed Forces Medical Services, Oslo, Norway

Kenneth J. Hoffman, MD, MPH
Assistant Professor, Departments of Preventive Medicine, and Psychiatry, Uniformed Services University of the Health Sciences, F. Edward Hebert School of Medicine, Bethesda, Maryland

Harry C. Holloway, MD
Professor, Department of Psychiatry, Deputy Dean, Uniformed Services University of the Health Sciences, F. Edward Hebert School of Medicine, Bethesda, Maryland

Krzysztof Kaniasty, PhD
Assistant Professor, Department of Psychology, Indiana University of Pennsylvania, Indiana, Pennsylvania

Jacob D. Lindy, MD
Associate Dean, Cincinnati Psychoanalytic Institute; Associate Professor, Department of Psychiatry, University of Cincinnati, Ohio

Craig H. Llewellyn, MD
Professor and Chairman, Department of Military and Emergency Medicine, Uniformed Services University of the Health Sciences, F. Edward Hebert School of Medicine, Bethesda, Maryland

Ulrik F. Malt, MD, PhD
Professor of Psychiatry, Department of Psychosomatic and Behavioral Medicine, University of Oslo, National Hospital, Oslo, Norway

John M. Mateczun, MD, MPH, JD
Force Surgeon, Headquarters Marine Forces Pacific, Hawaii

James E. McCarroll, PhD
Research Psychologist, Department of Military Psychiatry, Walter Reed Army Institute of Research, Washington, DC

Brian G. McCaughey, DO
Head, Medical Corps Programs, Naval Health Sciences Education and Training Command, Bethesda, Maryland

Fran H. Norris, PhD
Assistant Professor, Department of Psychology, Georgia State University, Atlanta

Roger J. Pentzien, MD
Associate Professor, Department of Psychiatry, Uniformed Services University of the Health Sciences, F. Edward Hebert School of Medicine, Bethesda, Maryland

James F. Phifer, PhD
Assistant Professor and Clinical Neuropsychologist, Department of Rehabilitation Medicine, University of Alabama Medical School, Birmingham

Beverley Raphael, AM, MBBS, MD, FRANZCP, FRC
Professor and Head, Department of Psychiatry, University of Queensland, President Designate, Australasian Society Traumatic Stress Studies

Robert Rosenheck, MD
Director, VA Northeast Program Evaluation Center, Evaluation Division of the National Center for PTSD, Westhaven, Connecticut; Clinical Professor, Department of Psychiatry, Yale University School of Medicine, New Haven, Connecticut

Arieh Y. Shalev, MD
Director, Center for Traumatic Stress, Hadassah University Hospital, Jerusalem, Israel

Jon A. Shaw, MD
Professor and Director, Division of Child and Adolescent Psychiatry, University of Miami School of Medicine, Florida

Elizabeth M. Smith, PhD
Associate Professor, Department of Psychiatry, Washington University School of Medicine, St Louis, Missouri

Susan D. Solomon, PhD
Chief, Violence and Traumatic Stress Research Branch, National Institute of Mental Health, Rockville, Maryland

Peter Steinglass, MD
Director, Ackerman Institute for Family Therapy, New York

Robert J. Ursano, MD
Professor and Chairman, Department of Psychiatry, Uniformed Services University of the Health Sciences, F. Edward Hebert School of Medicine, Bethesda, Maryland

Lars Weisaeth, MD, PhD
Professor and Head, Division of Disaster Psychiatry, Medical Faculty, University of Oslo; Head, Department of Psychiatry, Joint Norwegian Armed Forces Medical Services, Norway

Kathleen M. Wright, PhD
Deputy Chief for Science, Department of Military Psychiatry, Walter Reed Army Institute of Research, Washington, DC

Foreword

In drawing together the themes of trauma and disaster that appear in this volume, the authors have provided a valuable and creative stimulus to our knowledge of the human chaos that occurs when individuals and communities are exposed to horrific and life threatening situations. This work makes a unique contribution in its integration of disaster, war and other trauma studies. In identifying common themes such as the nature of traumatic stress in accidents, disasters, and technological incidents, and the impact of such traumatic encounters with death, some of the aetiological processes underlying the effects of such trauma can be understood. These findings, integrating the contributions of many of the senior workers in the field, set in place a framework for the understanding of the trauma per se and its management. Each contributor brings not only a sound scientific appraisal but the wisdom and compassion of clinical understanding.

Psychosocial contexts, as well as culture, are identified as important modulating processes – they may be reflected in: the support which may buffer and facilitate working through and integration of the stressor experience; the form and pattern of community responses and their effects; the secondary trauma of relocation; the dislocation and disruption of social frameworks; and the social movements of professional support and debriefing.

Traumata are best understood when the responses are considered across individual, group, family and community perspectives; and from the vantage point of developmental systems from childhood to older adult life. Each level of description leads the reader to a more in-depth understanding with implications for research, service provision and policy and planning. Trauma reactions are described in terms of their phenomenology and occurrence in different trauma settings, and in different developmental contexts, from childhood through to older adult life.

The title of this book is aptly chosen – chaos does symbolize and reflect the response of individuals and communities to massive and overwhelming trauma. It is the mastery and structuring of this chaos that is the way to recovery.

Making meaning, making structure of chaos, is a vital human response, a return to functioning human systems. This exciting work will provide structure, meaning and pathways to guide researchers, clinicians and community disaster planners. The expertise and the humanity of the contributors who help to formulate this structure have produced an excellent and exciting volume – one that adds substantially to the field of trauma and disaster studies and moves these efforts to new heights.

Beverley Raphael, AM, MBBS, MD, FRANZCP, FRC

Professor and Head, Department of Psychiatry
The University of Queensland
Member, International Board of Traumatic Stress Studies
President Designate, Australasian Society
   Traumatic Stress Studies

Preface

Traumas and disasters throw lives into chaos and fill individuals with the terror of the unexpected and the fear of loss, injury and death. Trauma is always a catalyst for change and adjustment; for some it also becomes a life long wound. A surprisingly high number of people are exposed to traumatic events each year. The effects of such events extend well beyond the direct victims to include their families, their communities, and those who try to help. All become part of the trauma and disaster community.

Much can be learned from these groups to better understand the human experience of trauma and to help those who are its victims. These are the goals of this volume. This book spans a wide array of traumas and disasters – from technological and natural disasters to the manmade disaster of war. There are many unique aspects of these various disasters, but also, frequently unnoticed common threads. All traumas and disasters stir terror; often they include exposure to death and the experience of physical injury. Fears of contamination, loss of home and the resulting relocation can further complicate recovery. Manmade and natural disasters differ in the degree to which they are felt to be preventable and controllable. When one asks who are the victims of trauma, there are no excluded groups. The victims of trauma span all ages and include groups and communities which may be far distant from an immediate disaster site. From biology to sociology, the acute and chronic effects of traumatic stress can be profound.

The format and content of this volume are designed to highlight the commonalties as well as the unique factors among traumatic events. The book brings together both observational reports and empirical studies in order to make the findings convey their own story and make them usable to the researcher, the clinician and the administrator. Both the practical implications and the areas in which we need more understanding are emphasized.

Many people have made this work possible and to them we owe our thanks. Of course, this includes the outstanding group of contributors to this volume. They represent the cutting edge of thinking in the area of traumatic stress and disasters and in the application of this knowledge to the real world. We also greatly appreciate the support of Drs Harry Holloway, James Zimble, David Marlowe and Jay Sanford. Their support has provided both the opportunity and the vision for much of the effort that has gone into this volume. Finally, and most importantly, are those individuals and communities who, by sharing their experience of trauma and disaster, remind us all of the depth of the human experience, and educate us in how to help others who may suffer the effects of traumatic events.

Part I
Introduction

1

Trauma and disaster

ROBERT J. URSANO, CAROL S. FULLERTON and
BRIAN G. McCAUGHEY

You spoiled it: why did you spoil it? I'd like everything to be normal. Michael
Jackson ... wanted everyone to be normal. I was in the hospital as a psychiatric
patient, but I am not a psychiatric patient at all. I don't have any complaints ...
seems my brain is too much concentrated on. I love my father ... I'd like you to be
healthy. I'd like me to be healthy and to be sent to America.
  Our, our, our Yerivan. My mother did her hair like this. First and foremost I must
become like my mother ... I am ashamed. This is my secret. It is not a secret.
(Quote from a 16 year-old girl shortly after the 1988 Armenian earthquake.)

Trauma and disasters are a part of our everyday lives, despite our wishes.
With the advent of mass communications, we are more aware than ever of
the frequency of these events; we see and hear both manmade and natural
disasters from around the globe rather than only in our own community. In
the modern political world, the manmade traumas of war, chemical
weapons, terrorism, hostage events, and nuclear accidents are of particular
concern. These traumatic events often have widespread and devastating
impacts on health and national and community stability, even when only a
few individuals are primary victims.

The human chaos of disasters is not random. Rather traumas and
disasters are structured by the complex feelings, thoughts and behaviors
which are part of every disaster and trauma. For most individuals these
feelings, thoughts and behaviors are transitory. For some, they linger long
after the traumatic event has passed, recalled in memory by new experiences
which serve as a reminder of the past trauma.

Traumas and disasters affect hundreds of thousands every year: victims,
their relatives, their friends, disaster workers, and witnesses. In recent
years, there has been a significant increase in mortality in nearly all types of
disasters. In the 1960s the mortality rate per event was 750 for earthquakes,

3

158 for floods and 88 for cyclones. In the decade of the 1970s these rates rose to 4871 for earthquakes, 213 for floods and 2291 for cyclones. The increase appears to be due to increasing population density, urbanization and climatic change. When examined across countries, less developed countries have a greater morbidity and mortality from disasters than do more developed countries, even when population density is controlled (Guha-Sapir, 1989). The long-term and chronic effects of famine, water-borne diseases and disability are rarely included in these estimates.

Records in the United States indicate that a large proportion of the nation is regularly affected by disasters (Federal Emergency Management Agency, 1984; Rubin & Nahavandian, 1987). In 1987, over 120000 individuals died of trauma and violence. Between 1965 and 1985, 31 states experienced five or more presidentially declared disasters. Between 1974 and 1980, 37 major catastrophes occurred in the United States. From October 1979 to September 1980, over 688000 persons and 90000 different families received emergency care following a disaster. In the 99th and 100th United States Congress, over 175 Bills were introduced to deal with disasters, terrorism, and war victims. In 1990 alone, there were 35 presidentially declared disasters which involved 585 counties; over $2 billion were obligated by the Federal Emergency Management Agency to assist the victims of these disasters. Breslau et al. (1991) estimated the lifetime prevalence of exposure to traumatic events as 39.1% in a random sample of 1007 young adults from a large health maintenance organization in Detroit, Michigan. Norris (1988) estimated that 6–7% of the United States population are exposed to a disaster or trauma each year – ranging from motor vehicle accidents and crime to hurricanes and tornadoes. In a representative sample of women over the age of 18 in the United States, Kilpatrick (1992) found 68.9% had been exposed to a traumatic event at some time in their lives.

The financial cost of traumas and disasters is enormous. The actual cost of any disaster is difficult to estimate, but certainly it includes the cost of property loss, disaster relief efforts, lost income, and the cost of health care. Although records are incomplete and inaccurate, international agencies estimate that disaster relief efforts cost over one trillion US dollars each year (Guha-Sapir, 1989). In the United States, direct federal assistance from the Federal Emergency Management Agency (FEMA) totaled over $6 billion from 1965 to 1985. In 1989, the American Red Cross spent $14057000 for the victims of Hurricane Hugo, and $19500000 for the victims of the 1989 Loma Pretia earthquake in San Francisco, California. It is estimated that, in the year 2000, over 1700 deaths will occur in the United

States owing to major disasters and property and income loss will total more than $17 billion.

The psychological responses of individuals to trauma vary greatly. The meaning of any traumatic event is a complex interaction of the event itself and the individual's past, present, and expected future as well as biological givens and social context (Ursano, Kao, Fullerton, 1992). The meaning of the trauma affects not only how the trauma is experienced initially, but also the way in which recovery occurs and life is reestablished. Overall, most individuals exposed to traumatic events and disasters do quite well and do not suffer prolonged psychiatric illnesses. But for some, psychiatric illness, behavioral change, or alterations in physical health result. Certainly, no one goes through profound life events unchanged.

Communities also suffer the ravages of trauma and disasters. In the modern world, communities extend well beyond their geographic borders. Families and work ties can spread throughout a country, a nation or the world. Rapid transportation and communication have made the global village a reality which is evident in every disaster situation. The ability of communities to plan for, and recover from, a disaster must be the focus of a community's leadership and rescue services. If disaster plans do not consider the psychological effects of trauma, the consequences can overwhelm all available services and resources, exhausting rescue workers as well as victims. In Israel at the time of the first SCUD missile attack during the Persian Gulf War, over 200 people reported to the emergency room having injected themselves with atropine thinking they had been exposed to chemical gas. Over 500 admissions occurred owing to acute anxiety (Solomon, 1992). The psychological effects of a disaster, manmade or natural, can quickly overwhelm the medical and social rehabilitation resources if they are not recognized and managed.

Defining traumatic events and disasters

A traumatic event is recognized by the nature of the event, by the effects of the trauma on individuals and groups, and by the responses of individuals and groups to the event. In general, traumatic events are dangerous, overwhelming, and sudden (Figley, 1985). They are marked by their extreme or sudden force, typically causing fear, anxiety, withdrawal, and avoidance. Traumatic events have high intensity, are unexpected, infrequent, and vary in duration from acute to chronic. They may affect a single individual, e.g. a motor vehicle accident or a violent crime, or they may affect entire communities, e.g. an earthquake or a hurricane. Disasters, by definition, are both traumatic, and overwhelm the available community resources, further threatening the individuals' and the community's ability to cope.

The American Psychiatric Association (1987) defines a traumatic event as '... a psychologically distressing event that is outside the range of usual human experience (i.e. outside the range of such common experiences as simple bereavement, chronic illness, business losses, and marital conflict).... would be markedly distressing to almost anyone, and is usually experienced with intense fear, terror, and helplessness.... either a serious threat to one's life or physical integrity; a serious threat or harm to one's children, spouse, or other close relatives or friends; sudden destruction of one's home or community; or seeing another person who has recently been, or is being seriously injured or killed as a result of an accident or physical violence. In some cases, the trauma may be learning about a serious threat or harm to a close friend or relative, e.g. that one's child has been kidnapped, tortured, or killed. The trauma may be experienced alone (e.g. rape or assault) or in the company of groups of people (e.g. military combat). Traumatic events include natural disasters (e.g. floods, earthquakes), accidental disasters (e.g. car accidents with serious physical injury, airplane crashes, large fires, collapse of physical structures), and deliberately caused events (e.g. bombing, torture, death camps). Sometimes there is a concomitant physical component of the trauma, which may even involve direct damage to the central nervous system (e.g. malnutrition, head injury)' (pp. 247–8). Recent discussions which will result in new psychiatric diagnostic nomenclature (DSM-IV) have emphasized the life threatening nature of traumatic events.

Disasters are either natural or manmade. Natural disasters include hurricanes, tornadoes, floods, earthquakes and avalanches. Manmade disasters include airplane crashes, personal assaults, serious motor vehicle accidents, war, terrorism, and hostage and prisoner of war events. Psychological responses to traumatic events vary depending on the type of disaster (for a detailed discussion, see Weisaeth chapter). The impact phase of a disaster may last seconds, hours or days. Disasters cause social disruption, loss and damage to property, and mass casualties. The effects on individuals and communities are physical, psychological, and social; both immediate and long term. The time course of recovery can vary greatly.

Trauma and psychological health

The study of psychological responses to trauma began with observations of the emotional reactions to one of the oldest manmade traumas – war. Early interest in the concept of posttraumatic disorders is found in the literature on reactions to the American Civil War when 'nostalgia' was used to describe the symptoms of combat stress. Later, in the First World War, terms such as 'shell shock', 'battle fatigue', and 'war neurosis' were common descriptors of the emotional responses to war (Trimble, 1985). The 'thousand mile stare' described the exhausted foot soldier on the verge of collapse. The symptoms of combat stress varied with the individual and the context but included anxiety, startle reactions and numbness (Grinker & Spiegel, 1945).

Studies of the responses of various populations to traumatic experiences broadened our understanding of the psychological effects of trauma, e.g. concentration camp survivors (Eitinger & Strom, 1973; Matussek, 1971; Chodoff, 1963; Krystal, 1968), and rescue workers following the Hiroshima devastation (Lifton, 1967). Several modern disasters have been studied in detail: the Coconut Grove Nightclub fire (Adler, 1943; Lindemann, 1944), the 1972 Buffalo Creek flood (Erikson, 1976; Gleser, Green & Winget, 1981; Rangell, 1976; Titchener & Kapp, 1976), the Chowchilla kidnappings (Terr, 1983), and the Mount St Helen's volcanic eruption (Shore, Tatum & Vollmer, 1986; Shore, Vollmer & Tatum, 1989). Early systematic studies across different types of traumas note two types of responses: intrusive and denial-avoidant symptoms. Horowitz (1976) made an important contribution by elaborating on these two types of responses. He identified several themes reported by patients: fear of a repetition of the stressful event, shame over helplessness or emptiness, rage at the source of the stress, guilt or shame over aggressive impulses, fear of identification or merger with the victims, and sadness over loss.

An important advance in the scientific study of responses to trauma was the formal recognition of stress syndromes, 'traumatic neuroses', in the *Diagnostic and statistical manual of mental disorders* (DSM-I) (American Psychiatric Association, 1952). Later, posttraumatic syndromes were referred to as 'transient situational disturbances' and 'adjustment reactions' (American Psychiatric Association, 1968). The diagnosis of posttraumatic stress disorder (PTSD) first appeared in the psychiatric nosology in DSM-III (American Psychiatric Association, 1980). The description of PTSD was refined in DSM-III-R (American Psychiatric Association, 1987) by operationally defining the stressor criterion and providing information about symptoms in a broader range of populations including traumatized children.

There are now numerous studies which have examined the emotional, behavioral, and physiological consequences of catastrophic events. Yet many aspects of the health effects of trauma are not well understood. Many individuals who are exposed to a traumatic event will have some symptoms. However, for most this will be 'a "normal" response to an abnormal event'. For most, these symptoms are transitory. The symptoms appear to be metabolized – digested – and the individual suffers no long-term effects. For some, however, the symptoms are more enduring.

The effects of traumatic events are not always bad. Although many survivors of the 1974 tornado in Xenia, Ohio experienced psychological distress, the majority described positive outcomes: learning that they could handle crises effectively, feeling that they were better off for having met this type of challenge (Taylor, 1977; Quarentelli, 1985). One victim of the Oakland fires of 1992 told reporters 'I value my family so much now. Its amazing how the little "things" [in life] matter. The fire taught me that and I owe it a debt of gratitude for teaching me this lesson.' Trauma may also bring a community closer together or reorient an individual to new priorities, goals or values. Sledge, Boydstun and Rahe (1980) found that approximately one-third of US Air Force Vietnam era prisoners of war (POWs) reported having benefited from their prisoner of war experience. These POWs tended to be the ones who had suffered the most traumatic experiences.

Trauma acts as a psychic organizer, producing a clustering of specific affects, cognitions, and behaviors that can be released under certain symbolic, environmental, or biological stimuli (Holloway & Ursano, 1984) For some, trauma facilitates a move toward health (Card, 1983; Sledge et al., 1980; Ursano, Boydstun & Wheatley, 1981). A traumatic experience can become the center around which a victim reorganizes a previously disorganized life, reorienting values and goals (Ursano, 1987).

Posttraumatic stress disorders

A number of psychiatric disturbances have been associated with exposure to traumatic events. Although PTSD has been the most studied traumatic disorder in recent years, it should be remembered that it is not the only psychiatric disorder to follow traumatic events. Major depression, generalized anxiety disorder, and substance abuse are also well documented after exposure to traumas and disasters (for review, see Davidson & Fairbank, 1992; Kulka et al., 1990; Karem, 1991; Rundell et al., 1989). The diagnosis of PTSD requires exposure to a traumatic event. In addition to exposure, there must be reexperiencing (intrusive), avoidant and arousal symptoms (see Table 1.1). The symptoms must also have been present for at least one month.

Table 1.1. *Posttraumatic stress disorder*

A. Exposure to a traumatic event

B. Reexperiencing symptoms (at least one of the following)
   1. Intrusive recollections
   2. Dreams
   3. Acting or feeling as if the traumatic event were recurring
   4. Distress at exposure to events that symbolize or resemble trauma

C. Avoidant symptoms (at least three of the following)
   1. Avoid thoughts or feelings associated with the trauma
   2. Avoid activities or situations that arouse recollections
   3. Inability to recall important aspects of the trauma
   4. Diminished interest in significant activities
   5. Feelings of detachment or estrangement from others
   6. Restricted range of affect
   7. Sense of foreshortened future

D. Arousal symptoms (at least two of the following)
   1. Difficulty falling asleep
   2. Irritability or outbursts of anger
   3. Difficulty concentrating
   4. Hypervigilance
   5. Exaggerated startle
   6. Physiologic reactivity upon exposure to events that symbolize or resemble the trauma

One of the best predictors of psychiatric illness after a traumatic event is the severity of the trauma. Psychopathology before trauma is neither necessary nor sufficient to the diagnosis of psychiatric illness after trauma. This is not to say that it is unrelated. Most studies show that those with psychiatric illness prior to a traumatic event or disaster may be at increased risk. However, it is also clear that those with no previous psychiatric illness are also at risk. In studies of World War II, the frequency of psychiatric casualties was highly correlated with the rate of wounded and killed in action and, therefore, with battlefield intensity. The more intense the battle, the greater the rate of psychiatric casualties. Studies of USAF prisoners of war from the Vietnam era also contribute to our understanding of the relationship of trauma and illness. These prisoners of war were highly screened pilots, nearly all of whom were college graduates, selected and trained for combat. Those who were shot down prior to 1969 experienced substantially worse conditions, with greater torture, maltreatment and solitary confinement than did those shot down after 1969 (Ursano, 1981; Ursano et al., 1981). The two groups were very comparable on all other measures. The pre-1969 group showed greater rates of psychiatric disturbance over the five year follow-up period after return. A small group of these prisoners of war had incidentally been seen for psychiatric evaluation prior to being shot down. Of this group, some had been diagnosed as having no psychiatric illness after an exceptionally thorough assessment. Some of these fliers developed psychiatric illness after captivity. Others who had a history of psychiatric illness prior to shootdown, did not develop psychiatric illness after being prisoners of war. These data support the view that, in severe trauma, the greater the trauma the greater the risk of psychiatric illness. In addition, the small group in the case study indicates that psychiatric illness prior to a traumatic event is neither necessary nor sufficient to the development of psychiatric illness after severe trauma.

Another set of data which emphasize the importance of the degree of trauma is a study of twins discordant for service in Vietnam (Goldberg et al., 1990). Using mail and telephone interviews, 715 twin pairs discordant for service in Vietnam were examined. Of this group, 16.8% of those who served in Vietnam had current PTSD; 5.0% of those who had not served had the diagnosis. Among those with high levels of combat exposure, there was a ninefold increase in the prevalence of PTSD compared to their matched, nonexposed twin. Combined with the World War II and the Vietnam prisoner of war studies, these data highlight the importance of the degree of trauma rather than preexisting psychiatric illness or even biology in the development of psychiatric illness after traumatic events.

Prevalence and incidence of PTSD

Several studies have examined the prevalence of PTSD in the general population, and in groups at risk, i.e. those exposed to extreme stressors such as war and combat, mass casualty disasters such as plane crashes, and natural disasters such as earthquakes, floods, and tornadoes (for review, see Davidson & Fairbank, 1992). Prevalence is the proportion of individuals in a population who have a particular disease. This rate provides an estimate of the probability (risk) that an individual in the population will have the illness at a given point in time (Hennekens & Buring, 1987). In contrast, incidence refers to the number of new cases of disease that appear over a specific period of time in a population of individuals at risk.

Prevalence in the general population Using the Diagnostic Interview Schedule (DIS) in the Epidemiological Catchment Area (ECA) survey, Helzer Robins and McEvoy et al. (1987) found a 1% lifetime prevalence of PTSD for adults in the St Louis area. In the North Carolina ECA survey site,

Davidson and Fairbank (1992) found a 1.3% lifetime prevalence of PTSD among adults in the Piedmont region. In a random sample of young adults from a health maintenance organization in the Detroit, Michigan area, Breslau et al. (1991) found a 9.2% lifetime prevalence of PTSD using the DIS. This higher rate may reflect the greater exposure to traumas in the inner cities. Shore et al. (1989) used the DIS to examine responses to the Mount St Helens volcanic eruption and found that the control group of individuals not exposed to the disaster had a lifetime prevalence rate of 3%. Kilpatrick (1992), using telephone interviews of a national sample of women over age 18, found a 12.8% lifetime prevalence of PTSD while 5.2% met diagnostic criteria for PTSD in the past 6 months.

Incidence in populations at risk In the St Louis study, Helzer et al. (1987) found the incidence of PTSD in combat veterans to be 6.3%. In wounded Vietnam veterans, the rate was 20%. Civilians exposed to physical attack showed a 3.5% rate. This study, however, had a very small number of trauma victims. A large study completed by the Center for Disease Control (1987) examined 2490 Vietnam veterans and found 14.7% of Vietnam theater veterans had combat related PTSD compared to 0.6% of those without Vietnam experience. There was no difference between the Vietnam and the NonVietnam Groups in noncombat related PTSD (1.8% vs. 2.6%).

The major study commissioned by the United States Congress and the Department of Veterans Affairs to look at Vietnam veterans used the Structured Clinical Interview as the primary diagnostic instrument (Kulka et al., 1991). This study found current PTSD in 15.2% of male and 8.5% of female Vietnam theater veterans. The lifetime prevalence rates in these groups was 30.9% for males and 26.9% for females. The rates were four times greater for males in the highest war zone stress areas, and seven times greater for females in the greatest war zone stress areas. The rates were higher for those who were injured.

Rates of PTSD in veterans of the Persian Gulf War appeared to be low immediately upon return (Ursano & Rosenheck, 1991). Initial systematic studies have generally supported these observations with rates of PTSD of approximately 9%, although these varied greatly (Rosenheck et al., 1992).

Winfield et al. (1990) found a 3.3% incidence of PTSD in sexual assault victims in North Carolina. Breslau et al. (1991) found that 23.6% of those exposed to a traumatic event developed PTSD. In Breslau's population, risk factors for PTSD following trauma were: early separation from parents, neuroticism, preexisting anxiety or depression, and family history of anxiety. Shore et al. (1989) found incidence rates of 3.6% in individuals exposed to the Mount St Helens volcanic eruption. Kilpatrick (1992) reported a 45.2% lifetime prevalence of PTSD among women who had experienced both a life threat and injury due to trauma. In this same sample Kilpatrick found 19.5% current PTSD.

Features of PTSD

Comorbidity is common with PTSD. Major depression, anxiety disorders, and alcoholism often coexist with PTSD in the general population (Breslau et al., 1991; Davidson & Fairbank, 1992; Helzer et al., 1987), and among veterans (Behar, 1984; Breslau & Davis, 1986; Escobar et al., 1983; Green et al., 1989; Helzer et al., 1987; Kulka et al., 1990; Roszell, McFall & Malas, 1991; Shalev, Bleich & Ursano, 1990; Sierles et al., 1983). Shalev et al.'s (1990) findings highlight the importance of cigarette abuse among individuals with PTSD, an often forgotten substance of abuse. Of those with PTSD, from 62% to 92% have a previous or concurrent psychiatric disorder (Davidson & Fairbank, 1992; Helzer et al., 1987; Shore et al., 1989), compared to only 15% to 33% of nonPTSD comparison groups (Davidson & Fairbank, 1992; Helzer et al., 1987).

Increasing attention has been given to the biological aspects of PTSD. The literature suggests that several biological systems are affected by PTSD, e.g. the central and peripheral sympathetic nervous system (SNS), the hypothalamic–pituitary–adrenocortical (HPA) axis, the endogenous opioid system, and the diurnal sleep cycle. Several recent review articles and books provide comprehensive reports of laboratory and clinical findings on the biological aspects of PTSD (Boehnlein, 1989; Burgeswatson, Hoffman & Wilson, 1988; Davidson & Nemeroff, 1989; Giller, 1990; Jones & Barlow, 1990; Kolb, 1988; Krystal et al., 1989; Van der Kolk, 1988; Wolf & Mosnaim, 1990).

Some biological aspects of PTSD have been examined using animal models (for review, see Bremner, Southwick & Chorney, 1991). The experimental model of inescapable stress may parallel the exposure to stress experienced by individuals with PTSD. Seligman & Beagley (1975) made an important early contribution with their animal findings that indicated behavioral and neurochemical changes resulting from inescapable stress. The behavioral outcome was termed 'learned helplessness'. Learned helplessness describes the situation in which animals previously exposed to inescapable shock no longer attempt to escape subsequent shock even if there is a way to escape the shock. Inescapable stress is associated with learning and memory impairments that are related to alterations in certain brain structures including the temporal lobe, amygdala, and hippocampus (Squire & Zola-Morgan, 1991). Inescapable stress is also associated with conditioned fear responses related to exposure to trauma (Davis, 1986), such as the fear and terror evoked in a rape victim who experiences a reminder of the trauma. Animal models can be used to identify neurobiological changes that occur in humans who develop PTSD.

Shalev (1991) identified the acoustic startle reaction as important to the physiologic responses seen in PTSD. Patients with PTSD show a lack of habituation to acoustic stimuli which in other subjects easily produces habituation and decreased startle response to acoustic stimuli. Further study is needed to replicate this finding and to determine whether it is a biological marker for PTSD or a conditioning effect of the trauma.

Features of posttraumatic stress disorders are often seen in disaster and rescue workers (Bartone et al., 1989; Durham, McCammon & Allison, 1985; Fullerton, McCarroll, Ursano & Wright, 1992; Raphael, 1986; Wright et al., 1990). These individuals are often hidden victims of disasters and traumas. Disaster and rescue workers are repeatedly exposed to mutilated bodies, mass destruction, and life threatening situations while doing physically demanding work which itself creates fatigue, sleep loss, and often risk to one's life. They also experience the stresses of their role as a help provider (Raphael, 1986). Repeated exposure to trauma can put rescue workers, especially first responders such as fire fighters and police officers, at increased risk of developing posttraumatic stress disorders (Durham, McCammon & Allison, 1985; Keating et al. 1987; Breslau et al., 1991; McFarlane, 1988a, 1988b; McFarlane & Raphael, 1984).

Over 650 fire fighters are forced to retire each year due to occupational illness – including psychological stress (Hildebran, 1984). Lifton (1967) described the psychological distress of rescue workers in Hiroshima. He found that feelings of fear, anger, hatred, and resentment often interfered with effective functioning. Rescue workers in the Granville, Australia, 1977 rail disaster reported feeling helpless and overwhelmed by the magnitude and unexpectedness of the disaster, the sight and smell of the dead bodies, the anguish of the relatives, the suffering of the injured, and the extreme pressure of the work (Raphael, 1986). Approximately 20% of the rescue workers reported feelings of depression, anxiety, and insomnia one month following the disaster. McFarlane (1986) conducted a long-term study of psychiatric morbidity in fire fighters exposed to the Ash Wednesday bushfires in South Australia in 1983. Twenty-nine months after the bushfires, 21% of the 459 fire fighters were still experiencing recurring imagery that interfered with their lives.

Research on trauma and disaster

Despite these advances, many aspects of the posttraumatic stress disorders remain obscure. Present research includes studies of the etiology, taxonomy, and validity of PTSD (e.g. Goldberg et al., 1990; Jones & Barlow, 1990; Laufer, Brett & Gallops, 1985; March, 1990; Oei, Lim & Hennessy, 1990; Wolfe & Keane, 1990), and examination of disorders other than PTSD which may follow trauma (Karem, 1991; for review, see Rundell et al., 1989; Shalev et al., 1990). Current research has also examined: cooccurring diagnoses with PTSD (Breslau & Davis, 1986; Green et al., 1989; Roszell et al., 1991; Sierles et al., 1983); examination of the stressor criterion (Breslau & Davis, 1986; Brett, Spitzer & Williams, 1988; Feinstein & Dolan, 1991; Green et al., 1990; Lindy, Green & Grace, 1987; Ursano, 1987); and the relationship between indicators of chronic stress and symptoms of PTSD (Davidson & Baum, 1986).

The scientific study of trauma involves numerous conceptual, practical, and methodological dilemmas (for reviews, see Green, 1982; Baum, Solomon & Ursano, 1990). Understanding the salient issues in the study of trauma is important to researchers and can make the findings of this literature more helpful to community leaders and disaster planners.

Research in a trauma community

Research on trauma is often conducted in the field. Unlike laboratory research, field research allows only limited control over variables. Since disasters often strike suddenly and without warning, disaster sites are usually chaotic and resources are stressed beyond their limits. In order to study immediate responses to trauma, research teams must mobilize quickly, often without prior warning. The initial tasks of a research team are to gain an understanding of the unique aspects of the disaster environment, and to establish contacts for future collaboration. The research team must integrate smoothly into the disaster environment, an environment in which outsiders are often experienced as intrusive. Researchers are often experienced as 'wanting something' from an environment in which the resources are already insufficient. Researchers must be knowledgeable of the culture and customs of the groups they wish to study in order to be accepted by their 'coinvestigators', i.e. victims of the trauma and disaster workers.

Members of a research team, like other disaster workers, also experience the stresses of the traumatic event. Keeping alert to the signs of stress in the team is important to the health and functioning of the team (Brand et al., 1993). Team members need adequate rest and respite. The team leader must regulate the working hours. Excessively long working hours must be avoided. Dedication to the mission is important, however, overdedication can be a problem. It is useful to alert team members of the potential for overdedication. Recognizing this in oneself may be difficult, so training should emphasize being alert to overdedication in other team members. The team leader should implement any action to be taken and be aware that overdedication is often related to feeling important to the team. At times, being asked to take a timeout may result in feeling devalued, but it may be necessary.

Research methodology

Sampling (who to study?) Determining the type and extent of exposure to a traumatic event is complex. An epidemiologic perspective is critical to identifying the at-risk population and the probability of disease. The primary victims are those who directly experience a disaster. Others who may be effected by the disaster include disaster and rescue workers, mental health workers, clergy, witnesses to the disaster, relatives and friends. Some of these people may not even have been at the disaster site. Groups with differing degrees of exposure to the trauma can provide a 'dose response' variable to study the effects of the disaster or trauma. Control groups, i.e. individuals who were unexposed to the trauma and matched with trauma victims on certain characteristics, allow the researcher to examine the effects of the trauma by comparing the trauma victims to a similar group who did not experience the disaster.

Assessment (when to measure?) It is important to study the anticipatory, acute, and long-term responses to trauma. Some traumatic events have a warning phase prior to the actual event, such as volcano eruptions or the anticipation of a war deployment. Assessment of the anticipatory responses has important implications for coping with trauma. Acute responses to trauma must be measured soon after the traumatic event. Timing is essential and a rapid response by the research team is required in order to study these responses. For long-term follow-up studies, tracking subjects over time is costly, difficult and at times near impossible. Tracking is problematic with mobile populations such as the military, and in communities that have been uprooted by disasters such as floods or hurricanes. A plane crash usually involves following individuals who live in multiple locations.

Attrition – the loss of subjects over time – occurs for a variety of reasons: lack of interest or time, migration, illness, death, and fear of troublesome reminders of the traumatic event. Migration itself is important to study following community disasters in which some people move away and some choose to stay in a potentially unsafe environment. Illness or death can occur; in some cases possibly resulting from the trauma. In disaster populations, people may not want to be reminded of the tragedy for a variety of reasons including fear that troublesome images may return if they think back over the event. Those who drop out may be the ones who are having the most difficulty and are afraid to reveal their problems. Alternatively, the ones who are having difficulty may choose to remain in the study, hoping to receive help for troublesome symptoms. Potential sampling biases may thus be created. Therefore, it is important to follow-up individuals who drop out and at least find out their reasons. Assessment of reasons for dropouts can help determine whether a sampling bias is occurring. This is important to decisions about data analysis and should be reported in the write-up of the study.

Measurement (what to study and how to measure it?) Determining what and how to measure responses to trauma is a major research task. The use of standardized instruments facilitates the generalization of findings. Event specific questions can be used to describe aspects that are unique to a particular disaster event. A balance of standardized measures and event specific questions facilitates the study of generic as well as unique aspects of a traumatic event.

The measurement of psychological, physiological, and sociocultural responses to trauma is important to assessing health outcome. It may be difficult to determine problems that resulted specifically from a traumatic event. Some difficulties may have existed prior to the trauma and were made worse by the event. Baseline information often is collected retrospectively, except when data prior to the event are available. Symptom assessments should measure PTSD and other posttraumatic stress disorders.

Stress mediators are variables that influence the response to a trauma: background variables, social supports, preexisting illness, and sociocul-

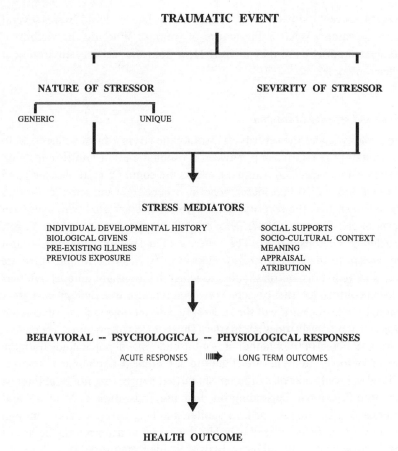

Fig. 1.1. Traumatic stress model.

tural context. Other life events also affect responses to trauma, or may occur as a result of trauma.

Trauma and health: a working model

Responses to trauma vary. Despite commonalities, no two individuals or traumas are exactly the same. In order to understand responses to traumatic events, it is important to consider the individual and his or her context. Our working model (Fig. 1.1) illustrates the relationships between traumatic events, stress mediators and health. The model addresses several basic questions. What is the nature of trauma? Who are the victims of traumas, and why are they at risk? How does the recovery environment affect outcome?

Type and severity of trauma

Both the type and the severity of a traumatic stressor must be assessed to understand the relationship between a traumatic event and its effects on health. Some aspects of traumatic events are common to all disasters and trauma and can be considered generic; others are event specific. Studies have shown that the severity of the stressor is correlated with symptom severity (Helzer et al., 1987; Penk et al., 1981; Shore et al., 1986; Yager, Loafer & Gallops, 1984). The severity of a stressor, however, is not equivalent to the type of stressor (Ursano, 1987). For example, there are stressors (e.g. pins, needles, nails) to which balloons are uniquely vulnerable in contrast to other objects. However, it is also true that, given a great enough force, the nature of the stressor (e.g. blunt object, sharp object, flat object, round object) does not matter. The balloon will pop no matter what. The best predictors of whether or not the balloon will pop include both the degree of force and the nature of the stressor. Some balloons may not pop at all and may only take on a different shape that may or may not be of interest or more functional, depending on their use and future. Individuals and trauma can be thought of in a similar manner. Given a severe enough trauma, its characteristics may be less important to determining the risk of psychiatric illness. But all individuals have their unique vulnerabilities.

Social supports

Social supports directly and indirectly contribute to the behavioral and mental health outcomes of individuals exposed to disasters. Social support is the comfort, assistance, and information an individual or group receives from others. Research findings on the relationship between social supports and health outcome are mixed (for review, see Wallston et al., 1983), suggesting the need to further examine social supports. Families can be an important source of emotional and instrumental support to the primary victims of trauma (Figley, 1983). They can provide comfort and understanding to disaster workers (Raphael, 1986). The spouse/significant other is likely to be an important part of the recovery environment following trauma (Fullerton et al., in press). The length of time one has lived in a disaster community can be an important contributor to the degree of distress experienced when disaster strikes (Fullerton et al., 1992)

Providing support during times of stress can be rewarding to the support provider, but it may also be stressful (Shumaker & Brownell, 1984; Solomon et al., 1987; Taylor, 1990; Fullerton et al., 1992). The support provider may become overwhelmed if the demands are experienced as excessive or burdensome. Although women may be more likely than men to respond in a supportive manner during times of stress (Kessler & McLeod, 1984), women may experience strong social supports as burdensome during these times (Solomon et al., 1987). Solomon (1992) found increased somatic and psychiatric distress among wives of veterans of the Lebanon war suffering from combat stress reactions and posttraumatic stress disorder. Solomon found evidence of stress associated with increased responsibility on the wife, and possible identification with her husband's symptoms. McCarroll et al., in press observed that spouses of mortuary workers were at times unwilling or unable to listen to worker's experiences of working with the dead. Fullerton et al. 1992 reported significant levels of intrusive and avoidant symptoms in significant others of mortuary workers even though they had no direct contact with the mortuary or the dead.

Appraisal, attribution and meaning

Appraisal has generally been construed as the process of evaluation of the meaning or significance of an experience in terms of its relationship to one's well-being (Lazarus & Folkman, 1984). Primary appraisal is the evaluation of the perceived threat to well-being and safety, as well as the perceived challenge and the potential for gain and growth (Lazarus & Folkman, 1984). Secondary appraisal is an individual's assessment of what, if anything, can be done to prevent or decrease harm (Folkman et al., 1986). This generally includes an individual's perception of how to reconstitute one's life and community, and how to understand what has happened. Understanding what has happened after a disaster often includes attribution of responsibility, i.e. the assigning of a cause to the events. Generally, causes are seen as either under one's control or outside of one's control. Events which are seen as controllable are usually experienced as less stressful.

The meaning or significance of an experience is another aspect of appraisal. In Yerivan, a city hard hit by the 1988 Armenian earthquake, the 16 year-old woman quoted at the opening of the book developed a delirium, possibly secondary to a pneumonia after the earthquake. Her psychotic thinking continued, however, after her infection had been cured. Psychotic delusions after a trauma are unusual but illustrate the attempt to recover, to reconstitute the world through fantasy, and to develop a cognitive map of the traumatic events, and what must be done to go on. The young woman's mother had died in their home when it collapsed in the disaster. The young woman continuously brushed her hair, as her mother had done for her. Her comments were dismissed by her care providers as delirious. In fact, they reveal a poetic description, mixing her experience of her lost city and her lost mother along with her plan to reclaim her life, to make everything normal and bring it back the way it was.

Individuals and groups actively construct the meaning of traumatic events (Dollinger, 1986; Green, Wilson & Lindy, 1985; Holloway & Ursano, 1984). The construction of meaning is an active process which affects the outcome of traumatic experiences and appears itself to be affected by trauma (Ursano, Kao & Fullerton in press). A traumatic event may serve as a stimulus that evokes or 'turns on' certain of the mechanisms by which meaning is constructed, such as thinking by similarity (Ursano & Fullerton, 1990). Meaning is a rich and varied concept which is not static but results from the interaction of past history, present context and physiological state. Thus, the meaning of a traumatic event changes over time with the individuals' ever changing psychosocial context. For example, immediately following the crash of an Air Force C-141 cargo plane, the remaining members of the squadron were convinced that the crash must have been caused by aircraft failure. But, soon they had to start flying the plane again. By that time, the squadron believed the crash had been caused by human error. 'I would never do that', was the prominent belief. The meaning of a traumatic event both constrains and facilitates certain behaviors, in this case the ability to fly again.

The loss of a child in a disaster carries a particular meaning. Singh and Raphael (1981) observed that parents who lost children did the least well of any bereaved following a rail accident in Australia. During a satellite 'telemedicine' consultation following the December, 1988 Armenian earthquake, victims of the earthquake described the loss of their children as the loss of 'the future', a very particular type of threat. These fears were further evident in a rumor which spread through the community that children were being kidnapped. Child victims of any trauma carry powerful and far reaching meanings to those exposed.

Another aspect of appraisal is the perception of risk, i.e. the expectation of injury and the fear of loss of life. These perceptions may be unique to an individual or shared by groups or communities. The actual risk may be very different from the perceived threat. The distinction between perceived threat and actual risk can identify different cognitive styles evident in the face of traumatic events. The dimensions of perceived threat and actual risk (exposure) can be used in a 2×2 matrix to identify four basic groups of perceived threat and actual risk perceptions: high perceived threat/high actual risk; high perceived threat/low actual risk; low perceived threat/high actual risk; and low perceived threat/low actual risk. (A similar model was used by Schwartz (1984) in studies of physiologic arousal. He used the Marlowe–Crowne Scale of Social Desirability (Crowne & Marlowe, 1960; Evans, 1982) to group individuals based on their level of physiologic response compared to their level of reported anxiety.) These four groups can be expected to vary in the cognitive mechanisms they use to manage the experience of threat.

These cognitive styles have consequences for health behaviors which can alter the risks of morbidity and mortality. Of particular interest are those individuals who see threat when little risk is present and those who see no threat when actually high risk is involved. Studies are needed to assess the psychological and behavioral effects of disaster on these subpopulations. A tendency to deny the risk that is present will affect the ability or willingness of a trauma victim to take the time needed for respite, rest and recovery. Conversely, a tendency to identify oneself as a victim will affect the individual's willingness to return to work, a necessary part of the normalization of the trauma experience and of long-term recovery. For example, a physician who was hit by a car while riding a bicycle, despite knowing he was bleeding, got up immediately to direct traffic, knowing there was substantial risk of injury secondary to his own movement. This counter-phobic activity increased his risk of morbidity and mortality. Individuals with the two extreme cognitive styles, described by the 2×2 matrix, may be high risk subpopulations.

Our journey begins . . .

Although there has been increased interest in examining the emotional, behavioral, and physiological consequences of catastrophic events, many aspects of the health effects of trauma are not well understood. In this book we explore individual and group responses to trauma; we journey through lives thrown into chaos by trauma. In the chapters that follow, the understanding that emerges imparts an order and predictability to the experience of trauma and disasters. Through understanding this order, this structure, we can better help those exposed to traumatic events.

References

Adler, A. (1943). Neuropsychiatric complications in victims of Boston's Coconut
    Grove disaster. *Journal of the American Medical Association*, **123**, 1098–101.
American Psychiatric Association. (1952). *Diagnostic and statistical manual of
    mental disorders*. Washington, DC: American Psychiatric Association.
American Psychiatric Association. (1968). *Diagnostic and statistical manual of
    mental disorders*. 2nd edn., Washington, DC: American Psychiatric
    Association.
American Psychiatric Association. (1980). *Diagnostic and statistical manual of
    mental disorders*. 3rd edn., Washington, DC: American Psychiatric
    Association.
American Psychiatric Association. (1987). *Diagnostic and statistical manual of
    mental disorders*. 3rd edn. Revised, Washington, DC: American Psychiatric
    Association, pp. 247–51.
Bartone, P. T., Ursano, R. J., Wright, K. M. & Ingraham, L. H. (1989). The
    impact of a military air disaster on the health of assistance workers. *Journal
    of Nervous and Mental Disease*, **177**(6), 317–28.
Baum, A. (1987). Toxins, technology, and natural disasters. In G. R. Vanden Bos
    & B. D. Bryant (eds.), *Cataclysms, crises, and catastrophes: psychology in
    action*. Washington, DC: American Psychological Association, pp. 5–54.
Baum, A., Solomon, S. D. & Ursano, R. J. (1990). Emergency/disaster studies:
    practical, conceptual, and methodological issues. In J. P. Wilson (ed.), *The
    international handbook of traumatic stress syndromes*. New York, NY:
    Plenum Press Inc.
Behar, D. (1984). Confirmation of concurrent illnesses in post-traumatic stress
    disorder (ltr). *American Journal of Psychiatry*, **141**, 1310.
Boehnlein, J. K. (1989). The process of research in posttraumatic stress disorder.
    Perspectives in Biology and Medicine, **32**, 455–64.
Brandt, G. T., Fullerton, C. S., Ursano., R. J. & Noward, A. E. (1993, May).
    Psychiatric Consultations to Disaster. Presented at the 146th meeting of the
    American Psychiatric Association, San Francisco, CA.
Bremner, J. D., Southwick, S. M. & Chorney, J. S. (1991). Animal models for the
    neurobiology of trauma. *PTSD Research Quarterly*, **2**(4), 1–3.
Breslau, N. & Davis, G. C. (1986). Chronic stress and major depression. *Archives
    of General Psychiatry*, **43**, 309–14.
Breslau, N., Davis, G. C., Andreski, P. & Peterson, E. (1991). Traumatic events
    and posttraumatic stress disorder in a urban population of young adults.
    Archives of General Psychiatry, **48**, 216–22.
Brett, E. A., Spitzer, R. L. & Williams, J. B. W. (1988). DSM-III-R criteria for
    post-traumatic stress disorder. *American Journal of Psychiatry*, **145**, 1232–6.
Burgeswatson, I. P., Hoffman, L. & Wilson, G. V. (1988). The neuropsychiatry
    of post-traumatic stress disorder. *British Journal of Psychiatry*, **152**, 164–73.
Card, J. J. (1983). *Lives after Viet Nam*. Lexington, MA: Lexington Books.
Chodoff, P. (1963). Late effects of the concentration camp syndrome. *Archives of
    General Psychiatry*, **8**, 323–33.
Crowne, D. P. & Marlowe, D. (1960). A new scale of social desirability
    independent of psychopathology. *Journal of Consulting Psychology*, **24**,
    349–54.
Davidson, J. R. T. & Fairbank, J. A. (1992). The epidemiology of posttraumatic
    stress disorder. In J. R. T. Davidson & E. B. Foa (eds.), *Posttraumatic stress
    disorder: DSM-IV and beyond*. Washington, DC: American Psychiatric
    Press, pp. 147–72.

Davidson, J., Swartz, M. & Storck, M. et al. (1985). A diagnostic and family study of post-traumatic stress disorder. *American Journal of Psychiatry*, **142**, 90–3.

Davidson, J. R. T., Hughes, D. & Blazer, D. et al. (in press). Post-traumatic stress disorder in the community: an epidemiological study. *Psychological Medicine*.

Davidson, J. R. T. & Nemeroff, C. B. (1989). Pharmacotherapy in posttraumatic stress disorder: historical and clinical considerations and future directions. *Psychopharmacology Bulletin*, **25**, 422–5.

Davis, M. (1986). Pharmacological and anatomical analysis of fear conditioning using the fear-potentiated startle paradigm. *Behavioral Neuroscience*, **100**, 814–24.

Dollinger, S. J. (September, 1986). The need for meaning following disaster: attributions and emotional upset. *Personality and Social Psychology Bulletin*, **12**(3), 300–10.

Durham, T. W., McCammon, S. L. & Allison, E. J. (1985). The psychological impact of disaster on rescue personnel. *Annals of Emergency Medicine*, **14**, 664–8.

Eitinger, L. & Strom, A. (1973). *Mortality and morbidity after excessive stress.* New York: Humanities Press.

Erikson, K. T. (1976). Loss of communality at Buffalo Creek. *American Journal of Psychiatry*, **133**, 302–6.

Escobar, J. I., Randolph, E. T. & Puente, G. et al. (1983). Post-traumatic stress disorder in Hispanic Vietnam veterans: clinical phenomenology and sociocultural characteristics. *Journal of Nervous and Mental Disease*, **171**, 585–96.

Evans, R. G. (1982). Clinical relevance of the Marlowe–Crowne Scale: a review and recommendations. *Journal of Personality Assessment*, **46**, 415–24.

Federal Emergency Management Agency (1984). *Program guide, disaster assistance programs.* Washington, DC: US Government Printing Office.

Feinstein, A. & Dolan, R. (1991). Predictors of post-traumatic stress disorder following physical trauma: an examination of the stressor criterion. *Psychological Medicine*, **21**, 85–91.

Figley, C. R. (1983). Catastrophes: an overview of family reactions. In C. R. Figley and H. I. McCubbin (eds.) *Stress and the family, Vol. II: Coping with catastrophe.* New York: Brunner/Mazel, pp. 3–20.

Figley, C. R. (ed.) (1985). *Trauma and its wake: traumatic stress theory, research and intervention*, New York, NY: Brunner/Mazel.

Folkman, S., Lazarus, R., Dunkel-Schetter, C., DeLongis, A. & Gruen, R. (1986). Dynamics of a stressful encounter: cognitive appraisal, coping and encounter outcomes. *Journal of Personality and Social Psychology*, **50**, 992–1004.

Fullerton, C. S., Wright, K. M., Ursano, R. J. & McCarroll, J. E. (in press). Social support for disaster workers after a mass-casualty disaster: effects on the support provider. *Nortic Journal of Psychiatry*.

Fullerton, C.S., McCarroll, J. E., Ursano, R. J. & Wright, K. M. (1992). Psychological responses of rescue workers: fire fighters and trauma. *American Journal of Orthopsychiatry*, **62**(3), 371–8.

Fullerton, C.S., Ursano, R. J., Kao, T. & Bhartiya, V.R. (1992, June). *Community bereavement following an airplane crash.* Paper presented at the meeting of the International Society of Traumatic Stress World Congress, Amsterdam, The Netherlands.

Giller, E. L. (1990). *Biological assessment and treatment of posttraumatic stress disorder*. Washington, DC: American Psychiatric Press.

Gleser, G. C., Green, B. L. & Winget, C. N. (1981). *Prolonged psychosocial effects of disaster: a study of Buffalo Creek*. New York: Academic Press.

Goldberg, J., True, W. R., Eisen, S. A. & Henderson, W. G. (1990). A twin study of the effects of the Vietnam War on posttraumatic stress disorder. *Journal of the American Medical Association*, **263**(9), 1227–32.

Green, B. L. (1982). Assessing levels of psychosocial impairment following disaster: consideration of actual and methodological dimensions. *Journal of Nervous and Mental Disease*, **17**(9), 544–52.

Green, B. L., Grace, M. C. & Lindy, J. D. et al. (1983). Levels of functional impairment following a civilian disaster: the Beverly Hills Supper Club fire. *Journal of Consulting and Clinical Psychology*, **51**, 573–80.

Green, B. L., Wilson, J. P. & Lindy, J. D. (1985). Conceptualizing post-traumatic stress disorder: a psychological framework. In C. R. Figley (ed.), *Trauma and its wake: the study and treatment of post-traumatic stress disorder*. New York, NY: Brunner/Mazel, Inc, pp. 53–69.

Green, B. L., Lindy, J. D., Grace, M. C. & Gleser, G. C. (1989). Multiple diagnosis in posttraumatic stress disorder: the role of war stressors. *Journal of Nervous and Mental Disease*, **177**(6), 329–35.

Green, B. L., Grace, M. C., Lindy, J. D. & Gleser, G. C. (1990). War stressor and symptom persistence in posttraumatic stress disorder. *Journal of Anxiety Disorder*, **4**, 31–9.

Grinker, R. & Spiegel, J. (1945). *Men under stress*. Philadelphia, PA: Blakiston.

Guha-Sapir, D. (1989). Rapid assessment of health needs in mass emergencies: review of current concepts and methods. *World Health Statistics Annual*, **43**, 171–81.

Helzer, J. E., Robins, L. N. & McEvoy, L. (1987). Post-traumatic stress disorder in the general population. *New England Journal of Medicine*, **317**, 1630–4.

Hennekens, C. H. & Buring, J. E. (1987). *Epidemiology in medicine*. Boston: Little, Brown & Co.

Hildebran, J. F. (1984). Stress research: a perspective of need, a study of feasibility. *Fire Command*, **51**, 20–1.

Holloway, H. C. & Ursano, R. J. (1984). The Vietnam veteran: memory, social context, and metaphor. *Psychiatry*, **47**, 103–8.

Horowitz, M. J. (1976). *Stress response syndromes*, 2nd edn. Northvale, NJ: Aronson.

Jones, J. C. & Barlow, D. H. (1990). The etiology of posttraumatic stress disorder. *Clinical Psychology Review*, **10**, 299–328.

Karem, E. G. (1991, October). *The Lebanon wars: more data*. Presented at the Annual Meeting of the International Traumatic Stress Society, Washington, DC.

Keating, J. P., Blumenfield, M., Reilly, M., Pine, V. R. & Mittler, E. (1987). Post-disaster stress in emergency responders. Paper presented at the American Psychiatric Association meetings, Chicago.

Kessler, R. C. & McLeod, J. D. (1984). Social support and mental health in community samples. In S. Cohen & S. L. Syme (eds.) *Social support and health*. New York: Academic Press, pp. 219–40.

Kilpatrick, D. (1992). *Etiological factors in the development of crime-related post-traumatic stress disorder*. Presented at the World Conference of the International Traumatic Stress Society, Amsterdam, The Netherlands.

Kolb, L. C. (1988). A critical survey of hypotheses regarding posttraumatic stress disorders in light of recent findings. *Journal of Traumatic Stress*, **1**, 291–304.

Krystal, H. (1968). *Massive psychic trauma.* New York: International Universities Press.

Krystal, J. H., Kosten, T. R., Southwick, S., Mason, J. W., Perry, B. D. & Giller, E. L. (1989). Neurobiological aspects of PTSD: review of clinical and preclinical studies. *Behavior Therapy,* **20,** 177–98.

Kulka, R. A., Schlenger, W. E. & Fairbank, J. A. et al. (1990). *Trauma and the Vietnam War generation.* New York, NY: Brunner/Mazel.

Kulka, R. A., Schlenger, W. E., Fairbank, J. A., Jordan, B. K., Hough, R. L., Marmar, C. R. & Weiss, D. S. (1991). Assessment of posttraumatic stress disorder in the community: prospects and pitfalls from recent studies of Vietnam veterans. *Psychological Assessment: A Journal of Consulting and Clinical Psychology,* **3**(4), 547–60.

Laufer, R. S., Brett, E. & Gallops, M. S. (1985). Dimensions of posttraumatic stress disorder among Vietnam Veterans. *Journal of Nervous and Mental Disease,* **173**(9), 538–45.

Lazarus, R. S. & Folkman, S. (1984). *Stress, appraisal and coping.* New York: Springer.

Lifton, R. J. (1967). *Death in life – survivors in Hiroshima.* New York: Random House.

Lindemann, E. (1944). Symptomatology and management of acute grief. *American Journal of Psychiatry,* **101,** 141–8.

Lindy, J., Green, B. & Grace, M. (1987). The Stressor criterion and post-traumatic stress disorder: commentary on Breslau and Davis. *Journal of Nervous and Mental Disease,* **175,** 269–72.

March, J. S. (1990). The nosology of posttraumatic stress disorder. *Journal of Anxiety Disorders,* **4,** 61–82.

McCarroll, J. E., Ursano, R. J., Wright, K. M. & Fullerton, C. S. (in press). Coping with the handling of the dead after traumatic death. *Victimology.*

McFarlane, A. C. (1988*a*). The longitudinal course of posttraumatic morbidity: the ranges of outcomes and their predictors. *Journal of Nervous and Mental Disease,* **176,** 30–9.

McFarlane, A. C. (1988*b*). The phenomenology of post-traumatic stress disorders following a national disaster. *Journal of Nervous and Mental Disease,* **176,** 22–9.

McFarlane, A. C. (1986). Long-term psychiatric morbidity after a natural disaster. *The Medical Journal of Australia,* **145,** 561–3.

McFarlane, A. C. & Raphael, B. (1984). Ash Wednesday: the effects of a fire. *Australian NZ Journal of Psychiatry,* **18,** 341–53.

Matussek, P. (1971). *Die Konzentrationslagerhaft und ihre Folgen.* New York: Springer.

Norris, F. H. (1988). Toward establishing a database for the prospective study of traumatic stress. Presented at the National Institute of Mental Health Workshop: Traumatic stress: defining terms and instruments, Uniformed Services University of the Health Sciences, Bethesda, Maryland.

Oei, T. P. S., Lim, B. & Hennessy, B. (1990). Psychological dysfunction in battle: combat stress reactions and posttraumatic stress disorder. *Clinical Psychological Review,* **10,** 355–88.

Penk, W. E., Robinowitz R., Roberts, W. R. et al. (1981). Adjustment differences among male substance abusers varying in degree of combat experience in Vietnam. *Journal of Consulting and Clinical Psychology,* **49,** 426–37.

Quarantelli, E. L. (1985). An assessment of conflicting views on mental health: the consequences of traumatic events. In C. R. Figley (ed.) *Trauma and its*

Wake, NY: Brumner Mazel, pp. 173–215.

Rangell, L. (1976). Discussion of the Buffalo Creek disaster: the course of psychic trauma. *American Journal of Psychiatry*, **133**, 313–16.

Raphael (1986). Victims and helpers. In B. Raphael. *When disaster strikes: how individuals and communities cope with catastrophe.* New York: Basic Books, Inc, pp. 222–44.

Robins, L. N., Helzer, J. E. & Croughan, J. L. et al. (1981). *NIMH diagnostic interview schedule: Version III.* Rockville, MD: NIMH. Public Health Service. (Publication No. ADM-T-42-3 [5–8] [8–81]).

Rosenheck R., Becnel, H., Blank, A. S. et al. (1992). Returning Persian Gulf troops: first year findings. Report of the Department of Veteran's Affairs to the United States Congress on the psychological effects of the Persian Gulf War.

Roszell, D. K., McFall, M. E. & Malas, K. L. (1991). Frequency of symptoms and concurrent psychiatric disorder in Vietnam veterans with chronic PTSD. *Hospital and Community Psychiatry*, **42**(3), 293–6.

Rubin, C. B. & Nahavandian, M. (1987). Details on frequency of disasters, incidents for federally declared disasters, 1965–1985. *Program in science, technology and public policy.* Washington, DC: George Washington University.

Rundell, J. R., Ursano, R. J., Holloway, H. C. & Silberman, E. K. (1989). Psychiatric responses to trauma. *Hospital and Community Psychiatry*, **40**(1), 68–74.

Schwartz, G. (1984). Psychobiology of health: a new synthesis. In B. L. Hammonds & C. J. Scheirer (eds.), *Psychology of health.* Washington, DC: American Psychological Association, pp. 149–93.

Seligman, M. E. P. & Beagley, G. (1975). Learned helplessness in the rat. *Journal of Comparative and Physiological Psychology*, **88**, 534–41.

Shalev, A. (1991). Recent biological findings in PTSD and their potential clinical applications, presented to the International Traumatic Stress Society Annual Meeting, Washington, DC.

Shalev, A., Bleich, A. & Ursano, R. J. (1990). Posttraumatic stress disorder: somatic comorbidity and effort tolerance. *Psychosomatics*, **31**(2), 197–203.

Shore, J. H., Tatum, E. L. & Vollmer, W. M. (1986). Psychiatric reactions to disaster: the Mount St. Helens experience. *American Journal of Psychiatry*, **143**, 590–5.

Shore, J. H., Vollmer, W. M. & Tatum, E. L. (1989). Community pattern of post-traumatic stress disorders. *Journal of Nervous and Mental Disease*, **177**, 681–5.

Shumaker, S. A. & Brownell, A. (1984). Toward a theory of social support: closing conceptual gaps. *Journal of Social Issues*, **40**(4), 11–36.

Sierles, F. S., Chen, J. J. & McFarland, R. E. et al. (1983). Post-traumatic stress disorder and concurrent psychiatric illness: a preliminary report. *American Journal of Psychiatry*, **140**, 1177–9.

Singh, B. & Raphael, B. (1981). Postdisaster morbidity of the bereaved: a possible role for preventive psychiatry. *Journal of Nervous and Mental Disease*, **169**, 203–12.

Sledge, W. H., Boydstun, J. A. & Rahe, A. J. (1980). Self-concept changes related to war captivity. *Archives of General Psychiatry*, **37**, 430–43.

Solomon, S. D., Smith, E. M., Robins, L. N. & Fischbach, R. L. (1987). Social involvement as a mediator of disaster-induced stress. *Journal of Applied Social Psychology*, **17**(12), 1092–112.

Solomon, Z. (1992). *Psychological effects of the Gulf War on high risk sectors of the Israeli population.* International Symposium on Stress, Psychiatry and War, World Psychiatric Association, Paris, France.

Squire, L. R. & Zola-Morgan, S. (1991). The medial temporal lobe memory system. *Science,* **253,** 1380–6.

Taylor, S. E. (1990). Health psychology: the science and the field. *American Psychologist,* **45**(1), 40–50.

Taylor, V. (1977). Good News About Disaster. *Psychology Today,* (OCT) 93–126.

Terr, L. C. (1983). Chowchilla revisited: the effects of psychic trauma four years after the school-bus kidnapping. *American Journal of Psychiatry,* **140,** 1543–50.

Titchener, J. L. & Kapp, F. T. (1976). Family and character change at Buffalo Creek. *American Journal of Psychiatry,* **133,** 295–9.

Trimble, M. (1985). Post-traumatic stress disorder: history of a concept. In C. Figley (ed.), *Trauma and its wake.* New York: Brunner/Mazel, pp. 5–14.

Ursano, R. J. (1981). The Vietnam era prisoner of war: precaptivity personality and the development of psychiatric illness. *American Journal of Psychiatry,* **138**(3), 315–18.

Ursano, R. J. (1987). Comments on: 'Post-traumatic stress disorder: the stressor criterion.' *Journal of Nervous and Mental Disease,* **175**(5), 273–5.

Ursano, R. J., Boydstun, J. A. & Wheatley, R. D. (1981). Psychiatric illness in US Air Force Vietnam prisoners of war: a five-year follow-up. *American Journal of Psychiatry,* **138,** 310–14.

Ursano, R. J., Kao, T. & Fullerton, C. S. (1992). PTSD and meaning: structuring human chaos. *Journal of Nervous and Mental Disease* **180**(12), 756–9.

Ursano, R. J. & Fullerton, C. S. (1990). Cognitive and behavioral responses to trauma. *Journal of Applied Social Psychology,* **20**(21), 1766–75.

Ursano, R. J. & Rosenheck. R. (1991). Report of Joint Department of Veterans Affairs and Department of Defense Working Group; Public Law 102–25: post-traumatic stress disorder in operation desert storm returnees.

Van Der Kolk, B. A. (1988). The trauma spectrum: the interaction of biological and social events in the genesis of the trauma response. *Journal of Traumatic Stress,* **1,** 273–90.

Wallston, B. S., Alagna, S. W., DeVellis, B. M. & DeVellis, R. F. (1983). Social support and physical health. *Health Psychology,* **2**(4), 367–91.

Winfield, I., George, L. K. & Swartz, M. et al. (1990). Sexual assault and psychiatric disorders among women in a community population. *American Journal of Psychiatry,* **147,** 335–41.

Wolf, M. E. & Mosnaim, A. D. (1990). *Posttraumatic stress disorder: etiology, phenomenology, and treatment.* Washington, DC: American Psychiatric Press.

Wolfe, J. & Keane, T. M. (1990). Diagnostic validity of posttraumatic stress disorder. In M. E. Wolf & A. D. Mosnaim (eds.). *Posttraumatic stress disorder: etiology, phenomenology, and treatment.* Washington, DC: American Psychiatric Press, Inc, pp. 49–63.

Wright, K. M., Ursano, R. J., Bartone, P. T. & Ingraham, L. H. (1990). The shared experience of catastrophe: an expanded classification of the disaster community. *American Journal of Orthopsychiatry,* **60**(1), 35–42.

Yager, T., Loafer, R. & Gallops, M. (1984). Some problems associated with war experience in men of the Vietnam generation. *Archives of General Psychiatry,* **41,** 327–33.

Part II
The nature of traumatic stress

through their threat to life, bodily integrity, security, and self-image (Fields, 1980). Mass victimization has occurred in the two world wars, the Holocaust, Vietnam, Cambodia, and other war torn areas.

In order to understand the psychological responses to trauma it is important to understand the terror response. In this chapter, we describe how terror is a part of our lives. We examine individual and group needs for safety, the childhood experience of terror through fairy tales, and the role of terror in literature and film. The process of victim stigmatization and recovery from terror are described.

The experience of terror

Safety and childhood tales of terror

People want to feel safe, to experience the environment as stable and predictable. We are often not aware of feelings of safety until something happens to threaten our feeling safe (Sandler, 1987). Most living organisms seek safety when exposed to dangerous and threatening situations (Cantril, 1950; Hebb & Riesen, 1943, Hebb, 1946; Hudson, 1954). Some people respond to the loss of safety during times of traumatic stress by moving towards the familiar (Ursano & Fullerton, 1990). Harlow & Harlow (1965) observed that in times of danger individuals often seek the shelter of their home environment, their 'haven of safety'.

Groups establish and maintain feelings of safety through shared beliefs. Individuals attach meaning to traumatic events in order to make them comprehensible, predictable and under control. Rituals and symbols organize a traumatic experience by providing meaning to the events (Ursano & Fullerton, 1990). Rumors often develop during times of stress (Young et al., 1989). Rumors created and maintained by a group, provide a shared belief that places a traumatic event in a familiar context.

Groups protect themselves by developing boundaries. Boundaries are created by consensus in order to separate the safe from the dangerous and to keep danger outside the group (Bion, 1965; Douglas, 1966, 1985, Douglas & Wildavski, 1982). Failure to keep dangers out creates terror expressed by suspicion, paranoia, and anger towards group members (Bion, 1965). Terror caused by an outsider breaches the boundary of the group, inducing loss of feelings of safety and security. The responses of the group may be flight, fright, or an overwhelming sense of deprivation and dependency. Terror created by a group leader can be used to induce group

2

The psychology of terror and its aftermath

HARRY C. HOLLOWAY and CAROL S. FULLERTON

Traumatic events create terror – before, during, and after the trauma. This state of extreme fright is evoked by the experience of vulnerability, helplessness, loss of control, uncertainty, and threat to life. Often threats of violence are used to induce terror (Symonds, 1983). Recently, the world was reminded that terror is also induced in both individuals and groups by weapons, such as biological and chemical warfare, that cause shock, horror, helplessness, and panic. The psychological trauma of chemical and biological weapons is based on their capacity to contaminate and insidiously destroy an individual's sense of security and trust in the environment (Fullerton & Ursano, 1990). In Tel Aviv, Israel, 60 individuals sought emergency care after a SCUD missile explosion, thinking they had been exposed to chemical and biological warfare agents. No exposure had occurred but the terror of these weapons led them to a wrong belief. Soldiers in Saudi Arabia reportedly slept in their protective masks and gear for both protection and psychological comfort. In earlier wars when the threat of chemical and biological warfare was low protective gear had been rapidly discarded.

Terror is associated with human induced traumas: personal attacks, rapes, hostage takings, and terrorism to name a few. Violent crimes, in particular, affect millions of people each year. Thirty-seven million Americans were victims of crime in 1984 (Herrington, 1985); six million of these were victims of violent crime. Russell (1984, 1986) studied a random sample of 930 women. Twenty-four percent reported at least one experience of rape and 31% reported an attempted rape. The frequency of hostage events has increased dramatically over the past two decades (Jenkins, 1983; Hatcher, unpublished observations; McCann, Sakheim & Abramson, 1988; Ochberg, 1978; Rothberg et al., 1986). Acts of terrorism against individuals, institutions, and revered cultural symbols create feelings of vulnerability conformity. McCarthyism in the 1950s used threats to induce terror and assure control by the leader and conformity of the group.

Children by their nature are small, frail and subject to domination and mistreatment by adults (parents and others) at will. They live in a world of terror in which the fragile illusion of safety provided by the family is always at risk. From this perspective, children's affirmations of omnipotence are, on the whole, defensive. Fairy tales contribute to the child's understanding and experience of safety, competence, and growing autonomy. Bruno Bettelheim (1977) suggested that fairy tales provide the opportunity for children to experience evil and terror as a part of life. A child can identify with the characters in a fairy tale and feel reassured that although evil and feelings of terror are an integral part of life they can be controlled. The themes of these children's' fairy tales teach us about the experience of terror: how it is experienced and where it begins.

Consider the story of 'Hansel and Gretel'. Two children deserted in the forest by their parents, come upon a house made of goodies and begin to eat it. A woman inside the house takes them in and feeds them. The woman turns out to be an evil witch who is planing to devour the children. Hansel and Gretel ultimately fight off the witch, shoving her into the oven. The story of Hansel and Gretel stirs terror through fear of abandonment and vulnerability. But the story ultimately provides solace. The children save each other and become independent despite the evil intent of their parents. The young reader is reassured that terror is a manageable part of the world.

The story of 'Jack and the Bean Stalk' illustrates another aspect of terror. In the story, Jack acquires magical beans; he plants the beans and a large bean stalk grows. Jack climbs the bean stalk high into the sky where he finds a giant living. Jack steals valuables from the giant and brings them to his mother. The two of them then become rich and powerful members of their community. Bettelheim suggested that this story illustrates how children use magic and their own intelligence to manage large forces in the world that threaten them.

Fairy tales expose children to the evils of the world and communicate information about the origins and resolution of terror through fictional characters with whom children can identify. The terror of vulnerability and the loss of safety are prominent themes in fairy tales. As children experience the inevitable threats to their illusion of safety, they develop confirmation that, although feelings of terror are a part of life, they are also manageable. Through fairy tales, the parent exposes the child to terror, and the child learns that terror can be relieved and a sense of mastery achieved.

Terror in film and literature

Terror in film and literature brings the fairy tale into the world of adults and emphasizes the universality of evil. Such films threaten our view that the world is safe, but nonetheless, reassure us of conventional outcomes. Many individuals voluntarily expose themselves to terror by going to horror movies and reading terrifying novels. They often achieve a sense of mastery and control by watching films of terror (Terr, 1989). Vicarious exposure to terror may help us deny actual terrors – we can watch a horror movie from a distance and not be destroyed. According to Terr, the fear is loss of control; knowing is controlling. Terr (1989, p. 388) illustrates the point with the example of a 13 year-old boy who slept through an earthquake in Northern California. The boy explained, 'If I slept through it, I could die in my sleep in an earthquake. And then I'd never have a chance to do anything to save myself.'

Films stir terror in a variety of ways. Stephen King (1981) distinguishes terror from other emotions (horror and revulsion) evoked by horror films and literature. In tales that use terror to frighten, we actually see nothing that is nasty or grotesque. Each person is invited to remember their worst nightmare, to conjure up their most frightening fantasy. King (1981) illustrates his definition of terror through a basic tale of terror entitled, 'The Hook': A young couple in their teens are out on a date. While driving up to Lover's Lane, the radio interrupts with an urgent bulletin. A homicidal maniac named 'The Hook' has just escaped from the nearby asylum for the criminally insane. The Hook got his name because in place of his right hand is a razor-sharp hook. His old hang-out was Lover's Lane, where he would attack couples making-out and slice off their heads with his hook. After hearing the bulletin, the girl is frightened and wants to go home, but the guy reassures her and they stay, continuing to make-out. Shortly, the girl begins to hear noises coming from outside the car and insists on leaving. The guy, angry about leaving so soon, peels out of the parking spot and drives her home. He goes to open her car door and is stunned, frozen in his tracks – there hanging from the doorhandle is the razor-sharp hook!

The terror evoked by 'The Hook' originates in the imagination. In a similar way, the classic tale of terror, 'The Monkey's Paw' invites our imagination to create its own terrifying fantasy. As the old woman rushes to answer the knocking at the door we begin to fear what she will find on the other side. Although nothing is there when she opens the door, we imagine what might have been there if her husband had been slower to make the

Table 2.1. *Sources of terror depicted in film*

The madman (or madwoman)
The unholy
Contamination
Breaking taboo
Entering environments where we do not belong
Offending the powerful
Disaster events

third wish. We are never allowed to see what is behind the door. We see only that which exists in our imagination. In the fable 'The Tell-Tale Heart', terror results from the frightening images evoked by the sound of the heartbeat as well as the sense of participating in the madness of another.

King (1981) divides tales of terror into two groups: those which result from an intended act or conscious decision to do evil, and those which are caused by nature, for example, a stroke of lightning. It is interesting to note that actual traumatic events can be divided into the same two groups: human induced trauma such as terrorism and rape, and natural disasters such as floods and earthquakes.

The sources of terror depicted on film are manifold (see Table 2.1). One of the common sources is the madman (or madwoman). The insane killer is out of control in films such as 'The Cabinet of Dr Calgari', 'Psycho', and 'Halloween'. These terror films stigmatize the emotionally ill. The victim, however, may also be perceived as partially to blame. The silent terror movie, 'Bride of Frankenstein', involves a mental patient who kills people upon the direction of an insane doctor. In one scene, Frankenstein becomes concerned that the monster is trying to mate. The terror is enhanced by the suggestion that the monster will be created over and over again.

Vampire movies create terror by depicting the unholy. The vampire is both attractive and sinister. The vampire steals not only sexual favors but life itself. Sex is depicted as scary and dangerous. The vampire's evil is a perverse sexual evil. According to King's (1981) taxonomy, the evil is outside, human-like, but not under human control. Vampire movies use the spoiling of the sacred and those things which protect us to stir terror in their audience.

Contamination by infection is another theme frequently used to create terror. The film, 'Rabid', involves a young woman who is infected by a

virus. The virus is created while treating the young woman for a severe burn
that she sustained while riding with her boyfriend on a motor bike.
Subsequently, others become infected who, in turn, infect still others.
Death is the result of the contamination.

'Night of the Living Dead', and 'Dracula' evoke terror by breaking
taboos. Both films deal with the forbidden: cannibalism, pollution, and
infection. Much of the effect of 'Night of the Living Dead' comes from the
graphic depiction of decay; 'Dracula' uses seduction to attract and repel. In
'Night of the Living Dead' we break a fundamental taboo – the separation
of the living and the dead. The world of the dead invades that of the living
because science has gotten out of control. The trouble begins when
organisms return from outer space via a satellite, another boundary
breached by man attempting what he should not. One scene in the uncut
version of the movie is of a child who kills his mother, and then eats her –
still another taboo broken.

People entering environments where they do not belong is another form
of breaking a taboo which is often depicted in films to induce terror. In the
movie 'Deliverance', four men from an urban area venture deep into the hill
country on a white water canoe trip. They are curious about a world
different from their own. Their curiosity results in the public rape of one of
the men and the murder of a stranger from the hill country. The trip
becomes filled with guilt and haunting fear. The film achieves an unsettling
realism, that threatens the viewer's denial, creating a sense of living in a
world of strangers who might do one in. The paradox is that the viewer is
threatened with the core of truth in the paranoid delusion – perhaps our
own sense of safety and concept of health and normality are a delusion. As
the shared group beliefs of safety, health and normality collapses, terror
threatens.

The individual who offends a powerful someone or something is another
source of film terror. Often the individual is not aware of the offense.
Unfortunately, a terrible revenge may await him or her. The film 'Carrie'
illustrates the potential terror in human relationships. Carrie, an adolescent
girl with supernatural powers, becomes the victim of a cruel joke by her
peers. On stage to be crowned at a high school dance, Carrie is drenched
with animal blood. Her anger and rage evokes her destructive supernatural
powers. In an act of vengeance she destroys the culprits and the entire town.

In most of these films the author, the actors, and the director terrify us in
a controlled manner. No matter how disastrous the outcome of these
fantasies, we know they are mere fictions. Our norepinephrine rush does

not overwhelm us; surviving the fright strengthens our sense of denial and our delusion of control.

Over the past two decades there have been numerous films depicting actual disasters and catastrophes: 'The Poseidon Adventure', 'Towering Inferno', 'Airport' (and its sequels 'Airport 75' and 'Airport 77'), 'Avalanche', 'Earthquake', 'City on Fire', 'The Titanic', and 'The Hindenburg', to name a few. Quarentelli (1985) examined the content of American disaster films and found a disproportionate number of them dealt with disasters caused by human error. Some aspects of these disaster films, however, do not mirror the reality of disasters. For example, little attention is given to disaster planning and long-term recovery. Quarentelli concluded that misperceptions and distortions about disasters can originate from disaster films themselves. By terrifying and establishing blame, disaster films create a sense of moral order. This supports the belief that disasters are avoidable rather than an expectable outcome of the failure of complex systems over which human control is very imperfect.

The individual who uses terror as a tool on the city streets, or in our airports, or directs his agents and soldiers to bring terror into the homes of citizens, uses the same approach as the dramatist. Alfred Hitchcock learns his trade from Robespierre, the French revolutionist, and from Don Carlos, infante and pretender to the Spanish throne. In turn, 'the Jackal' learns from Hitchcock. The difference, however, is that Hitchcock provided an opportunity for his audience to recover their belief in safety while Carlos through his terrorist acts discourages any such recovery. Both intentionally induce transitional regressive states which put one in touch with a sense of personal and social hopelessness. The political terrorist uses terror as a tool for behavioral control and to enforce followership in the same way as the prototypic abusive parent. The abusive parent, like the terrorist, is frequently convinced that s/he is acting for the good of the victim. Given the complexities of this interpersonal relationship, it is not surprising that the victims sometimes have grave difficulties making sense of their victimization. Jon Shaw's paper on the illusion of safety (1987) describes additional developmental effects of trauma's impact on its victims.

Victim stigmatization

The victims of human induced trauma – terrorism, hostage taking, rape, personal attack – are frequently seen as responsible for their fate (Beigel & Berren, 1985; Frederick, 1980; Janoff-Bulman, 1985; Krupnick &

Table 2.2. *Mechanisms of stigmatization of the trauma victim*

Human induced traumas facilitate stigmatization
The victim's feelings facilitate stigmatization:
  Guilt
  Self blame
  Humiliation
  Shame
  Idealization of the terrorist
The group/community's feelings facilitate stigmatization:
  Victim seen as causing or deserving the trauma
  Wish to avoid 'contamination'
  Wish to maintain a sense of personal invulnerablity
  Wish to maintain a view of the just/moral world
  Wish to see the world as predictable, orderly and controllable

Horowitz, 1980; Lerner, 1970; Ryan, 1971; Symonds, 1975). The victims
are often considered deviant and possibly deserving of what has happened
to them (see Table 2.2). Several authors have hypothesized that, by making
the victim to blame, we maintain our feelings of personal invulnerability
(Janoff-Bulman, 1982; Lerner, 1980). The sense of a moral, ordered
universe is maintained at the price of blaming the victim. Often, the victims
of violent acts are subtly excluded from their groups and avoided. The
victim is left isolated at a time when s/he most needs social supports (Coates
& Winston, 1983; Symonds, 1980). People avoid the victim out of fear of
guilt by association (Frederick, 1980), or contamination (Symonds, 1975).
The word, *victim*, originally meant a beast selected for sacrifice or driven
out (as a scapegoat) in a symbolic dispelling of evil.

Self-blame is common following victimization (Janoff-Bulman, 1979;
Simon & Blum, 1987; Wortman, 1976). Victims of violence frequently feel
humiliated and ashamed (Krupnick & Horowitz, 1980), and may experience themselves as worthless and debased (Simon & Blum, 1987). Janoff-
Bulman (1979) suggests two types of self-blame. Behavioral self-blame is
adaptive and targets certain behaviors that can be changed, such as
hitchhiking in the case of a rape victim. These behaviors are modifiable and
controllable. In contrast, characterological self-blame is maladaptive, for
example, the rape victim who believes she is a bad person.

Hostages often feel guilt and self-blame at being unable to avoid capture
(Hatcher, 1981). The hostage situation recapitulates in many ways the
experience of the helpless child. The hostage can thus experience the source

of their terror as also their protector. The bond between victim and victimizer serves the defensive function of decreasing the victim's fear and helplessness (Simon & Blum, 1987). This same bond can be experienced by the hostage taker as a reason to keep his/her victim alive. The identification of the hostage victim with the captor is known as the Stockholm Syndrome, named after a hostage-taking incident in Stockholm during which a captor and captive became lovers.

Similarly, there are stereotyped roles for the victims of disaster and disaster helpers. The disaster helper is seen as powerful, strong, and resourceful; the victim as powerless, weak, resourceless, and ineffective (Short, 1979). Disaster victims may feel weak, inadequate and obligated to accept the help of others. They may feel that, once they accept help, their recovery should be complete. This expectation can make it difficult for them to express distress, grief, and anger. As a consequence of these stereotypes, the vulnerabilities of the disaster rescuer/helper are often overlooked, leading to a failure to provide appropriate support for the disaster worker who is repeatedly exposed to trauma.

In his book, *Belief in a Just World: a Fundamental Delusion*, Lerner (1980) describes assumptions that people make in order to keep the world manageable and predictable. Individuals need to maintain the belief that the world is predictable, orderly, and controllable. This illusion, according to Lerner, enables people to achieve their goals and avoid becoming overwhelmed. Lerner conducted experiments in which subjects observed another person being hurt. Observers indicated that they most admired the individuals inflicting the pain. The victim was seen as bad or spoiled, even when the victim was the more physically admirable than the perpetrator.

Lerner's findings suggest that the victims of terror are stigmatized, in part, by the process of being seen as spoiled or bad. When this occurs, others then feel it is unlucky to associate with them. The victim becomes a castout of the community, carrying the burden of having been a victim which others want to disown and disavow.

Cultures and groups stigmatize those who break taboos and cross forbidden boundaries. Mary Douglas (1966) demonstrated that people who go into forbidden areas become carriers of a 'blight', a cultural evil. As evil befalls these individuals, they themselves become taboo. Sometimes they are seen as witches, sometimes as heros; in either case they are seen as possessing special powers.

In some societies the special power of victims is seen in their nobility and greatness in suffering (Raphael, 1986). The victimized individual feels special, reflecting their powerful cultural significance. Many hostages feel a

Table 2.3. *The recovery environment following trauma*

1. Provide rest and respite
2. Provide a safe environment
3. Protect against further stigmitization
4. Allow for the expression of anger
5. Be aware of preexisting psychiatric disturbances or life events
6. Provide the opportunity to regain self-esteem
7. Avoid 'second injury'
8. Validate feelings – 'normal response to abnormal situation'
9. Provide the opportunity to reassess life goals

sense of entitlement and special fortune following escape from their captivity. This is as important a part of their experience as is survivor guilt. Their sense of being exceptional is reinforced if they are also acclaimed as heroes. For some, memories of captivity support a heroic vision of themselves, while for others the memories recall a frightened fragile self. Conflicted and conflicting emotions develop as time passes as the now free victim attempts to understand his or her experiences.

Recovery from terror

The experience of terror has implications for the treatment of victims of trauma (see Table 2.3). Traumatized individuals feel unsafe and terrified. The victims of terror experience vulnerability, helplessness, loss of control, uncertainty, and a possible threat to life. The trauma can cause feelings of guilt, shame, low self-esteem, distrust, and self-blame. In addition, the victims of human induced violence are often stigmatized. The recovery of those who experience terror requires addressing these aspects of the experience.

Provide rest and respite Meeting the physical needs of the individual is extremely important and should be done immediately. This includes providing food and water, warmth, and respite. Medical treatment should be given as needed. Other interventions may be experienced as an intrusion if the individual is exhausted, hungry, and cold. Care must be taken to assume physical needs have the first priority.

Provide a safe environment Providing a safe environment is critical. Many victims of terror have experienced an overwhelming loss of safety

(Symonds, 1983). They must restore their sense of safety. Reuniting individuals with family and friends is important to regaining feelings of safety. When reunion is not possible, information about family and friends should be made available, particularly if the family and friends were also in danger or affected by the trauma. When to begin to talk about the loss of family or friends must be carefully considered.

Avoid further stigmatization The social milieu and its support functions should protect against further trauma by stigmatization. The recovery environment should provide support, protection, containment, and structure and must avoid the further stigmatization of converting the victims of trauma into 'patients' or 'permanent' victims. Stigmatization isolates victims at the time they most need social support (Coates & Winston, 1983; Symonds, 1980). Privacy without isolation is important (Symonds, 1980). Another kind of stigmatization – that of being labeled a hero – may have to be addressed when the former victim accepts the role of hero, potentially reinforcing the group's denial of the changes in their world. The role of hero or savior can be quite seductive, but it is also isolating and in the long run may lead to the individual being treated as 'damaged'. The hero may have to hide 'unworthy' but real emotions; the hero comes to fear that his or her less attractive aspects will become public. The rescue worker and the therapist must aid the victim in the development of sufficient self-acceptance to support the living of a relatively complex life, one in which he or she has both good and bad aspects. The effects of trauma cannot be undone, but they can be used by the former victim to support a sound psychological adjustment (Ursano, Boydstun & Wheatley, 1981).

Allow for the expression of anger Feelings of fear, hatred, and hostility are common in victims of human-induced trauma (Simon & Blum, 1987). It is important to provide the opportunity for victims to recognize and express these feelings.

Be aware of preexisting psychiatric disturbances or life events Preexisting psychiatric conditions may affect recovery and place individuals at increased risk following traumatic events. Major life events or stressors can also influence recovery. The victim and his or her family needs to prepare for the return home. For example, if the individual returns to a home situation where avoidance and denial characterize the style of the family, or if the victim is outright rejected, problems will occur.

Provide the opportunity to regain self-esteem Victims of trauma frequently experience a sense of helplessness and powerlessness. Victims of human

induced violence may feel particularly valueless and debased (Simon &
Blum, 1987). These victims often experience shame (Symonds, 1980) and
humiliation (Simon & Blum, 1987). It is critical to provide an opportunity
for the victim to regain a sense of self-esteem and control over their life.
Assumptions about personal invulnerability, the existence of a meaningful
world, and positive self-perception may have been shattered (Janoff-
Bulman, 1985). Equally likely is that the victim's sense of entitlement may
be perceived as too demanding. A family or work group may cast out, or
isolate the shattered or the entitled victim. Return to a realistic view of one's
self marks an important transition in the victim's return to 'normal' life.

Avoid 'second injury' Symonds (1980) defined 'second injury' as the
victim's perceived rejection and lack of support from others following the
victimization experience. Feelings of fright and helplessness may lead
victims to cling to helpers following trauma. Victims experience a heightened sensitivity to the interpersonal distance of others. They may easily
perceive the helper as indifferent or unfeeling. Some disaster workers
nurture and comfort victims, however, others remain detached and avoid
excessive interpersonal interaction with victims. A difficult, and often
overlooked, aspect of the recovery process is terminating relationships with
those who have provided assistance during times of terror such as rescue
workers and hospital staff.

Validate feelings – normal response to abnormal situation It is important to
expect recovery following trauma and to acknowledge a range of reactions
that are a normal response to an abnormal life situation. Validation of
feelings is very important in the acute recovery phase following trauma.
Individuals need to share their traumatic experience including feelings of
powerlessness and helplessness. Debriefing groups, as discussed later in the
book, provide an opportunity to share the disaster experience. The
debriefing must be done in a supportive setting and timed so to not interfere
with the provision of respite.

Provide the opportunity to reassess life goals Some individuals have used
the experience of terror after a trauma to move toward health (Card, 1983;
Sledge, Boydstun & Rahe, 1980; Ursano et al., 1981). The trauma experience can provide an opportunity for individuals to reassess values and gain
a new appreciation for life (Ochberg, 1980).

Conclusions

Terror is a universal human experience. In order to remind ourselves that we can control evil forces and overcome feelings of terror, we repeatedly expose ourselves to terror and escape from terror through film and literature. Our need to view the world as safe and predictable begins in infancy and continues throughout our lives. We belong to groups that develop boundaries and rituals to contain our fears and anxieties. At times, these fears are projected onto other groups.

Others may stigmatize the victim of trauma in order to maintain their feelings of personal invulnerability. The terror filled victim is blamed, devalued, and seen as flawed and deserving of his or her fate. The victim is rejected by others in order to avoid contamination or, alternatively, because the victim's sense of entitlement is felt as too demanding. The victim may be recast as a hero. This may be rewarding, but it also creates a stereotyped role that can isolate the victim from his or her family and community.

Therapeutic interventions during the acute recovery phase affect long-term outcome. Interventions must emphasize the transitory nature of the problem and the expectation of recovery. The meaning given to the traumatic event by the victim will change the effects of the trauma over time. It is particularly important not to ignore the potential for growth and positive reorganization of one's life as a potential outcome of terror, trauma and disasters.

References

Beigel, A. & Berren, M. R. (1985). Human-induced disasters. *Psychiatric Annals*, **15**(3), 143–50.

Bettelheim, B. (1977). *The uses of enchantment.* New York: Vintage Books.

Bion, W. (1965). Selections from 'Experience in Groups'. In A. Colman & H. Bexton (eds.) *Group relations reader.* Sausolito: Grex.

Brickman, P., Rabinowitz, V. C., Karuza, J., Coates, D., Cohn, E. & Kidder, L. (1982). Models of helping and coping. *American Psychologist*, **37**, 368–84.

Cantril, H. (1950). *The 'why' of man's experience.* New York: The MacMillan Company.

Card, J. J. (1983). *Lives after Viet Nam.* Lexington, MA: Lexington Books.

Coates, D. & Winston, T. (1983). Counteracting the deviance of depression. *Journal of Social Issues*, **39**, 171–96.

Douglas, M. (1966). *Purity and danger: an analysis of the concepts of pollution and taboo.* London: Routledge and Kegan Paul.

Douglas, M. (1985). *Social research perspectives.* New York: Russell Sage Foundation.

Douglas, M. & Wildavski, A. (1982). *Risk and culture*. Berkeley: University of California Press.

Fields, R. M. (1980). Victims of terrorism: the effects of prolonged stress. *Evaluation and Change* (special issue), 76–83.

Frederick, C. J. (1980). Effects of natural vs. human induced violence upon victims. *Evaluation and Change* (special issue), 71–5.

Fullerton, C.S. & Ursano, R.J. (1990). Behavioral and psychological responses to chemical and biological warfare. *Military Medicine*, **155**, 54–9.

Harlow, H. & Harlow, M.K. (1965). The affectional system. In A. Schrier, H. Harlow & I. Stollnitz (eds.) *Behavior of nonhuman primates (Vol. 2)*. New York: Academic Press.

Hebb, D.O. & Riesen, A.H. (1943). The genesis of irrational fears. *Bulletin of the Canadian Psychological Association*, **3**, 449–50.

Hebb, D.O. (1946). On the nature of fear. *Psychological Review*, **33**, 259–76.

Herrington, L. H. (1985). Victims of crime: their plight, our response. *American Psychologist*, **40**, 99–103.

Hudson, B.B. (1954). Anxiety in response to the unfamiliar. *Journal of Social Issues*, **10**, 53–60.

Janoff-Bulman, R. (1979). Characterological versus behavioral self-blame: inquiries into depression and rape. *Journal of Personality and Social Psychology*, **37**, 1798–809.

Janoff-Bulman, R. (1985). The aftermath of victimization: rebuilding shattered assumptions. In C. R. Figley (ed.) *Trauma and its wake: the study and treatment of post-traumatic stress disorder*. New York: Brunner/Mazel, pp 15–35.

Jenkins, B. (1983). Research in terrorism: areas of consensus, areas of ignorance. In B. Eichelman, D. A. Soskis & W. H. Reid (eds.). *Terrorism: interdisciplinary perspectives*. Washington, DC: American Psychiatric Association, pp. 153–77.

King, S. (1981). *Danse macabre*. London: Futura.

Krupnick, J. & Horowitz, M. (1980). Victims of violence: psychological responses, treatment implications. *Evaluation and Change* (special issue), 42–6.

Lerner, M. (1970). The desire for justice and reactions to victims: social psychological studies of some antecedents and consequences. In J. Macaulay & L. Berkowitz (eds.), *Altruism and helping behavior*. New York: Academic Press.

Lerner, M. (1980). *The belief in a just world: a fundamental delusion*. New York: Plenum Press.

McCann, I. L., Sakheim, D. K. & Abramson, D. J. (1988). Trauma and victimization: a model of psychological adaptation. *The Counseling Psychologist*, **16**(4), 531–93.

Ochberg, F. (1978). The victim of terrorism: psychiatric considerations. *Terrorism*, **1**, 147–67.

Ochberg, F. (1980). Victims of terrorism. *Journal of Clinical Psychiatry*, **41**, 73–4.

Quarentelli, E. L. (1985). Realities and mythologies in disaster films. *Communications*, **11**, 31–44.

Raphael, B. (1981). Personal disaster. *Australian and New Zealand Journal of Psychiatry*, **15**, 183–98.

Raphael, B. (1986). *When disaster strikes: how individuals and communities cope with catastrophe*. New York: Basic Books, Inc.

Rothberg, J. M., Jones, F. D., Fong, Y. H., Harris, P. H. (1986). Terrorism and other disasters: mental health aspects. Presented at the Symposium on Military Psychiatry and Civilian Populations, Military Section, World Psychiatric Association, Washington, DC (May).

Russell, D. E. H. (1984). *Sexual exploitation: rape, child sexual abuse, and workplace harassment*. Beverly Hills, CA: Sage.

Russell, D. E. H. (1986). *The secret trauma: incest in the lives of girls and women*. New York: Basic Books.

Ryan, W. (1971) *Blaming the victim*. New York: Vintage Books.

Sandler, J. (ed.) (1987). *From safety to superego: selected papers of Joseph Sandler*. New York: The Guilford Press.

Shaw, J. (1987). Unmasking the illusion of safety. *Bulletin of the Menninger Clinic*, **51**, 49–63.

Short, P. (1979). Victims and helpers. In R. L. Heathcote & B. G. Tong (eds.), *Natural hazards in Australia*. Canberra: Australian Academy of Science.

Simon, R. I. & Blum, R. A. (1987). After the terrorist incident: psychotherapeutic treatment of former hostages. *American Journal of Psychotherapy*, **XLI**(2), 194–200.

Sledge, W. H., Boydstun, J. A. & Rahe, A. J. (1980). Self-concept changes related to war captivity. *Archives of General Psychiatry*, **37**, 430–43.

Symonds, M. (1975). Victims of violence: psychological effects and aftereffects. *The American Journal of Psychoanalysis*, **35**, 19–26.

Symonds, M. (1980). The 'second injury' to victims. *Evaluation and Change* (special edition), 36–8.

Symonds, M. (1983). Victimization and rehabilitative treatment. In B. Eichelman, D. A. Soskis & W. W. Reid (eds.), *Terrorism: interdisciplinary perspectives*, Washington, DC: American Psychiatric Association.

Terr, L. C. (1989). Terror writing by the formerly terrified: a look at Stephen King. *Psychoanalytic Study of the Child*, **44**, 369–90.

Ursano, R. J., Boydstun, J. A. & Wheatley, R. D. (1981). Psychiatric illness in US Air Force Vietnam prisoners of war: a five-year follow-up. *American Journal of Psychiatry*, **138**, 310–14.

Ursano, R. J. & Fullerton, C. S. (1990). Cognitive and behavioral responses to trauma. *Journal of Applied Social Psychology*, **20**(21), 1766–75.

Wortman, C. B. (1976). Causal attributions and personal control. In J. H. Harvey, W. J. Ickes & R. F. Kidd (eds.), *New directions in attribution theory*, vol. 1, Hillsdale, NJ: Erlbaum.

Young, J. J., Ursano, R. J., Bally, R. E. & McNeill, DC (1989). Consultation to a clinic following suicide. *American Journal of Orthopsychiatry*, **59**, 473–6.

3

Exposure to traumatic death: the nature of the stressor

ROBERT J. URSANO and JAMES E. McCARROLL

Trauma and disasters, both manmade and natural, are frequent occurrences in the present day world: terrorism, plane crashes, earthquakes, industrial accidents, combat and poison gas attacks to name but a few. Common to the occurrence of nearly all disasters and combat is the likelihood of violent death and the presence of human remains – burned, dismembered, mutilated, or relatively intact. Exposure to mass death as well as individual dead bodies is a disturbing and sometimes frightening event. The nature of the stress of exposure to traumatic death and the dead and its relationship to posttraumatic stress disorder and other posttraumatic psychiatric illnesses is not well understood (Breslau & Davis, 1987; Lindy, Green & Grace, 1987; Rundell et al., 1989; Ursano, 1987; Ursano & McCarroll, 1990).

The tasks of body recovery, identification, transport, and burial may require prolonged as well as acute contact with mass death. Recent research has shown that victims, onlookers, and rescue workers are traumatized by the experience or expectation of confronting death in disaster situations (Jones, 1985; Miles, Demi & Mostyn-Aker, 1984; Schwartz, 1984; Taylor & Frazer, 1982). Exposure to abusive violence (Laufer, Gallops & Frey-Woulters, 1984) and to the grotesque (Green et al., 1989) significantly contributes to the development of psychiatric symptoms in war veterans, particularly intrusive imagery (Laufer, Brett & Gallops, 1985; Lifton, 1973).

Despite the widespread recognition that exposure to dead bodies is one of the major stressors in disasters, few studies have examined the psychiatric effects of exposure to dead bodies and body parts. The major psychiatric textbooks do not mention the topic (Kaplan & Sadock, 1985; Talbot, Hales & Yudofsky, 1988). Hersheiser and Quarantelli (1976) reported that, as of the time of their study, there were no empirical studies of the handling of the

46

Table 3.1. *Mediators of the stress of traumatic death*

Anticipated stress of exposure to traumatic death
Previous experience
Gender
Volunteer status

dead in disasters. Jones (1985) found little information on the psychological effects on rescuers of recovering live victims and almost nothing on the effects of exposure to the dead. Regardless of profession or past experience, exposure to violent death can create additional victims in those who assist after a disaster (Miles et al., 1984).

How individuals and groups prepare for, behave during, and respond after, witnessing traumatic death has received little scientific scrutiny. Hersheiser and Quarantelli (1976) reported on how the dead were treated by the living following a flood. They observed increasing respect for the body through the phases of search, recovery, identification, and preparation for burial. Taylor and Frazer (1982) reported that about a third of the volunteers who recovered bodies from the Mount Erebus air crash in Antarctica experienced transient problems of moderate to severe intensity. Further, at three months, one-fifth continued to report high levels of stress-related symptoms. In a survey of 592 US Air Force personnel involved in the recovery, transport, and identification of the bodies of the Jonestown, Guyana mass suicide, Jones (1985) found that youth, inexperience, lower rank, and the greater exposure to the dead were associated with higher levels of emotional distress. Higher rates of dysphoria were also found in blacks compared to whites, possibly due to greater identification with the black victims by the black body handlers.

Mediators of the stress of exposure to mass death

Anticipation and previous experience

The stress of anticipation can itself be debilitating, affecting performance, behavior, and health (Table 3.1). Research on the effects of exposure to death and the dead, however, has focused on rescue workers after a disaster. The period prior to exposure has rarely been examined. Ersland, Weisaeth and Sund (1989) reported that waiting time was a frequently reported stressor among professional fire fighters. The disaster worker anticipates the stress of upcoming work before it actually begins and may already begin work with a substantial stress burden. The work with the disaster casualties may be more or less stressful than what was anticipated. Disaster workers may wait minutes to days after notification before they actually begin their rescue work. In interviews of disaster workers, we have heard stories of extended periods of waiting and high levels of stress. For example, novice rescue workers recruited to remove bodies from a plane which had caught fire and burned after landing had to wait several hours while wooden supports were put under the wings of the plane so it would not collapse.

The stress of anticipation has important psychological and physiological effects. Mitchell, Sproule & Chapman (1958) showed that the physiological responses to anticipated exercise were qualitatively the same as those to exercise itself, differing only in magnitude. The stress of anticipation has also been found to cause changes in human skin conductance and heart rate (Susnowski, 1988). Arthur (1987) reported that adrenocortical hormones were secreted mainly during the anticipation of stressful events rather than during confrontation. Complex patterns of cortisol secretion have been found in patients prior to surgery. The highest levels were seen in the pre-operative preparation of the patients (Czeisler et al., 1976). Sumova & Jakoubek (1989) found that, in rats conditioned to receive a painful foot shock, anticipated stress acted as a specific trigger. The anticipation produced stress induced analgesia which could be blocked by naloxone (an opioid blocking agent). They hypothesized that the endogenous opioid system played an important role in decreasing the self-destructive effects of stress. To our knowledge, gender differences in anticipated stress have not been studied. There is a large body of scientific literature on gender differences in illness reporting and in the use of health care services by disaster victims (Cleary, Mechanic & Greenley, 1982; Solomon et al., 1987).

Previous experience with a stressful event has been shown to reduce the effects of the stressor. Inexperienced persons generally report higher levels of fear or anxiety then do experienced persons. This has been shown in studies of parachute jumpers (Fenz & Epstein, 1967) and in pilots (Drink-water, Cleland & Flint, 1968; Mefferd et al., 1971). The contributions of experience to psychological responses to disaster work have been noted by several authors but how experience specifically contributes has not been examined. Experienced disaster workers consistently show lower stress responses following a disaster than do nonexperienced workers. Ersland and colleagues (1989) found that a higher proportion of nonprofessional rescuers than professionals reported poor mental health nine months after recovering victims from an oil rig collapse at sea. The more experienced rescuers were less likely to have poor mental health than the less experienced rescuers. Weisaeth (1989) observed that a high level of disaster training or experience was significantly correlated with optimal behavior during the disaster. Hytten and Hasle (1989) found that fire fighters experienced in mass disasters had lower stress responses after the event than did nonprofessional fire fighters. The long-term effects of past experience and training are less clear. Lundin (1990) found that during the first week after a disaster, professional rescue workers had significantly greater unpleasant feelings than nonprofessionals. However, after nine months, the reverse was true. Weisaeth's (1989) study of disaster behavior among survivors of an industrial explosion suggested that training and experience were extremely powerful variables in predicting health outcome. Norris and Murrell (1988) reported that persons who had experienced severe flooding in southeastern Kentucky had fewer symptoms than those who had not experienced floods. They reported these findings as evidence for stress inoculation and emphasized the advantages of prior experience with a stressor.

We were interested in the effects of gender and past experience on the anticipated stress of disaster workers who would handle the dead of a disaster. We measured anticipated stress in male and female soldiers, a group with and without prior experience, and in college students, who were inexperienced in handling the dead. In both groups, we measured the anticipated stress of handling bodies using a questionnaire. Inexperienced females had higher anticipated stress scores than inexperienced males. Experience lowered the grand mean (62.34) by 8.32 points while inexperience raised it by 1.98. Being male lowered the grand mean by 2.83 points; being female raised it by 11.61. The gender difference was replicated in the college students. There were no gender differences when experienced groups were compared. We found no relationship between anticipated stress scores and age, race, or education in either of the two populations.

A second measure of anticipated stress was used in the soldier population. This second measure consisted of ratings of the anticipated stress of handling bodies which were presented in slides depicting traumatic death. Inexperienced male soldiers had a higher mean anticipated stress score (slides) than did the experienced males. There was a significant correlation $r(108) = .66$, $< .001$, between the mean anticipated stress score on the questionnaire and the mean anticipated stress score measured by the slides. The significant correlation between the two methods of measuring anticipated stress provides some support for the construct validity of the concept of anticipated stress (McCarroll et al., in press).

Although these data are cross-sectional, they suggest that at least part of the 'inoculation' effect of experience, is achieved by lowering anticipated stress prior to a disaster. Such lowered stress may itself decrease the trauma of a disaster and increase successful disaster behavior and coping. Predisaster counseling (Myers, 1989) may also be effective in part through its effects on anticipated stress. High levels of anticipated stress may also contribute to fatigue and thus to other disease conditions. Lower anticipated stress may be a mechanism through which experience and training contribute to decreased fatigue, increased performance, and decreased risk of adverse psychological effects in experienced disaster workers.

Volunteer status, previous experience, and anticipated stress

Prior to Operation Desert Storm, the four military services were required to provide a contingent of personnel to staff the mortuary where the war dead would be identified and prepared for shipment home to their families for burial. Pre- and post-Desert Storm, questionnaires were given to military personnel who worked in the mortuary, and who were support personnel whose duties did not involve contact with remains. In the pregroup, we were able to study the stress of anticipation of working with the fatalities from the war, for the mortuary workers, and the stress of deployment to a wartime mortuary for everyone. Those who agreed to participate in the study were asked to complete questionnaires as soon as possible after arriving and prior to leaving at the end of their duty. These questionnaires included demographic and background information and a number of standard psychometric instruments designed to measure the stress of working with the fatalities, psychological distress, social support, interpersonal relationships, and self-presentation. Two instruments were used to measure distress: the Impact of Events (IES) Scale (Horowitz, Wilner & Alvarez, 1979) and the Brief Symptom Inventory (BSI) (Derogatis & Melisaratos, 1983), a shorter version of the SCL-90-R (Derogatis, 1983). We used the Global Severity Index (GSI) as an overall indicator of psychological distress, and the five subscales of theoretical interest as responses to trauma: anxiety, depression, somatization, hostility, and interpersonal sensitivity (Green et al., 1989; Rubonis & Bickman, 1991; Rundell et al., 1989). A total of 562 people worked in the mortuary; 87% agreed to participate in the study (86% of the mortuary workers and 93% of the support workers).

Only 18% of the total group had previously participated in a mass casualty experience or a disaster; 37% had worked with dead bodies; and 52% had seen someone who had died by violent means. Sixty-four percent were volunteers. The difference between male volunteers (65%) and female volunteers (59%) was not statistically significant.

This study provided a unique opportunity to study nonvolunteers. When all subjects were examined (mortuary workers and support workers, both males and females), individuals who were not volunteers for this assignment had significantly higher scores than volunteers on the Global Symptom Inventory (GSI) of the BSI, as well as for the subscales of somatization, anxiety, and depression. This was also true for mortuary workers alone; there were no significant differences between scores for volunteers and nonvolunteers in the support worker group (McCarroll et al., 1992).

Experience was statistically significant only on measures of the stress of anticipation of handling bodies. Inexperienced mortuary workers had higher mean total IES scores compared to those with previous experience handling the dead. The same pattern was shown for IES intrusion scores, and IES avoidance scores.

Both volunteer status and experience were significantly related to the IES total, intrusion and avoidance for male mortuary workers. Mean scores of females were not statistically significant for either variable. The means of the nonvolunteers were always higher than the volunteers and the means of the inexperienced males were always higher than those who were experienced (McCarroll et al., 1992).

Thus, both experience and volunteer status predicted lower psychological distress and intrusive and avoidance symptoms in military personnel anticipating working with the dead of the Persian Gulf War. The findings on volunteer status are unique since this variable can rarely be studied. Anticipated stress is an important aspect of all disaster and rescue work. The stress burden clearly begins well before actual exposure.

Nature of the stress of exposure to traumatic stress

In order to better understand the nature of the stress experienced by exposure to traumatic death, we collected observations, interviews, and empirical data from various disaster body handlers (Ursano & McCarroll, 1990).

Our first observations were made at the Dover Air Force Base Mortuary following the military air disaster of December 1985 in Gander, Newfoundland where 256 people were killed. Over 400, mostly inexperienced, volunteers served as body handlers. Their duty often required close contact with severely burned and dismembered bodies over a period of days to months. Observations began at Dover within 48 hours of the plane crash and continued throughout the arrival of the bodies and body parts, including the most intense period of body identification (2 weeks). Interviews with individuals involved in the body identification process were conducted during the process and several months thereafter. These included the individuals responsible for mental health consultation to the volunteer body handlers (Robinson, 1988), those providing support from the hospital and chapel, the mortuary workers (Cervantes, 1988), and those responsible for the overall body recovery and identification processes (Maloney, 1988a, b). Subsequent to these observations, extensive longitudinal observations, interviews and empirical data have been collected on other individuals exposed to traumatic death: the USS Iowa turret explosion in 1989; Ramstein Air Base Flugtag disaster of 1988 (Ursano et al., 1990); United Airlines Flight 232 air crash in Sioux City, Iowa in 1989; and Operation Desert Storm casualties of 1991 (Ursano et al., 1992). In most of these studies, the longitudinal follow-up has extended over 1 to $1\frac{1}{2}$ years.

A final data set was obtained from group and individual interviews with approximately 50 civilian and military personnel with extensive experience with and exposure to handling bodies in rescue, recovery, identification, burial preparation and transport. These included hospital and forensic pathologists, military body handlers from the Viet Nam era, police and fire department personnel, emergency medical technicians, and Red Cross disaster relief workers. Participants were asked to describe the nature of their jobs, experiences, and their observations of the stress of handling dead bodies. Everyone was asked or spontaneously volunteered material on the following questions: 'What types of bodies are the most troublesome to you?'; 'What is it about dead bodies that affects your functioning or that of others?'; 'How do you get yourself through rough spots?'; 'How long does it take and how do you prepare yourself to go back to work after an exposure?'; 'How do you deal with the stress of such incidents?'; 'Have you seen people who were unable to function in the field and what seemed to happen?'

Disturbing bodies

Nearly everyone experiences viewing and contact with children's bodies as stressful regardless of the age or sex of the body handler or whether he/she had children (see Table 3.2). Children's bodies were reported as difficult because they 'appeared innocent', were 'complete victims' or they had 'untimely deaths'. 'They have not yet lived'. 'They had no control over it'. Pathologists hated doing autopsies on children. In the Gander, Newfoun-

Table 3.2. *Nature of the stress of*
exposure to traumatic death

═══════════════════════════════

Children's bodies
Natural looking bodies
Sensory stimuli
Novelty, surprise, and shock
Identification and emotional involvement
Personal effects
Friendly fire death
Female combat deaths
Accidental deaths
Enemy dead

═══════════════════════════════

dland, US Army plane crash of 1985, the discovery of toys in the wreckage
sent waves of anxiety and concern through the disaster workers as they
worried that children had been on the plane. None, in fact, were on board.

Natural looking bodies and ones with no apparent cause of death were
also reported as disturbing. Bodies that were fully clothed and not
obviously injured were described as 'eerie'.

I would say that it was probably more difficult for me to deal with remains that had a
single gunshot wound or single penetration that we knew were going to go home
viewable; more so than an air crash where the remains were severely charred or
decomposed. I think we key on the face of that person. If there isn't a face or a head,
... it seemed like the whole focal point of expression was gone. In the case of ____
who had a single shrapnel wound to the neck, we knew he was going home, out of
the war, because of a little damn piece of metal, a fragment. I think it probably
bothered me to see how sensitive life is to foreign objects compared to a hell of a
crash or an explosion which tears you up.

Pine (personal communication, 1988) reported that in cases of the
'untouched, but dead, everybody stops'. He reported a case in which a
beautiful young woman, who had died in a plane crash, appeared natural to
a recovery worker. However, her feet had been underneath the seat rack
and had been torn off leaving only two stumps for legs. When the disaster
worker saw this, he yelled, 'Jesus Christ!' Badly burned bodies, 'floaters'
(bodies that had lain in water for a long time), and decapitated bodies were
vivid in people's memory.

Rescuers may consciously avoid the fact of being in contact with a dead
body. A police harbor unit diver recalled his first underwater contact with
the foot of a body:

'I hoped it was just a sneaker' . . . feeling the ankle I thought, 'Let it be just a boot' . . . feeling the leg, 'Please, God, let it just be a wader'.

This concern was also expressed by a fireman,

A lot of firemen don't want to recognize a dead infant. One fireman went into a room full of smoke and felt around, touched the dead infant, and said it was a dog.

Wearing gloves to handle the bodies, even by rescue workers unlikely to touch bodies, was reported by many. It seemed to serve both a real and an imagined protective role. The gloves, in some settings, also became a symbol of being a member of this special group – the body handlers.

Sensory stimulation

Profound sensory stimulation is an extremely bothersome aspect of body handling. The smell of the body(ies) was often noted; visual and tactile sensitivity were also reported. One body handler at Dover AFB was concerned about not being able to 'wash the smell away'. He wondered if the odor was real or 'in my head'. In fact, there was very little odor with these bodies since they were frozen due to the snow and cold in Gander. Individuals who reported working with the bodies from the Jonestown mass suicide and those who worked with the Marine bodies from the Beirut bombing in 1985 felt greatly disturbed by the overwhelming odor of these already decaying bodies. The rescuers frequently tried to mask the odor with burning coffee, smoking cigars, working in the cold or using fragrances such as peppermint and orange oil (Cervantes, 1988).

Even when a volunteer escorted only a single body through all the stages of an identification process, he or she was exposed to many more bodies. This contributed to the stress of the experience. The sight of a large number of bodies was described by some volunteers as 'overwhelming', including those who had had experience with traumatic death in police or emergency service work. One man reported, 'The bodies just kept coming and coming. It felt like you were surrounded', and another said, 'It's hard not to look when you are surrounded; you are too tense to be bored. There were 15 dead bodies looking at me with their jaws cut open.'

The preparation and consumption of food was frequently difficult after exposure to traumatized bodies. Badly burned bodies were reported to look and smell like roast beef. After exposure to burned bodies, many individuals, including members of our research team, reported avoiding eating meat for several months. To one body handler, rice in brown gravy looked like maggots. In Sioux City, one rescue worker reported that he had lost all sexual interest in women because he could not look at their bodies without being reminded of the dead females he had recovered. Security police guarding the dead at Sioux City felt great discomfort when the wind blew blankets off the dead, exposing parts of the bodies.

One emergency medical service worker reported being particularly disturbed by the loud sound of a body thrown on a hard examining table, especially if the head struck the surface. She complained about the way the morgue workers handled the bodies of people she brought in. Many individuals reported persistent images of dead bodies or body parts, particularly if the bodies were burned or mutilated.

Novelty, surprise, and shock

In addition to the raw, offensive sensory stimulation, surprise, shock and fear of the unexpected are disturbing aspects of handling dead bodies. When we asked a group of experienced military body handlers how they would train a group of inexperienced people to retrieve bodies if they only had a day to do so, we were told, 'Tell them the worst. Make it so there are no surprises. Let them know what they are getting in for.'

The surprise and shock of seeing the victim's face when the body bag is opened was described by one subject: 'When our soldiers open that bag, they don't know what they are going to see!' Another man who handled bodies in Vietnam recalled that he was always upset when bodies were lying face down in body bags. The back of the head is very strong and usually intact regardless of the condition of the face. He was always frightened of what he might see when he turned the body over. Pathologists at Dover Air Force Base X-rayed the body bags before opening them in order to lessen the initial shock and surprise. They reported that seeing bodies at a crime scene was generally more difficult than seeing the same bodies in a laboratory where the setting was familiar and surprises were unlikely.

The opening of the first body bag at the mortuary after a disaster is nearly always a quiet, anxiety-filled event. One group of inexperienced body handlers during Operation Desert Storm physically moved 15–20 feet away from the body when the bag was opened, without anyone having spoken a word. When the body bag was fully open and there were no 'surprises', they moved closer. One individual described having to recover a child's body for burial. When he initially picked up the body, he was disturbed by the way it felt in his arms because it reminded him of recently carrying one of his own children.

Identification and emotional involvement

Identification or 'emotional involvement' with the deceased produces a high degree of distress. Identification, a sense of kinship with the body, was described by many subjects in different ways. Some reified identification in a magical way with guidance of how to act: in the same way that a body handler took care of a body from the battlefield, someone would take care of him. A common reaction was, 'It could have been me.' Children's bodies often stimulated a sense of emotional involvement. The viewers frequently reported thoughts such as, 'I remember when my kids were about that age.'

In the body identification process, one of the most difficult jobs is working with the personal effects of the dead (Maloney, 1988b). It was reported that, during the Vietnam war, handling the personal effects of the dead was more stressful for soldiers than working in the area that processed the remains for shipment home. As in other wars, some soldiers carried extensive collections of letters and photographs from loved ones. Graves registration personnel had to screen these items for objectionable material and the presence of blood or body fluids before they could be sent home. In reading these letters, some workers became disturbed, bothered by the feeling of knowing the family and the fact that they knew the soldier was dead and the family back home did not.

In Vietnam, we lost more of our people who dealt with personal property, that had to read the letters and screen the personal effects, than the ones who actually worked with the hands on side of it . . . with human remains. That's something that a lot of people find hard to believe, but after you explain it to them, that a guy would sit there day after day reading those letters from a loved one. That would probably be more of a mental stress than those who worked with the deceased human remains from combat.

Say a guy got zapped after 11 months, he had 11 months worth of letters. Somebody had to sit down and physically read every one of those letters because they would be sent back to the next of kin. Those guys who worked on the personal property side, they would have to sit there and do that day after day, month after month, and finally, for some of them, the stress of getting emotionally involved with those people . . . anybody could. You know, you sit there day after day and read through a guy's stuff, especially if you've got children and if you've got any kind of feeling within you whatsoever. . . . But some of them just couldn't cope with it. Some had to be sent back to the mortuary side and some had to be put back for reassignment.

And another reported:

We were just taking the personal effects off the remains and we had the soldier's billfold in our hands and here was a picture with his wife and two children. You know the impact that had on me! It just stopped me cold and I said something to the men. I said 'Isn't this God-awful that we know this soldier is dead and his wife and children are going to get that news in a matter of hours or days'.

A body handler who participated in the Grenada operation reported,

Most of us had horrendous nightmares about escorting a friend or family member home in a casket.

The dead bodies of friends and acquaintances, as well as 'brothers in uniform', were always disturbing. Pathologists had an unwritten rule that they would not do an autopsy on a friend. 'I wanted to remember him the way he was.' An officer in charge of a large graves registration facility in Vietnam reported, 'I always feared seeing somebody I knew.' A fireman said,

What makes the biggest impact is seeing a dead fire fighter – it brings it home. You have to deal with the realities: you're here and he is not.

A senior police official,

I had a cop die in my arms. I still cannot get it out of my head. I didn't know him. It was 19__, up in _____. He got shot in the back five times. I took him off the roof and got him down to the sixth floor and he died in my arms. I still can't get that out of my mind, still think about it once in awhile, if I hear a name or something comes out. But, I won't dwell on it. I just didn't like the idea that a brother I had worked with died in my arms.

At Dover Air Force Base, one group of body handlers became very upset after working for weeks with the personal effects of one victim. They developed the fantasy that they knew the victim and his family. Another group became anxious when they saw features of the body (soot in throat, posture) which they thought indicated the individual had been alive after the crash. Experienced personnel, professionals and nonprofessionals, cautioned newcomers against becoming 'emotionally involved'. Most experienced workers could describe how they avoided emotional involvement. These body handlers gave tips to new personnel such as 'Don't look at the face' or 'Don't get emotionally involved.' 'Don't think of it as a person.'

At Sioux City, rescue workers reported distress when they saw handwritten materials in the wreckage. 'It meant someone wrote it. They had been alive.' Young workers, learning to work with the personal effects of Operation Desert Storm casualties, gingerly went through the personal effects, relaxing only when a more senior worker made it a standard routine with forms to complete.

Combat unique stresses

Death from friendly fire

The death of a soldier caused by an error of his/her comrades in arms is termed death by friendly fire. Such deaths occasionally also occur in civilian police work. Military commanders and troops generally realize that friendly fire deaths are an unavoidable part of war. However, that does not remove the shock, remorse, and trauma of the experience. During ground combat, artillery fire may be called in by the assault force to hit a target that is very close. The artillery fire may fall short of the target and hit the assaulting troops. In extreme cases, assault troops have called in fire knowing that it would certainly hit them; they sacrificed themselves to accomplish their mission. Air crew are never perfectly accurate in the engagement of their targets. Bombs can misfire or friendly forces be mistaken for enemy.

At times during Operation Desert Storm, body handlers reacted to friendly fire deaths as expected combat deaths, expressing that the fire was not intentional. The dead were comrades who had fallen in battle. A military officer who supervised body handlers at Dover Air Force Base during Operation Desert Storm expressed his anger by directing it at the fact that personnel killed by friendly fire did not receive the Purple Heart upon their death. His assumption expressed his feelings of the wastefulness of the death. In fact, these men did receive the Purple Heart. In other friendly fire deaths, troops had been clearly marked by clothing, position, or vehicles and the deaths 'should not have happened'. The body handlers reacted to these deaths with great anger and dismay.

Death of women in combat

The deaths of American military women in the Persian Gulf War stirred disquiet among the body handlers and supervisors. On looking back on the experience, one body handler remarked, 'The first woman casualty was the hardest to handle.' The body handlers had seen an interview with her on TV. This made her more real. The female's personal belongings were kept separate from the men's and were not handled through the usual procedures. Supervisors insisted that a female be present when the body of a dead female soldier was being identified. This angered the male body handlers. Female bodies were kept completely wrapped and personnel involved in the identification procedures were kept to a minimum. The bodies of the men, although always treated with respect, were not required to have a male escort and the bodies were always left uncovered during the identification procedures.

The body of a pregnant woman killed in Panama in 1989 was kept separate from the other dead. The body handlers treated her wooden casket as special. It was placed to the side and no bodies or boxes were stacked on top.

Accidental deaths

Accidental deaths which are due to avoidable accidents or clear misconduct were termed 'dumb deaths' by the observers. These deaths were reported to be particularly disquieting. The people had made it through combat and then were later killed while playing with munitions or handling weapons in an unsafe manner.

Enemy dead

American soldiers in Operation Just Cause in Panama reported few feelings about enemy dead. An exception was when several soldiers were going through the wallet of a dead Panamanian soldier and saw pictures of family, children, and a First Communion picture. They broke down and cried. They later went to see the chaplain to talk.

Coping

Coping strategies vary in the different stages of exposure to traumatic death and with the degree of experience of the body handler (Table 3.3).

Before the exposure

Few organizations practice their response to a disaster although such events are expectable. Only the timing is unpredictable. In the case of the crash of United Airlines Flight 232 in Sioux City, Iowa, in July 1989, an air crash disaster drill had been performed prior to the crash and was reported to have been very helpful. Inexperienced personnel who volunteer to help at a disaster site are rarely given more than a few hours to prepare themselves for what they will see and do. People often reported feeling frightened of their own reactions to the bodies, asking themselves, 'Will I be able to handle it?' People who volunteered in pairs or larger groups thought that

Table 3.3. *Coping strategies used in exposure to traumatic and disaster related death*

Stressor	Coping strategy
Before exposure (waiting)	
Lack of information regarding tasks and roles	Practice drills Briefings
Anticipating one's reaction to bodies	Inbriefing Gradual exposure
During exposure (on site)	
Sensory overload	Avoidance or attenuation of strong stimuli
Natural appearance of bodies	Disidentification and use of role
Handling victims' personal effects	Disidentification and use of role
Fatigue and overdedication	Work breaks, food, sleep, supervision
Intense personal feelings (*e.g. fear, aloneness*)	Pairing with experienced personnel Supervisory support Humor Talking
After exposure (postevent)	
Need for information	Debriefing Education
Intense feelings (*e.g. sadness, alienation*)	Debriefing Family and organizational support Awards

they could help each other get through the experience. Initial preparation by a supervisor, usually by an inbriefing, is essential for inexperienced volunteers. Our subjects were unanimous in saying that when volunteers enter a disaster scene, such as a mortuary, they should be 'told the worst' so as to minimize the surprises at the crash site or mortuary. In a recent disaster, a supervisor provided a sequence of short, staged preparation briefings in which he became more explicit as he moved volunteers from an initial assembly area to their eventual work site. This technique was reported afterwards to have been very helpful.

Little psychological preparation was reported by experienced personnel expecting to be sent on an operation. Nervousness was sometimes reported when they did not know what sort of trauma to expect, what condition the bodies were in, or how difficult it would be to extract or identify the victims. One experienced dental pathologist reported that, when he knew he had to go on a mission where he was the only professional, he had nightmares the night before; when he knew he was going with others, he slept soundly.

During exposure to the dead (on site)

Individuals defend against the multiple sensory stimuli associated with the dead: the sights of the bodies (grotesque, burned, and mutilated); the sounds during autopsy (heads hitting tables and saws cutting bone); the smells of decomposing and burned bodies; and the tactile stimuli experienced as bodies are handled.

Workers often reported that they did not see badly damaged bodies as human. Supervisors facilitated this process of 'disidentification' by telling inexperienced volunteers, 'Don't think of it as a body; think of it as a job.' Natural looking bodies were often seen as all too human. Such remarks as, 'He can't be dead; he hardly has a scratch on him', were common. People reported many internal, automatic strategies by which they distanced themselves from the bodies such as by not looking at faces.

As mentioned previously, many people attempted to mask odors by burning coffee, smoking cigars, working in the cold and using fragrances such as peppermint oil and orange oil inside surgical masks (Cervantes, 1988). Most reported that such strategies did not help much in reducing the odors. Some olfactory adaptation did occur and workers generally dropped these strategies over time. Gloves were worn by personnel who touched the bodies or the body parts. This decreased the tactile contact with the remains which was particularly difficult with decomposed and burned bodies.

Past experience was frequently reported as helpful but it did not make one invulnerable. Even very experienced personnel could be shocked or surprised by the sight of the grotesque. An experienced pathologist reported extreme discomfort at the sight of a body whose shoulder girdle had been cleanly sliced by a helicopter blade. When he first saw the body, he did not recognize what had happened. When he did recognize the injury, he wondered whether the individual had felt the cut, suffered, or lived long after the injury. He continued to have intrusive images of this scene. Even a nonhuman body can produce discomfort. Pine (personal communication, 1988) reported a person who was very distressed at finding a dead pet dog in the luggage compartment of a commuter aircraft crash. The person said that he 'could not handle' the dead dog and was distressed because he knew others would not take it seriously.

Physical fatigue was a frequent and significant stressor due to the long and irregular hours, little sleep, poor eating schedules, moving heavy loads, and minimal time to recuperate. The stress of the experience was reported to be reduced when the individual took frequent breaks or the supervisor acted to decrease the visual contact with bodies, such as by providing chairs that faced away from the bodies, or putting partitions between the identification stations. Overdedication contributed to the tendency to go on working under conditions that normally would not be tolerated. Even though breaks were seen as desirable, at the Dover mortuary following the Gander air crash, for example, many individuals worked up to 20 hours per day. Managers had to require some people to leave the area.

Some workers voluntarily left the scene because of nausea, fatigue or psychological discomfort. This did not always mean that the person was going to be ineffective. A senior noncommissioned officer (NCO) reported:

I talked to some of the guys who worked Gander. There were days when they'd go in there and they would pick up an arm or a leg and they'd start thinking about what that arm used to be attached to and the fact that it was all burned up. They would have to walk outside of those plastic tents that they were working out of and sit down and have coffee, smoke a few cigarettes and just walk away for a day because on that particular day their psyche was not enough to deal with what they were seeing that day. The next day they were OK.

In general, grief and upset per se are not often observed on site because of feelings about one's public image. Most workers were concerned about how they would look in front of the other workers, both supervisors and subordinates. No one wanted to look like they 'couldn't handle it'. In response to the question of 'What if the leaders are not able to be macho that day? Do you lose faith in them?' The answer from an experienced team leader was:

No, no, no! You *can't* lose faith in them. You have to talk to them and let them talk to you. 'What was it that bothered you on that case?' Tell them that it's OK to get sick or say 'Hey! I can't deal with it today.' Because their psyche won't allow them to deal with that body that day, we can't think any less of them because tomorrow it might be our turn.

Unfortunately, such an attitude is not always present. We heard stories of supervisors laughing when someone said they 'couldn't take it'.

Humor was recognized by everyone as a substantial tension reducer during and after operations. Humor was more common when the workers were out of public view. Most humor was very respectful. Some body handlers were frightened of 'black humor', feeling it reflected 'having gone over the edge', and become too hardened.

The professional role identity of individuals who handled the dead also facilitated coping with the psychological stress. The professional role was usually well defined. For nonprofessionals, roles had to be defined and reinforced by others. Often, a good time to define roles was during the inbriefing where the importance of each person's job was emphasized. For most volunteers, the idea that they were performing an important service for the dead, the families of the dead, and the community was very important.

The role of the medical examiner is well defined and of recognized importance. Curiosity and a sense of detective work helped sustain the medical examiners. They were frequently cautioned against becoming emotionally involved in their cases because their objectivity might be questioned in court. Their education to 'be objective' served a protective function. In some situations, however, they were not able to avoid emotional involvement. Most reported that they did not like to do autopsies on children, friends, family members or torture deaths in which the suffering of the individual was obvious.

The mortician strives to do everything right because of the families. He takes pride in the cosmetic treatment of the deceased. This goal reinforced the idea that something memorable would be ·given to the survivors. Cassem (1977) noted that feelings of helplessness in the face of death could be decreased by working to provide something memorable for the survivors.

The fire, police, and emergency medical service personnel we interviewed were strongly motivated by the opportunity to save lives. Deaths often caused them to question their competence. In a fire rescue company, when occupants of a house were found dead, the fire fighters said to each other, 'They were dead before the bells went off!', meaning that the victims had probably died before the fire alarm had even sounded and they were not to blame.

The leader and the work group were inevitably seen as sources of support during difficult operations. The professional work group was the primary source of support. The presence of an experienced coworker, especially for the uninitiated, was important. A new individual could share the tasks and the feelings with an experienced partner and decrease the shock and surprise of the initial exposure.

A large urban search and rescue fire company reported a very high level of social support and unit cohesion. During each shift, about 12 people lived together in a room that served as a kitchen, a dining room and a living room at the rear of the firehouse near the vehicles. They were proud of their comradery fact that:

We're like a family! We provide psychological first aid to each other – reassurance. All he [the guy next to you on the line] needs is the reassurance of someone else nearby.

The support or lack of support by senior leaders and the organization as a whole was always noticed by workers. Volunteer body handlers at Dover Air Force Base after the Gander disaster were alert to whether their supervisor visited or their senior commanders expressed support (Maloney, 1988*b*).

After exposure (postevent)

Often disaster workers needed help in the hours or days shortly after exposure to the dead. During this time, volunteers reported high levels of discomfort, both physical and psychological. Fatigue, irritability and a need for a transition 'back to the real world' were commonly expressed. Experienced persons described themselves as doing what they had to in their mortuary work in order to get the job done; however, it was often at a high personal cost. The experience of professional support frequently came from a 'critique' of the technical aspects of the work. One fireman pointed out that this sort of discussion had:

Two phases – an individual phase and a group phase. You find out months or years later that something had bothered someone and you never found out about it before – he never talked about it. You argue about what had been wrong.

For almost everyone, professional counseling or psychiatric assistance, even if available, was generally viewed as unacceptable. Often this was due to fears that the person would be fired, could not successfully testify in court, would be ridiculed by fellow workers or would lose their job. Most said they did not really feel the need for counseling, however, almost all of those interviewed said they could have benefited from a brief talk about the experience, particularly if it involved the work group. Some wished it had even been mandatory.

For the volunteer body handlers, unusual events often triggered intense feelings. While viewing a memorial service on television one man reported:

I felt the grief they [the families] were going through. They started naming names; when they came to mine [the body he had escorted through the identification process], I went in the bathroom and cried and cried.

Another reported:

Memorial services interfere with coping. At that point, it's no longer a job, it gets to be a name, a human being. You can't do both at the same time. You associate everything you do with each person. It all comes together.

Spouses of the body handlers were frequently unwilling to hear about the workers' experiences; other times, the workers themselves decided not to talk to their spouses about their disasters. One man reported that his wife required him to take his clothes off at the door and shower after any contact with remains. Others described their first (and sometimes only) attempt at telling their spouses how they felt about their work and reported that they were unlikely to repeat the experience.

The return to work was difficult for many, particularly when coworkers were not sympathetic or sensitive. Most workers appreciated some time off after the job was over. Some wanted to have time with their families; others wanted time alone. There was generally a feeling that those who had not been at the site could not understand what the volunteer had gone through. This contributed to the difficulty of talking about the experience. People who came by the mortuary for only a visit were called 'turistas'.

Consistent with other reports (Maloney, 1988*a*, *b*; Robinson, 1988), in the aftermath of an incident, alcohol use was widely reported. Some workers reported that large amounts were consumed without intoxication while others reported that 'getting smashed' was normal at the end of each day of an operation. Drinking also provided a social context for the work group, and an opportunity to receive and provide support to each other. Some military workers reported that when the troops were restricted to one beer per evening, the restriction did not apply to body handlers. When several individuals were ordered away from a disaster site for rest, they reported returning to their rooms and drinking alcohol.

Discussion

Exposure to traumatic death is common in natural and manmade disasters and is a significant psychological stressor that can make victims of rescuers. The rescue worker is traumatized through the senses: viewing, smelling and touching, experiencing the grotesque, the unusual, the novel and the untimeliness of the death. The stress of body handling begins prior to the exposure with the anticipation. Nonvolunteers and those with no previous experience appear to experience more distress during this time.

The extent and intensity of the sensory properties of the body such as visual grotesqueness, smell, and tactile qualities are important aspects of the stressor. It may be heuristically useful to consider exposure to human remains as a special category of toxic exposure in which such dimensions as the type of agent, frequency, intensity and duration of exposure all add to the risk of later stress reactions, (Bartone et al., 1989), breakdown, disease or even psychological growth. Exposure to a child's mutilated body appears to be extremely toxic regardless of the body handler's age or whether she/he has children.

Although all sensory modalities are involved in contact with a body, odor may have the highest potential to recreate significant past episodes in a person's life. The strength of memory appears to vary with the special involvement a person has with the odor (Engen, 1987). The amount of forgetting of olfactory recognition memory, both long and short term is very small and, thus, the accurate recognition of odors when encountered again is very high (Engen, 1987; Engen, Kuisma & Eimas, 1973). While odors are easily recognized, they are very difficult to recall at will which is fortunate for most persons exposed to the smells of death. One can easily remember the color and shape of an apple, but not its smell. There is a need for those who prepare food to be aware of the power of olfactory memory to vividly recreate a scene and for reliving some portion of the experience. Even though the recall of olfactory memory is relatively poor, we were informed of two cases of individuals who had served as body handlers at the Jonestown disaster who later received medical discharges from the military for posttraumatic stress disorder. A complaint common to both individuals was waking up at night with a vivid recollection of the smells of the bodies at Jonestown (Orman, personal communication, 1989).

The meaning or social context of a death is an additional dimension of the stress felt by the individual body handler. For example, the death of a drug dealer arouses less sympathy among policemen or medical examiners regardless of the condition of the body. The innocent, who are seen as victims, almost never fail to arouse feelings among those who deal with the remains. Interviewees who were body handlers during the Vietnam War talked about the stress of handling a large number of bodies of soldiers killed in action in an unpopular war. Deaths caused by friendly fire were similarly stressful. The deaths of these soldiers often seemed to have been a tremendous waste which contributed to feelings of depression and hopelessness among the disaster workers.

The role of identification and emotional involvement in the production and resolution of the stress of handling dead bodies requires further study. Working with personal effects is an infrequently recognized, powerful stimulus for identification and subsequent distress. Identification and feelings of 'knowing' the dead appear to heighten the trauma of the experience. Identification may serve to eliminate the unfamiliar and the unknown qualities of the dead – changing what is new and novel into something familiar and part of the past (Ursano & Fullerton, 1990). The 'switching on' of these cognitive mechanisms – identification, personalization and emotional involvement – by the trauma of dead bodies requires further study. Whether certain individuals are more prone to this perceptual style or whether it represents a basic biological mechanism which all individuals activate to a various degree is unknown. Ways of decreasing identification and emotional involvement may be effective preventive measures for those who must be exposed to this traumatic stressor.

The coping strategies used by rescue personnel differ in the pre, on site, and poststages of the disaster work. An informative and role-setting inbriefing is critical to the adjustment of the volunteer. This briefing helps form the context for much of what is later felt and seen. When it is not provided, individuals have greater difficulty coping and often fare poorly. But no matter how well volunteers are briefed, there is always some shock to the reality of the situation.

The overwhelming nature of the sensory stimulation usually leads participants, particularly volunteers, to develop cognitive and behavioral distancing (avoidance) strategies. Failure to protect against emotional involvement with the victim is recognized by most workers as putting a person at risk for psychological distress. Scheduling is the job of the supervisor. Before fatigue sets in, which can contribute to emotional vulnerability, it is essential that managers establish schedules and insure that rescue workers follow them. While there is little that supervisors can do about alcohol abuse off site, they can inform participants that the potential for alcohol abuse is high following exposure to trauma.

Transition out of the rescue work after exposure appears to be facilitated by an outbriefing (debriefing) where the workers can ask questions and information can be provided about the event, the body identification process, and community reactions. Statements of appreciation and recognition made at this time aid recovery. Family and organizational support is central during the transition period. When sensitivity and caring are shown by both the family and the primary work group, the participant appears more likely to verbalize his or her feelings regarding what has been seen and done. Many rescue workers and volunteers will not share everything with people who were not present with them through the ordeal.

Numerous strategies are used to cope with the stresses of body handling. Most appear to be effective in the short run; however, it is unclear which are more effective and what their long-term consequences are. Avoidance strategies appear to be effective during the initial exposure to the bodies. We do not know the effect of using such strategies over a longer time period. Reports from volunteers, as well as from experienced personnel, indicate that, at some point, they can no longer avoid reminders of previous disasters. For example, names of the victims or the sight of an object bring the experience back. It is unclear whether such an experience is helpful or harmful. The triggering of memories may help to 'metabolize' the experience. On the other hand, the recall of unwanted memories can be disturbing and interfere with the present tasks. It remains an open question when and under what circumstances the individual should be encouraged to talk or think about aspects of the disaster that she/he wishes to avoid.

Spouses of disaster workers need to be educated about their loved ones' experiences. Many workers claimed that they wished their spouses had been informed of the nature of their work. Information can be provided to spouses in order to allay their concerns. This will also reinforce this naturally occurring support system. Brief groups held for spouses can also be a useful intervention.

Nonexperienced workers may be at higher risk for acute effects than experienced personnel. The latter, however, are not immune from suffering the same psychological discomforts as the volunteers. Some experienced personnel reported becoming somewhat calloused through repeated exposure, but no one believed it possible to be totally desensitized.

Additional research of this powerful stressor is needed to further describe its components and better understand the role of sensory stimulation in recall, particularly in posttraumatic stress disorder, and the normal 'metabolism' of traumatic events. Finally, it should be noted that not all effects from disaster rescue work and handling dead bodies are negative. Volunteers almost unanimously report that they would volunteer again if another disaster occurred. People were proud of their contribution and of having done an important job that others either could not do or would never have the opportunity to do. It has been previously reported that most people do quite well following exposure to massive trauma. An important theoretical as well as practical question is how people use trauma to move toward health (Ursano, 1987).

References

Arthur, A. Z. (1987). Stress as a state of anticipatory vigilance. *Perceptual and Motor Skills*, **64**, 75–85.
Bartone, P. T., Ursano, R. J., Wright, K. M. & Ingraham, L. H. (1989). The impact of a military air disaster on the health of assistance workers: a

prospective study. *Journal of Nervous and Mental Disease*, **177**, 317–28.
Breslau, N. & Davis, G. C. (1987). Posttraumatic stress disorder – the stressor criterion. *Journal of Nervous and Mental Disease*, **175**, 255–64.
Cassem, N. (1977). Treating the person confronting death. In A. M. Nicholi, Jr. (ed.), *Harvard Guide to Modern Psychiatry* (p. 599). Cambridge, MA: The Belknap Press of Harvard University Press.
Cervantes, R. (1988). Psychological stress of body handling, Part II and Part III: debriefing of Dover AFB personnel following the Gander tragedy and the body handling experience at Dover AFB. In R. J. Ursano & C. Fullerton (eds.) *Exposure to death, disasters and bodies*. Bethesda, Maryland: F. Edward Hebert School of Medicine, Uniformed Services University of the Health Sciences (DTIC: A 203163, pp.).
Cleary, P. D., Mechanic, D. & Greenley, J. R. (1982). Sex differences in medical care utilization: an empirical investigation. *Journal of Health and Social Behavior*, **23**, 106–19.
Czeisler, C. A., Ede, M. C. M., Regestein, Q. R., Kisch, E. S., Fang, V. S. & Ehrlich, E. N. (1976). *Journal of Clinical Endocrinology and Metabolism*, **42**, 273–83.
Derogatis, L. R. (1983). *Hopkins Symptom Checklist-90-Revised*. Baltimore: Clinical Psychometrics, Inc.
Derogatis, L. R. & Melisaratos, N. (1983). The brief symptom inventory: an introductory report. *Psychological Medicine*, **13**, 595–605.
Drinkwater, B. L., Cleland, T. & Flint, M. M. (1968). Pilot performance during periods of anticipatory physical threat stress. *Aerospace Medicine*, **39**, 944–99.
Engen, T. (1987). Remembering odors and their names. *American Scientist*, **75**, 497–503.
Engen, T., Kuisma, J. E & Eimas, P. D. (1973). Short-term memory of odors. *Journal of Experimental Psychology*, **99**, 222–5.
Ersland, S., Weisaeth, L. & Sund, A. (1989). The stress upon rescuers involved in an oil rig disaster. 'Alexander L. Kielland' 1980. *Acta Psychiatrica Scandinavica Supplementum*, **80**(355) 38–49.
Fenz, W. D. & Epstein, S. (1967). Gradients of physiological arousal in parachutists as a function of an approaching jump. *Psychosomatic Medicine*, **29**, 33–51.
Green, B. L., Lindy, J. D., Grace, M. C. & Gleser, G. C. (1989). Multiple diagnosis in posttraumatic stress disorder. The role of war stressors. *Journal of Nervous and Mental Disease*, **177**, 329–35.
Hersheiser, M. R. & Quarantelli, E. L. (1976). The handling of the dead in a disaster. *Omega*, **7**, 195–208.
Horowitz, M., Wilner, N. & Alvarez, W. (1979). Impact of event scale: a measure of subjective stress. *Psychosomatic Medicine*, **41**, 209–18.
Hytten, K. & Hasle, A. (1989). Fire fighters: a study of stress and coping. *Acta Psychiatrica Scandinavica Supplementum*, **80**(355), 50–5.
Jones, D. J. (1985). Secondary disaster victims: the emotional effects of recovering and identifying human remains. *American Journal of Psychiatry*, **142**, 303–7.
Kaplan, H. I. & Sadock, B. J. (1985). *Comprehensive textbook of psychiatry*. Baltimore: Williams & Wilkins.
Laufer, R. S., Brett, E. & Gallops, M. S. (1985). Dimensions of posttraumatic stress disorder among Vietnam veterans. *Journal of Nervous and Mental Disease*, **173**, 538–45.

Laufer, R. S., Gallops, M. S. & Frey-Woulters, E. (1984). War stress and trauma. *Journal of Health and Social Behavior*, **25**, 65–85.

Lifton, R. J. (1973). *Home from the war*. New York: Simon & Schuster, Inc.

Lindy, J. D., Green, B. L. & Grace, M. C. (1987). The stressor criterion and posttraumatic stress disorder. *Journal of Nervous and Mental Disease*, **175**, 269–72.

Lundin, T. (1990). The rescue personnel and the disaster stress. In J. E. Lundeberg, U. Otto & B. Rybeck (eds.), *Proceedings of the Second International Conference on Wartime Medical Services*. Stockholm, Sweden: Frsvarets forskningsanstalt-FOA, pp. 208–16. (25–29 June)

Maloney, J. (1988a). The Gander disaster: body handling and identification process. In R. J. Ursano & C. Fullerton (eds.) *Exposure to death, disasters and bodies*. Bethesda, MD: F. Edward Hebert School of Medicine, Uniformed Services University of the Health Sciences (DTIC: A 203163), pp. 41–66.

Maloney, J. (1988b). Body handling at Dover AFB: The Gander disaster. In R. J. Ursano & C. Fullerton (eds.) *Individual and Group Behavior in Toxic and Contained Environments*. Bethesda, MD: F. Edward Hebert School of Medicine, Uniformed Services University of the Health Sciences (DTIC: A 203267), pp. 97–102.

McCarroll, J. E., Ursano, R. J., Fullerton, C. S. & Lundy, A. L. (June, 1992). Dimensions of stress among mortuary workers. Paper presented at the First World Conference, The International Society for Traumatic Stress Studies, Amsterdam, The Netherlands.

McCarroll, J. E., Ursano, R. J., Ventis, W. L. et al., (in press). *Effects of experience and gender on anticipated stress of handling the dead. British Journal of Clinical Psychiatry*.

Mefferd, R. B., Hale, H. B., Shannon, I. L., Prigmore, J. R. & Ellis, J. P. (1971). Stress responses as criteria for personnel selection: baseline study. *Aerospace Medicine*, **42**, 42–51.

Miles, M. S., Demi, A. S. & Mostyn-Aker, P. (1984). Rescue workers' reactions following the Hyatt Hotel disaster. *Death Education*, **8**, 315–31.

Mitchell, J. H., Sproule, B. J. & Chapman, C. B. (1958). The physiological meaning of the maximal oxygen intake test. *Journal of Clinical Investigation*, **37**, 538–47.

Myers, D. G. (1989). Mental health and disaster. In R. Gist & B. Lubin (eds.) *Psychosocial aspects of disaster*. New York: John Wiley & Sons, p. 198.

Norris, F.H. & Murrell, S. A. (1988). Prior experience as a moderator of disaster impact on anxiety symptoms in older adults. *American Journal of Community Psychology*, **16**, 665–83.

Penzien, D. B., Hursey, K. G., Kotses, H. & Beazel, H. A. (1982). The effects of anticipatory stress on heart rate and T-wave amplitude. *Biological Psychology*, **15**, 241–8.

Robinson, M. (1988). Psychological support to the Dover AFB body handlers. In R. J. Ursano & C. Fullerton (eds.) *Exposure to death, disasters and bodies*. Bethesda, MD: F. Edward Hebert School of Medicine, Uniformed Services University of the Health Sciences (DTIC: A 203163, pp. 67–90).

Rubonis, A. V. & Bickman, L. (1991). A test of the consensus and distinctiveness attribution principles in victims of disaster. *Journal of Applied Social Psychology*, **21**, 791–809.

Rundell, J. R., Ursano, R. J., Holloway, H. C. & Silberman, E. K. (1989).

Psychiatric responses to trauma. *Hospital and Community Psychiatry*, **40**, 68–74.

Schwartz, H. J. (1984). Fear of the dead: the role of social ritual in neutralizing fantasies from combat. In H. J. Schwartz (ed.) *Psychotherapy of the combat veteran*. New York: Spectrum Publications.

Solomon, S. D., Smith, E. M., Robins, L. N. & Fischbach, R. L. (1987). Social involvement as a mediator of disaster-induced stress. *Journal of Applied Social Psychology*, **17**, 1092–1112.

Sumova, A. & Jakoubek, B. (1989). Analgesia and impact induced by anticipation stress: involvement of the endogenous opioid peptide system. *Brain Research*, **503**, 273–80.

Susnowski, T. (1988). Patterns of skin conductance and heart rate changes under anticipatory stress conditions. *Journal of Psychophysiology*, **2**, 231–8.

Talbot J. A., Hales, R. E. & Yudofsky, S. C. (eds.) (1988) *Textbook of psychiatry*. Washington, DC: American Psychiatric Association Press.

Taylor, A. J. W. & Frazer, A. G. (1982). The stress of post-disaster body handling and victim identification work. *Journal of Human Stress*, **8**, 4–12.

Ursano, R. J. (1987). Commentary: Posttraumatic stress disorder: the stressor criterion. *Journal of Nervous and Mental Disease*, **175**, 273–5.

Ursano, R. J. & Fullerton, C. S. (1990). Cognitive and behavioral responses to trauma. *Journal of Applied Social Psychology*, **20**(21), 1766–75.

Ursano, R. J., Fullerton, C. S., Wright, K. M. & McCarroll, J. E. (eds.) (1990). *Trauma, disasters and recovery*. (DTIC: A225911: 104 pages) Uniformed Services University of the Health Sciences, Bethesda, MD.

Ursano, R. J., Fullerton, C. S., Wright, K. M., McCarroll, J. E., Norwood, A. E. & Dinneen, M. P. (eds.) (1992). *Disaster workers: Trauma and social support*. Uniformed Services University of the Health Sciences, Bethesda, MD.

Ursano, R. J. & McCarroll, J. E. (1990). The nature of a traumatic stressor: handling dead bodies. *Journal of Nervous and Mental Disease*, **178**, 396–8.

Weisaeth, L. (1989). A study of behavioral responses to an industrial disaster. *Acta Psychiatrica Scandinavica Supplementum*, **80**(355), 13–24.

4

Psychological and psychiatric aspects of technological disasters

LARS WEISAETH

The Greek inventor Daedalus was not concerned whether his inventions helped or harmed society. Icarus, his son, joyfully ascended on the wings his father invented. As he flew closer to the sun, however, the wings melted, sending Icarus plummeting into the sea, where he drowned. Man versus nature, man against himself, and man versus technology, is the topic of this paper.

Technology has a dual character. It is able to prevent disasters and to cause disasters. By definition, a technological disaster is the result of a failure of humanmade products. These include air crashes, large scale road accidents, train derailments and collisions, passenger ship and other maritime catastrophes, including oil rig destructions, industrial explosions, oil blowout, large fires of all sorts, mining disasters, nuclear plant accidents, leakages of hazardous substances from toxic waste disposal, etc. In contrast to war, another type of humanmade disaster, technological disaster, is not intended. In a technological disaster, a human action, or a product of human hand (a failed technology), results in the disruption of a community, and, at times, considerable death, injury and destruction.

Technology is certainly becoming safer. Road traffic, airlines, and railways are subject to stringent safety procedures. However, the absolute number of technological disasters is increasing. As technology develops, there are simply more things that can go wrong, even if unintended and uncalculated. When something does go wrong, or a mistake is made, there has been a human error and someone is always responsible. But is there always someone willing to assume the responsibility? Whether or not someone does assume the responsibility makes a substantial difference in the psychological reactions of those affected and of the public at large.

Since the industrial revolution, human beings have tried to harness the forces of nature by their inventions. In all walks of life, the last 200 years has seen amazing scientific progress. The pace of development itself, at times, seems to get out of control and nature, like the Greek gods, hits back. Ever since the Greek dramas, 'hybris' (arrogance, foolhardiness, and false pride) has meant the hero's downfall: 'Do not fly too close to the sun.' The 'experts' said that the Titanic was unsinkable and that nuclear reactors would only get out of control once every 5000 years. What is foolproof?

The aim of medicine has been to prolong life at nearly all costs, but it is increasingly evident that it is more important to add life to years rather than years to life. Our attempts to escape the unavoidable suffering inherent in the fragmentary nature of our present existence give rise to most of the avoidable sufferings in life [freely quoted from Hugh Kingsmill, 'The Genealogy of Hitler', in *The Poisoned Crown* (1944)]. Half a century later, one can observe our love affair with technology, and wonder to what extent it gave us a false sense of mastery and served to deny man's eternal existential problems of death and human frailty.

About 5% of all deaths in Western countries are violent or 'unnatural'. The vast majority are caused by accidents, primarily transport accidents. Very few of these violent deaths, about 5%, involve multiple deaths (more than five lives lost). Still, the large-scale accident or disaster is overwhelming when it strikes. For example, the 158 deaths caused by the ferry disaster off the Norwegian coast in April, 1990 made up 30% of the transport related deaths of the entire year in Norway.

The leak of poisonous gas from a Union Carbide Corporation plant in Bhopal, India, occurred in a densely populated suburb. It is now believed to have killed more than 3800 people. In addition, of the 300000 injured, 30000 were temporarily blinded by keratitis, and many were permanently disabled. The psychiatric morbidity has, of course, been striking (Sethi et al., 1987). The number of deaths which the nuclear radiation and fallout from the Chernobyl reactor accident caused, or contributed to, will never be known for certain.

Such incidents of mass death and injury overwhelm the emergency care services, at least in the initial phase. Helpers are likely to share the sense of powerlessness of the disaster victims. For this reason, disaster medicine and its subdiscipline, disaster psychiatry, are taught in medical schools as a part of emergency medicine.

This chapter will address recent developments which highlight the importance of technological disasters in our time. In addition, the chapter will describe both the classical technological disaster and the newer toxic type of disaster. Data from two recent technological disaster studies will be used to illustrate the major issues. The acute- and long-term psychosocial responses to a classical technological disaster are presented in a study of individuals exposed to an industrial explosion. In contrast to this familiar scenario, the much more alarming and newer type of technological failure, the toxic disaster, exemplified by the Chernobyl nuclear plant accident, and its short- and long-term psychosocial consequences, is presented.

Natural versus technological disaster: a blurred distinction?

Traditionally, the two types of disaster have been, 1) natural, i.e. an act of God, and 2) 'manmade'. Whereas in Western countries 'an act of God' has come to mean the power of the elements, a natural or accidental causation, in other parts of the world, divine intervention is still seen as a possible explanation for a disaster. Islamic fatalism, for example, explained the death of more than 1400 people in a tunnel, during the Haj in Mecca on 3 July, 1990, as God's will.

The United Nations General Assembly Resolution 42/169, adopted on 11 December, 1987, designated the 1990s as the decade of natural disaster reduction (WHO, 1988). Does the idea of reducing natural disasters seem surprising? Consider the following. Of the 109 worst natural disasters between 1960 and 1987, 41 occurred in developing countries (Berz, 1989). Furthermore, the number of deaths caused by disasters was far greater in the developing countries: 758 850 compared to 11 441 in developed countries! In general, the number of deaths and injuries caused by disasters is closely related to a country's level of economic development. This is how technology comes in. Preparedness, prevention and mitigation are the three key activities for coping with disasters and disaster risks. Earthquakes, windstorms, tsunamis, floods, landslides, volcanic eruptions, wildfires and other calamities have killed nearly 3 million people worldwide over the past two decades, and have adversely affected the lives of at least 800 million more (WHO, 1991). The vast majority of these lives could have been spared by better warning systems, more evacuation capacity, better building construction, etc. For example, the Netherlands has not suffered a major flood since the devastating 1953 flood, which claimed 1500 lives. One consequence of this disaster was the development of an intensive program of dam building. Technology can save lives.

If, however, technology can save lives by controlling natural hazards, failure or lack of technology increasingly is seen as responsible for deaths occurring in previously 'natural' disasters. As the world grows smaller, people in developing countries will probably alter their attitude about deaths from natural disasters, from a resigned and fatalistic outlook, to feelings of bitter despair: 'It could have been prevented.' The previous understanding and acceptance of the natural disaster through a general religious and fatalistic outlook may be lost. It is likely that this will increase the psychiatric morbidity of disasters.

In addition, disasters previously classified as natural are today considered, to an ever increasing degree, to be manmade. Mamiduzzaman Khan Choudhury, Professor of Meteorology from Bangladesh, commented at a 1990 meeting where representatives from 75 countries discussed the problem of global climatic changes: 'You quarrel while we drown.' He knew that 'manmade' future climatic changes which result in a rise in sea level may drown Bangladesh; floods used to be only natural disasters. The 1991 flood in Bangladesh claimed 200 000 lives. Still, there were 300 000 fewer casualties than there would have been without technological advances. How did the survivors interpret the causes of the flood? We do not fully know as yet, but there are reports that the educated citizens discussed the deforestation of the Himalayas, the weakening of the ozone layer, etc., as possible contributory causes, while the uneducated masses felt that God was angry with them.

The earthquake in Armenia, USSR, in December, 1988, claimed 30 000 lives. The majority died because their houses were poorly constructed. Was this a natural disaster or a technological failure? Similarly, after the San Francisco earthquake in 1989, harsh criticism was directed towards the method of road construction which had been used. Collapsing freeways had caused a number of deaths (see the chapter by McCaughey, Hoffman & Llewellyn in this book). The earthquake, however, was the same Richter magnitude as the Armenian quake. The effects of an earthquake in modern times depends, to a large extent, on the breakdown of manmade products.

Will man's changing perceptions of who is responsible, or who is to blame for disasters, have any psychological consequences? In all likelihood it will. Nature can do harm, but nature has no evil intent. Man has this capability. A dramatic example of the striking difference in response between a new technological threat and a permanent but natural threat is offered by the Chernobyl disaster. After the disaster, there was strong public reaction in several countries to the radioactive fallout from the Chernobyl reactor. In contrast to this is the moderate, or even absent, reaction to the normal background radiation from radon, which is a much greater risk to health. The former can be blamed on somebody, but the latter is more one's own responsibility since it depends upon where you choose to build your home.

The more human causation lies behind a disaster, the more pathogenic it seems to be in terms of psychiatric morbidity (Baum, 1986; see chapter by Davidson & Baum, this book). Manmade disasters are said to be more traumatic because of their unfamiliarity, unpredictability, uncontrollability and culpability. War may be an exception to this rule, since the suffering and death in war may take on a deep sense of noble sacrifice, perhaps increasing stress tolerance. However, this requires more direct study. Although there is a dearth of comparative studies (Frederick, 1986), the few findings available point to a more virulent effect of what man does to man than what nature does to man (Luchterhand, 1971), or what accidental trauma, for which no one is to blame, does to man (Weisaeth, 1989*a, c*). The man to man context differs from natural trauma in the pernicious and ever present attacks on an individual's integrity and self respect. Nature does not threaten man's self respect, even if it kills him. Thus human failure and violence are likely to produce more aggressive responses. In the words of Kai Erikson, technological disasters are not necessary. They are avoidable, therefore, they produce aggression rather than acceptance. They also produce more distrust and fear of other humans than do natural and accidental traumas. Because of this, manmade disasters frequently cause withdrawal and social isolation which is more detrimental to mental health than the limited phobias of natural disasters. (Weisaeth, 1989*a*). There are no available comparative studies of responses to a technological disaster which was perceived as truly accidental, and one which was seen as due to negligence, in which to examine this further.

Deadly 'survival' responses: is man a captive of his own evolution?

Through 4 million years of evolution the human race has had a long and intimate relationship with nature. In order to survive, the human race has had to cope with the natural dangers of the elements, wild animals and human enemies. One has good reason to believe that the genetic apparatus in the survivors, the people of today, has become uniquely adapted to cope with such threats. Some survival instincts can still be seen almost daily by semirealistic phobias such as fears of closed spaces, heights, darkness, etc. These atavisms sometimes still have life preserving effects.

It is interesting to speculate whether man's capacity to survive natural disasters and war is greater than his survival capacity when facing technological hazards. This hypothesis has not been systematically studied. But the fundamental question has been raised as to whether adaptive skills previously used with success in the pretechnological age have now become detrimental (Dixon, 1987). Every psychotherapist knows, and for that matter every psychotherapy patient perhaps knows even better, how extremely difficult it is for the human brain to rid itself of the effects of very early experiences. Is humankind even more at a loss when it comes to riding itself of the evolutionary effects of selection in the survival of the fittest?

While man's interaction with natural hazards has been going on for several thousand generations, his experiences with the breakdown of humanmade constructions can hardly be longer than a few hundred generations, i.e. a few thousand years. Perhaps this is not even enough time to give evolution a chance to work out its principles. Modern technology, dating back to the Industrial Revolution with power driven machines, trains, and manufacturing industry utilizing hundreds of potentially harmful materials, is scarcely 200 years old. A few examples will illustrate how, when facing a modern technological disaster, man's instinct at times, costs rather than saves lives.

In 1988, only six miners survived the coalmine disaster in Borken, Germany. Fifty other miners died. The only miners to survive were those who fled *into* the mine. All who tried to run out, to escape into the open air, perished because of toxic gases at the exit (Wolfram Schüffel, personal communication). Flight behavior in the natural environment, as well as when facing human enemies, has long been man's instinctive response to dangers with which he could not cope. Uncontrolled flight, as in individual or group panic, is characterized by overwhelming fear and the compelling thought of 'getting out' and 'getting away'. The consequences of such uncontrolled escape behavior can be fatal in manmade environments like mines, and also in high rise buildings, ships, oil rigs, etc. The fear of engulfment can precipitate premature jumping from a sinking ship. The fear of flames and smoke can elicit fatal jumping from high buildings.

Perceptually, humans are not only inclined to, but have no other choice than to react to cues of danger discovered with their limited senses. In a tunnel fire, for example, individuals will react to the sight of smoke, and its irritable and seemingly choking effect, provoking extreme fear and uncontrolled flight. At the same time, the effects of poisonous gases, like carbon monoxide, will not be noticed. When designing the physical layout of a construction site, to what extent is planning for survival in, for instance, a hotel fire, based upon technical calculations of toxic elements, rather than on the stimuli which are detected by the senses and probably contribute more to behavior?

If smoke moves faster than 7 meters per second, which it sometimes does, you cannot survive by running away from it. But your legs will probably try. It is a biological instinct, like the elk that tries to outrun your car by running ahead of it. The task, therefore may be to control one's basic survival patterns. Many died in Bhopal because they ran ahead of the approaching gas cloud. Certainly, many who were indoors died because they failed to shut the windows. Controlling natural responses is not enough. Problem solving is also needed. Under severe stress, man's basic, primitive response patterns tend to appear while learned responses tend to disappear. Drilled responses and overlearned procedures are the most stress resistant, while creativity which is so essential in complex problem solving, easily gives way to stereotypical responses. If this hypothesis is correct, that in some situations there is a conflict between man's natural behavior and necessary survival behavior, then the education, training and practice must be the decisive determinants of disaster response if one is to cope successfully with the dangers of a manmade disaster environment. By stress inoculation training (practice in simulated environments) and other techniques, industrial employees have been able to increase their problem solving capacity under stress (Hytten, Jensen & Skauli, 1990). Much work remains to be done in this promising research field.

The human brain is programmed for various types of adaptive behavior that are almost automatic. Fear helps man to discover danger and facilitates defensive strategies like flight behavior. However, the freezing response, adaptive when facing certain animals, is hardly helpful for the pedestrian who loses his mobility when seeing a car approaching.

Through its familiarity with natural dangers, the human perceptive apparatus has become suited to the discovery of danger. This is less so with the 'unnatural' dangers. Technological threats do not give the same warning. Frequently, some instrument is required to discover the danger in the early phase. Knowledge and information become more important, as well as trust in one's information sources. 'The position of man is obviously extremely insecure unless he can find out what is happening around him' (Rebecca West, *A Train of Powder*, New York, 1955). In his study of carbon monoxide leaks from a closed underground coalmine, Couch (1990) found that many exposed people refused to use the measuring instruments provided by the authorities. The population outside the risk area thought the problems of the affected population were exaggerated in order to increase compensation claims.

Fear and lack of fear

Responses to technological disasters are partly determined by the beliefs people had about the potential hazard before the disaster. The introduction of a new technology increases the risk of accidents, at least temporarily. About 4000 lives were lost on riverboats on the Mississippi River from 1810 to 1840, mainly due to boiler explosions. The novelty of the technology added to the trauma after the accidents. The military has had long experience in applying this knowledge. The psychological effect of a new weapon technology is always particularly horrifying, especially the first time it is used. When technology fails, and probably more so when the failing technology is new, it takes longer for the official inquiry about the causes to be published. The public's anxiety may be reinforced by this time lapse. Knowledge of the cause will also determine what can, and will, be done. This is of great public interest and is important to recovery. Frequently, the causes are so complex that the public is unable to comprehend the technicalities, leaving the feeling that the responsibility is dissolved, and that no one is to blame. As stated by Thomas Mann: 'The worst disasters are the ones for which there is no one to blame.'

The history of railway accidents is especially illustrative of how people respond to the failure of new technology. Initially, people were fascinated by, attracted to, and frightened of, the new and somewhat risky way of moving faster by machine power than by natural means. Soon after the railway was introduced in England, extremely destructive collisions with many deaths began to occur. The passengers' emotional reactions, particularly the anxiety responses after near misses and real accidents (they would be called posttraumatic stress reactions today), were misinterpreted by physicians. At the time, medicine had no real understanding of the relationship between the body and the mind. The physical signs of anxiety were misunderstood as symptoms of organic illness. A series of new diseases resulted, from 'tunnel disease' to 'railway spine'. In his influential book of 1866, the London surgeon John Ericksen (1866) gave seemingly convincing case stories of posttraumatic illness, which resulted in large compensation payments. This was neither the first, nor the last, time that the nature of anxiety responses to terrifying events would be misinterpreted. The dominant somatic interest and bias of modern medicine, the resistance in patients and society, have contributed to the slow growth in the understanding of these psychological problems.

Although not recognized in the disaster literature, the first systematic psychiatric disaster studies were undertaken by Eduard Stierlin (1909, 1911) of Zurich. He investigated 21 survivors of a mining disaster in 1906, and 135 persons two months after the earthquake in Messina, Italy in 1908. He compared the responses of technological and natural disasters. Stierlin identified cases of traumatic neurosis, as well as subjects who developed

Freudian 'anxiety neurosis'. He described a number of phenomena: a latency period in the psychological cases which was not seen in the cerebral organic cases; resiliency in children; vulnerability in the elderly; the rarity of classical hysteria; the triggering effect, as well as the curative shock effect, of trauma upon hysteria; the absence of compensation issues; frequent physiological disturbances; and posttraumatic sleep disturbances. Stierlin emphasized the etiological role of fright.

In a Norwegian population survey measuring fear of flying, 8% of adults (14% of females and 3% of males) suffered from flight phobia (Ekeberg, Seeberg & Ellertsen, 1989). However, as many as 54% stated they never were afraid of flying (67% of the men). But, when the answers from the men who had flown more than ten times in the last year were compared with a similar group of men actually on board a plane, the latter group reported more anxiety (Ekeberg, Seeberg & Ellertsen, 1988). The most likely explanation is that men deny some of their fears of flying when questioned outside the stressful situations. Fight or flight patterns are of no use to passengers on an airplane. In fact, the high arousal related to these patterns of reaction can cause additional problems. Denial is facilitated in passengers of jet airliners by the inability of humans to perceive forward movement, even at tremendous speed, during cruising. In contrast, downward movement, even if slight, is perceived. In fact, from the first days in life, sudden falling causes anxiety. Intensive information courses, and exposure training sessions can produce good treatment results for flight phobia (Ekeberg, Seeberg & Ellertson, 1990).

One may wonder whether lack of fear is just as irrational as too much fear. A rational fear is proportional to the external threat. The fear leads to vigilance and protective measures such as wise avoidance or a rational solution. Rational fear does not usually lead to psychiatric symptoms. Lack of fear, however, may signal denial of risk. An individual's capacity for denial is influenced by his or her developmental history. Shakespeare's statement in Hamlet, the 'best safety lies in fear', may be a wise statement. In pilot selection, the Defense Mechanism Test is used to identify and screen out candidates with a particularly high defense, i.e. the ability to block out danger signals. Such pilots tend to have more accidents. One explanation for this finding, may be that when denial is broken by a crisis, overreaction and more mistakes may occur. Similar findings were made in the study of the industrial explosion detailed below. Deniers of the risks involved at work had more severe shock and early reactions, and less adaptive responses when the blast occurred (Weisaeth, 1984).

What cannot be controlled can be denied. What cannot be seen is

Table 4.1. *Time phases of disaster*

Time phase	Proximity of the danger	Coping
Steady state	Distant	Preparedness
Crisis	Approaching	Crisis management
Disaster impact	Imminent/present	Survival/rescue

Afterperiods:
   Shock phase
   Reaction phase
   Repair phase
   New orientation
	Passed	Working through shock and posttraumatic stress reactions

especially easy to deny. Facing heavy pollution from nearby oil well fires in Kuwait in 1991, our consultation team experienced this same phenomenon. The polluted air could only be seen in the distance. There was the illusion that there was no pollution where we were standing.

Feelings of personal invulnerability reinforce denial. Today, man is in control of many risks that previously could not be influenced. Furthermore, today, man can unleash forces that have tremendous destructive potential. Denial in today's world may also have very different consequences than in earlier times.

When the primitive psychological defense mechanism of denial is challenged, a new and exaggerated awareness of vulnerability may be experienced. This, in turn, can easily create irrational fears, for example, of the invisible. An exaggerated fear of modern technology may also be a part of the NIMBY syndrome ('not in my back yard'). In the international arena, authorities are having great difficulty finding locations for detoxification plants. The public demands that such installations be built, but absolutely not close to where they live.

The phases of a technological disaster can be defined by the time since the disaster began. Each time phase of technological disasters has specific stressors that must be coped with (see Table 4.1).

Technological crisis situations

Technological crisis situations frequently pose the classic stress problems: 1) a severe threat to important values: human lives, finances, ecology, politics, etc.; 2) a combination of infrequent events; 3) reduced control. 4) high uncertainty; 5) lack of information; and 6) time pressure. These reduce the industrial employees'and the leaders' capacity for crisis management and, thereby, their ability to stop the disastrous chain of events from unfolding. The decision maker may himself be exposed to physical danger, the stress of responsibility, fear of failure, and reduced or even loss of control of a situation that perhaps is rapidly changing. The decision maker may make difficult decisions such as choosing the lesser of two evils because there is no solution that does not cause any harm. The decision maker intensely experiences the lack of information on which to base decisions. Disagreements and irrational interpersonal interactions with subordinates, colleagues, or superiors may increase the burden.

Modern technological crisis situations are complex and many factors must be considered. Decision makers experience information overload, and pressure to act very quickly and correctly in the face of impending danger. The problem solver must: 1) recognize the problem (i.e. critical event identification – the ability to discover that something has altered the steady state situation, and the capacity to interpret that change as a severe threat); 2) gather relevant information (which often is intensely threatening and therefore may be extremely unpleasant); 3) analyze alternative solutions (if there are any) 4) choose correct alternatives; and 5) implement the chosen solution.

Stress reactions may disturb each of these steps. Two response patterns seen in severe stress situations may disturb and significantly reduce problem solving capacity: defensive avoidance and hypervigilance. In addition, impairments in perceptual function occur: restricted and selectively reinforced perception of stimuli, a tendency to all-or-nothing perception of threatening aspects of the situation, and reduced information searching. The thinking capacity, or so called cognitive functions, may become more stereotypical, i.e. oriented to habitual themes, perseverating on selected items, or fixated to one or a few alternatives. Time perspective is frequently altered. Long-term thinking is reduced and priority is given to short-term thinking. The sense of time passing may be expanded or shortened, and the ability to think analytically is reduced. At the emotional level, surprise, anxiety (helplessness), depression (hopelessness), irritability, and reduced tolerance for disagreements are seen frequently. At the behavioral level, paralysis of action, or impulsive action may occur. Janis and Mann (1977) described a particular group dynamic, called 'group think', a collective pattern of defensive avoidance. Education is needed to teach these social psychological phenomena to every planner and operator in industry, defense, and other institutions which manage potentially destructive crisis situations.

Societal vulnerability to technological disaster

In some parts of the world, collective hazards are always present and represent a constant threat to survival. From the global perspective, both natural and manmade disasters constitute a major cause of death, as well as physical, psychological, and social distress and misery.

In the industrialized countries, the concentration of industrial complexes, advanced technology, and the density of population in urban centers have increased the possibility of disasters, and magnified their potential destructiveness. Although technology is becoming safer, the frequency of technological hazards is increasing owing to its large scale. The complex nature of modern technologies increases the risk of breakdown, e.g. thousands of dangerous substances are handled in the chemical industries and in the world's extensive transport systems. Although accidents may be less frequent, their consequences are more severe. Contrary to natural disasters in developing countries, peacetime technological disasters tend to be partial, limited in scope, and well circumscribed. Usually one's home or one's job, but not both, are destroyed. Although the destruction is devastating, the number of dead is less. These disasters are more intensive than pervasive. The larger social system is not directly affected and is willing, if not always totally able, to respond.

A toxic cooking oil disaster in Spain killed 600 and harmed another 25 000. More than 6000 people were referred to psychiatrists with toxic oil syndrome (Lopez-Ibor et al., 1985). The Zeebrugge ferry accident killed hundreds and exemplified the vulnerability of new ferry construction to human error. The Piper Alpha oil rig disaster in the North Sea during the summer of 1988 cost 167 human lives. The inquiry report listed 106 technical and organizational changes which the British authorities accepted. On older oil platforms in the North Sea, the Fatal Accident Rate (FAR), deaths per 100 million work hours, is approximately 21. New platforms must meet a new standard, 15 FAR. In comparison, the FAR values of bus travel have been estimated to be three, car driving 56, and mountain climbing about 4000.

'Modern' technological disasters may affect large areas, even several countries at once. As with other types of disasters, technological disasters cause death, injury, material destruction, financial losses, and have political implications. In addition, modern technology has the potential to cause tremendous environmental pollution. The Chernobyl nuclear plant disaster is illustrative of the extent of a modern technological disaster. The environmental consequences may be staggering. When toxic substances in the Sandoz chemical plant leaked into the Rhine, the cost resulting from poisoning the area was many times greater than the cost caused by destruction of the plant itself by the fire. On a larger scale, such toxic emission might have caused damage beyond anything seen in Europe in peacetime. After future technological disasters, the bill for cleaning up the environment may be truly formidable.

One technological disaster may be enough to stop an entire field of industry. The 'Hindenburg' airship fire in 1929 was the end of airship transport. The Three Mile Island nuclear power plant accident never developed into a disaster, except in a sociological sense (200 000 took to the roads). Although the accident stopped at the crisis level, it was very detrimental to further expansion of nuclear energy production in the United States. Chernobyl had even more extensive consequences in Europe. Nuclear energy production is relatively unique in that the whole population shares the risks. This is not so with coal mines, oil fields, etc. where production workers are alone in the area at risk.

As developing countries industrialize, technological disasters become an increasing threat. Gas leakage from the Union Carbide plant in Bhopal resulted in a substantial increase in patients seeking psychiatric help (Sethi et al., 1987). No exact figures on the psychiatric morbidity are available, but a series of studies have established morbidity in 20% to 50% of survivors one year after a disaster (Gleser, Green & Winget, 1981; Green et al., 1983; Sund, Holen & Weisaeth 1983; Weisaeth, 1985).

Even when there is only a brief duration of exposure, other manmade high shock disasters have shown persisting levels of morbidity in over 30% of the victims. Posttraumatic Stress Disorder (PTSD) is the most frequently reported disorder, followed by depression. Considering that some of the populations studied were in very good health prior to the disaster, and trained to cope with disaster, these morbidity rates are impressive. In addition, some groups had preventive and therapeutic interventions, e.g. industrial shift workers (Weisaeth, 1985), and offshore oil rig employees (Holen, 1990). Long-term psychiatric morbidity has also been reported (Ploger, 1977).

Some technological disasters, such as the accident at the Chernobyl nuclear power plant, are not acute, time-limited events. The accident, whether nuclear or other toxic waste, starts a sequence of events that continues to unfold over several years, thereby creating a situation of chronic stress. At times, these disasters have no definite 'low point', therefore the exposed population, does not know when 'the worst' is over (Baum 1986; see Davidson & Baum in this book). Disasters caused by a failure of technology imply a loss of control, i.e. although unintended, someone has failed. Feelings of betrayal and distrust of authorities and industries are common.

Risk factors and dimensions of disaster trauma

Those involved with technological disasters need to know predictors of the frequency of the disaster, the disaster type and severity, and the course of the resulting psychosocial disturbances. The psychosocial impact of a disaster is affected by the cause of the disaster, the amount of geographical displacement, the degree of threat to life, and the degree of loss and community disruption caused by the disaster. A disaster is the sum of numerous individual traumas. In times of war and peace, traumas include both physical and psychological components that vary greatly in their nature, severity, intensity, duration, and suddenness of onset.

The major psychological aspects of trauma are: 1) the overwhelming threat to one's own life, 2) the often severe and mutilating injuries – such as burns, 3) the experience of losing loved ones, and perhaps helplessly witnessing such deaths, and 4) facing impossible choices such as helping others at great risk to one's own survival. The dominant stressors at the periphery of a disaster zone may be high levels of uncertainty and little possibility of exerting control.

The lack of familiarity, anticipation, warning, control, predictability, and leadership increases the likelihood that the disaster will have shock effects that create paralysis and inhibition. Severe threats to life or the risk of being injured, trapped, or rendered helpless, also increase the risk. The likelihood of recurrence can prolong the stress of the disaster. Damage to, or destruction of, home, property or things of value are of secondary importance, as shown by the low psychiatric morbidity in disasters with less severe threats to life (Raphael, 1986).

In exposed individuals, the degree of preparedness, the severity of the threat, and the amount of mastery appear to be important determinants of the outcome, mediating between the stressors and psychopathological outcomes. The classic symptoms of traumatic exposure may result: helplessness, anxiety, emotional storm, hopelessness, inhibition, or conflict. Victims who were caught unaware ('shock trauma'), or in inescapable situations, appear to be at greater risk.

The amount of social support available during, and after, the disaster are also important. Community, company, and communication disasters ('The three Cs') have different social contexts. In Norway, different types of psychiatric interventions were used in these disasters (Weisaeth 1993). This classification of disaster types is related to Green's (1982) classification of a disaster as central or peripheral to the community. The agencies with which one must form a relationship in order to be effective in disaster consultation and support services vary in each case. For example, in communication disasters, people die, or are severely injured often far away from home. Their social network is not there. Relatives and friends must be brought in from the outside. The family comes in to give and also to take. They give what they have of social support. In cases of bereavement, they take what they can from those with first hand knowledge of the tragedy. On the other hand, a more central type of devastating disaster, e.g. the Buffalo Creek flood, changes the entire structure of the community, causes disruption of the kin network and loss of social support. More psychiatric morbidity can be expected in this type of situation (Erikson, 1976).

A disaster affects individuals, groups, and the community as a whole. The family unit is extremely important for disaster helpers. Were the family members together when the disaster struck? Were they split up? Were only some members affected? In the latter two cases, family members seeking to find each other (search behavior), is usually prominent during impact and the immediate aftermath of the disaster. The need to reunite may be so strong that individual evacuation may be difficult or even impossible. Most industrial disasters will hit employees and not whole families, destroying jobs not homes.

Some psychological aspects of technological disasters can best be illustrated by presenting findings from 'the impact, acute, subacute, and long-term postdisaster phases of a devastating industrial disaster (Weisaeth, 1984). Since many classic technological disasters are industrial and severely effect company employees, an intervention model for company disasters is briefly presented. Some consequences of the Chernobyl nuclear reactor accident are presented to illustrate psychological repercussions occurring far off as well as near, and short term as well as long term.

The paint-factory disaster

In 1976 a tremendous explosion hit the production plant of Norway's largest paint factory. The building collapsed and a series of explosions followed. A huge fire destroyed the production plant and the warehouses. Nearly 30000 square meters of buildings were engulfed in flames stretching up to a height of 400 meters. The fire was fed by millions of liters of chemicals and by 50 million cubic meters of air. A local windstorm was created by the combustion. The explosion shook the neighborhood and was heard kilometers away. The threat of spreading fire and further explosions necessitated the evacuation of 1000 people. Helped by earlier rain and fortunate wind direction, 150 fire fighters contained the fire within 12 hours and extinguished it after 36 hours. Six workers were killed. Of the 125 survivors, 21 had minor, and 2 had severe injuries. The community lost about 400 jobs as a result of fire.

This is the largest industrial disaster that has ever occurred in Scandinavia. Many aspects made this large scale technological accident a typical example of a 'modern disaster' and a psychic 'shock trauma': the lack of forewarning (90.4% received no warning), the brief but violent impact, the circumscribed but completely damaged area, and the great material destruction but limited number of casualties. The disaster was unprecedented, unanticipated, sudden, violent, uncontrollable and brief. Central to this disaster was the large number of people exposed to the shock trauma, and the narrow escape. Many individuals were exposed to severe danger but were not physically harmed.

While the factory was still smouldering, all employees were guaranteed continuous employment and assured that they would not suffer economic losses. Within two weeks the company improvised new jobs. The additional (secondary) disaster stressors, e.g. unemployment, economic difficulties, and compensation issues which usually occur following disaster were less than usual.

Exposure to the disaster stress

Everyone present at work when the explosion struck, was included in the follow-up study. The exact location of each subject at the time of the explosion could be established with a high degree of accuracy. Three danger zones were established, high, medium, and low stress exposure. The 66 subjects who were closest to the explosion made up the high stress exposure group (Group A). The 59 subjects in the outer locations at the time of the explosion made up the medium stress exposure group (Group B). The low stress exposure group (Group C) consisted of 121 employees not at work at the time of the explosion. Many of the Group C subjects witnessed the disaster at a distance. All of this group experienced a fantasy trauma ('it could have been me'). Several subjects participated in demanding rescue work.

The high exposure group consisted of 58 men, 6 women, and averaged 44.7 years of age (range 19–69, median 49). The medium exposure group was composed of 45 men, 14 women, and averaged 41.6 years old (range 17–70, median 43). The low exposure group had 115 men, 5 women, and averaged 48.5 years of age (range 21–67, median 51). Since the groups differed on age and sex, it was not surprising that more of Group A (41%) had high levels of disaster training and experience, compared to Groups B and C (25% and 38% respectively). The younger men and women frequently had low levels of disaster training and experience. Among the older employees, participation in WW II accounted for much of the intensive disaster training and experience. Of Groups A and B, 24% and 12%, respectively, had experienced life endangering situations lasting months or years. As many as 76% of Group A, and 66% of Group B had witnessed the violent injury or death of another person. The cohort was fairly representative of industrial employees in Norway, except for the unusually high frequency of disaster competent employees, mainly due to recruitment of those having maritime experience. Only 2.4% of the whole cohort had previously suffered 'severe' psychiatric impairment, i.e. total work incapacity. The three groups all represented a mentally healthy sample compared to the total population.

Follow-up

Interviewing began two days after the disaster. All 125 persons at the site when the explosion occurred were identified, contacted, and were willing to participate in the study. The interviews were conducted in the immediate vicinity of the disaster area. The subjects were interviewed again seven months postdisaster. Data about the acute disaster responses were collected in both interviews. Interviews with clinical cases were carried out one, two, three, and four years postdisaster. The four year postdisaster questionnaire included all of the 238 subjects still living.

Disaster behavior

The coping task during the impact phase is survival and rescue (see Table 4.1). The immediate responses frequently influence the chances of survival, ability to escape or be rescued and, thus the course of disaster events and the total losses. We hypothesized that successful coping during the disaster would reduce the risk of posttraumatic stress problems (Weisaeth, 1989b).

Based upon seven response variables, we categorized the impact behavior of the 123 industrial employees who had been exposed to the explosion and survived without suffering severe injuries. The seven variables were:

cognitive function, inadequate behavior, help received, leadership, cooperative activity, and absolute and relative rescue efforts. In the high stress exposure group, 37% showed 'optimal' disaster behavior, 34% showed 'adaptive' behavior, and 'maladaptive' behavior was present in 29%. In this group, severe inadequate behaviors were rare. Modelling and corrective social interactions may have played an important role, i.e. good examples of successful coping could be copied. Inhibited behavior and uncontrolled flight dominated the maladaptive responses, reflecting the effect of the shock trauma. These responses could easily have added to the number of deaths because the evacuation routes were complicated and demanded problem solving. The presence of good role models helped prevent greater loss of lives.

The following background variables correlated strongly with optimal disaster behavior: high level of disaster training/experience, male, age above 40, maritime occupational background, above average intellectual ability, and a life history without mental health problems. A discriminant analysis with eight variables predicted correctly whether the response was optimal or less than optimal in 84% of the 121 subjects tested in the analysis. A high level of disaster training/experience yielded an overall correct prediction rate of 63.6%, a sensitivity of 81%, specificity of 85.9%, and positive predictive power of 70.7% in predicting optimal disaster behavior. Judging from these findings, if a person is given adequate education and training he is very likely to be reliable and act rationally, even when facing extreme stress.

The acute aftermath

Many subjects experienced psychophysiological disturbances: shaking 69%, hyperventilation 11%, breathing difficulties 31%, palpitations 52%, sweating 45%, nausea/vomiting 16%, diarrhea 14%. Some wrongly interpreted these bodily symptoms of anxiety as the effect of toxic substance. Rumors about this began to spread, a predictable problem in chemical and nuclear disaster. Rapid and correct diagnosis of the nature of the responses helped stop an epidemic outbreak. The police calmed the sources of the rumors. Uncontrolled flight behavior at the impact phase resulted in some employees running home without being registered at the site as survivors. This created uncertainty about the exact number of missing persons.

Acute catastrophic stress reactions occurred in 43.8% of Group A, and in 23.8% of Group B. Two severely injured employees developed brief psychotic reactions. Up to 23% of Group A and 34% of Group B were

Table 4.2. *Frequencies (%) of seven posttraumatic stress reactions: early acute phase after an industrial disaster*

	Group A[a] (n = 66)	Group B[b] (n = 59)	Group C[c] (n = 121)
Anxiety	82%	71%	19%
Sleep disturbances	83%	76%	36%
Traumatic nightmares	61%	41%	14%
Startle response	86%	80%	34%
Fear of destroyed area	79%	69%	19%
Irritability	24%	2%	4%
Social withdrawal	38%	9%	2%

Notes:
[a] High stress group.
[b] Medium stress group.
[c] Low stress group.

judged to be fit for rescue work in the immediate aftermath. We have evidence that such endeavors function as reparative activities.

Reaction phase: acute posttraumatic stress reactions

In 48% of the subjects who experienced posttraumatic anxiety reactions, the reaction appeared immediately after their rescue. In 90.6%, anxiety was reported within five hours. The rapid anxiety reactions reflect typical reactions to exposure to shock trauma. The anxiety reactions were somewhat delayed in three subjects. In two of these subjects, anxiety developed after 21 days and 32 days, respectively, when both men were in situations which strongly reminded them of the disaster. The third subject developed symptoms of a heart neurosis after a few weeks.

Meeting at the gate of the company area was accepted as a full day's work during the first few days after the disaster. The goal was helping the employee return to the disaster scene without provoking excessive anxiety in those with phobic responses. During this period, several employees suffered unnecessary new stresses performing search and clean-up work, fire duty, etc. For most employees these jobs were useful activities in coping with stress reactions. Posttraumatic stress reactions in the three groups during the acute phase are presented in Table 4.2.

The findings show a clear dose–response relationship. Exposure in Groups A and B meets the stressor criterion for the diagnosis of PTSD in the DSM-III-R, in that the traumatic event was 'markedly distressing to almost anyone'. In general, Group C does not satisfy this criterion. Only a minority have posttraumatic stress reactions of significance. A few C-subjects did experience traumatic exposures doing rescue work, making it reasonable to use the PTSD diagnosis. Collective and individual interventions, based on clinical observations, contributed to a reduction of the psychosocial problems.

The frequency of irritability increased during the first seven months, in contrast to the other posttraumatic stress reactions which all decreased in frequency and intensity. Further analyses showed that neurasthenic symptoms were the likely explanation for the irritability, i.e. the irritability was driven by the severe anxiety and sleep disturbances.

Blame was not a prominent aspect of this technological disaster. The workers shared a sense of responsibility. The leadership assumed responsibility for the care and welfare of the workers without admitting guilt and without criticizing those who made errors. Thus the social system itself remained intact. If one accepts that the deeper meaning of a trauma is reflected in the nightmarish dreams that follow a trauma, the absence of themes of interpersonal threat in the dreams of the victims supports the view that it was seen as a truly accidental trauma. This is in strong contrast to the repetitive nightmares and sense of danger in the posttraumatic stress syndromes which we have seen in victims of the most dramatically manmade traumas, e.g. torture.

The long-term outcome is presented in Table 4.3. The dose–response relationship persisted over the long term. Central exposure was almost a necessary precondition for the presence of long-term PTSD, but it was not a sufficient factor. Of the PTSD cases diagnosed at seven months, one third had a significant psychosocial problem at another time in their lives. (There was no correlation with age, civil status, education, secondary disaster stressors, or life events after the disaster.) The data support the finding that the actual trauma is necessary to the pathogenetic cause of the PTSD. A severe exposure was sufficient to produce acute PTSD, and necessary to produce a disorder of long duration.

Personal experiences and training in how to cope with disasters or other dangers were significantly related to outcome. There was an unusually high frequency of disaster competent employees in all three groups. This was due to maritime background and, in part, to participation in the Norwegian Merchant Marines during World War II. No one with little or no disaster training responded optimally to the disaster. Half of the unprepared group

Table 4.3. *Prognosis and course of PTSD in subject groups A, B, and C: paint factory disaster*

Group	PTSD	1 week	7 months	2 years[a]	3 years[a]	4 years[b]
A	Severe	29%	11%	9%	8%	
	Marked	8%	20%	9%	5%	
	Moderate	6%	6%	9%	9%	
	Total	43%	37%	27%	22%	19%
B	Severe	7%	2%	2%	2%	
	Marked	7%	10%	2%	0%	
	Moderate	9%	5%	9%	2%	
	Total	23%	17%	13%	4%	2%
C	Severe	3%	0%			
	Marked	3%	1%			
	Moderate	4%	3%			
	Total	10%	4%			3%

Notes:
[a] Minimum numbers: Based on examination of risk group only.
[b] Numbers based on questionnaire study.

reacted inadequately. More important is the negative association between adequacy of disaster behavior and likelihood of PTSD. Those who coped well during the emergency were less likely to suffer posttraumatic shock and long-lasting reactions. This is an interesting finding, since it implies that we can reduce the frequency of PTSD by adequate training.

During the follow-up period, psychiatric morbidity, other than that related to the disaster, was quite low. In fact, the only two exceptions were, first a case of a cerebral tumor, and secondly, a case of manic depressive psychosis. This supports the idea that individuals with PTSD have a tendency to recover and usually the PTSD will not be replaced by another pathological reaction. But the posttraumatic stress syndrome was easily colored by existing disorders and responses to later stressors.

Based on our observations, subjects at risk of PTSD had the following characteristics:

1. Experienced high risk situations: exposure to particularly severe trauma the technological disaster.
2. Were high risk persons: the presence of high risk factors (vulnerability) in exposed persons predicted illness.

3. Exhibited high risk reactions: the early response to the disaster predicted later illness.

The combination of eight variables from numbers one and two above, predicted 91% of the PTSD cases after seven months. Early response variables were even better predictors. These findings serve as the foundation of our primary and secondary prevention intervention work.

From this industrial disaster, and from other large-scale accidents, we have developed a model for intervention in companies which suffer a disaster. It can be summarized in the following points. 1) A disaster support team should be a part of any company of sufficient size. It should be manned by key personnel from the company leadership (personnel department), the company health service, the industrial safety officers, and the labor union. The team is responsible for planning and implementing necessary actions after an accident. 2) A psychosocial intervention/treatment team should be available within larger companies. 3) When an accident occurs a meeting should be held immediately. The disaster team identifies groups at risk: next-of-kin, injured survivors and families, uninjured survivors, bystanders, workmates, rescue personnel (including search and identification workers), persons holding responsibility, the neighboring community of industrial companies, evacuees, etc. 4) Emotional first aid and crisis intervention are initiated. 5) Information is distributed. It is very important that information be given by authoritative sources to all groups involved. 6) Informal debriefings are begun. 7) Formal debriefings are conducted. 8) Company health services and union representatives must cooperate around those who need help. 9) Health checks are begun immediately postdisaster for all involved employees and, if need be, repeated at a later date, for example 3 and 12 months. 10) Initiate a visitors' plan. Promising rehabilitation results occur when the company maintains contact with hospitalized workers, i.e. having workmates and company representatives visit regularly over an extended period of time. This promotes a sense of belonging and prevents the employee from feeling forgotten.

The Chernobyl nuclear accident

On 26 April, 1986, at 1.23am, an accident at the fourth unit of the Chernobyl Nuclear Plant destroyed the reactor core and part of the building in which it was housed. Radioactive products which had accumulated in the core were released into the atmosphere producing a radioactive cloud. Gas and lighter particles were in the upper part of the cloud, and heavier particles were in the lower part. The height of the cloud reached several kilometers, decreasing as the intensity of the fire in the plant diminished. The upper part of the cloud, the first emissions, drifted speedily eastwards and was spread and dissolved over a large area, e.g. part of the radioactive cloud reached Japan and the USA.

The air currents containing most of the radioactivity drove north west towards the Nordic countries. This was an unusual wind direction for Scandinavia with the worst possible meteorological conditions, wind and rain. Within three days, the air masses spread over Mid-Scandinavia and patchy heavy rain fell.

Measurements indicated an enormous increase in the 'washout ratio' caused by the rainfall. Even one millimeter of light drizzle brought down particles that might have otherwise passed by. The radioactive cloud hit the mountain chain along the Swedish–Norwegian border, increasing the fallout in both countries. The rain caused fallout of Iodine 131, and Caesium 134 and 137. The halflife of Iodine 131 is 8 days. Caesium 134 and 137 have halflives of approximately 2.4 years, and 28 years, respectively. On April 28th, increased radioactivity was measured in the area of Oslo, Norway. The later air currents turned the radioactivity towards Poland, Czechoslovakia, Austria, and East Germany. The wind currents changed direction once more, and again brought considerable fallout over South Norway on May 4th, and a smaller amount as late as May 8th.

As part of a Scandinavian study (Weisaeth, 1990, 1991c), we developed a survey to study reactions to the Chernobyl accident when the first fallout was noted in Norway on April 28, 1986. A representative nationwide sample of 998 persons above 15 years of age was selected, and standardized interviews were carried out in their homes from May 21 to June 3, and from June 13 to June 24, the time period when concern about the fallout was the focus of everyone's attention. Results of the study indicated that the Norwegian population were neither knowledgeable nor prepared for nuclear fallout. There was insufficient understanding and confidence in the information that was given out, and it grossly failed to provide guidelines for the public. The data indicated that, although the majority of the population were psychologically affected by the crisis (all but a few had some thoughts or feelings about it), only a small proportion sought or required help. Compared to other severe crises, the Chernobyl disaster was rated somewhat less threatening; few protected themselves by changing habits.

Sex, age, educational level, perception of threat, and previous mental health were associated with both information and reaction variables and provided some indication of groups at risk. The data confirmed the impression that there was an information crisis during the first weeks following the Chernobyl disaster in which the public was discontent with the information and guidance provided by the authorities. The information crisis probably resulted from a combination of factors: shortcomings in previous public education; shortage of reliable and unambiguous data on the radioactive material; the diffuseness of the threat and ambiguity of the risks; the complexity of the subject; the seeming contradiction between the health authorities' assurances that the radiation level was not dangerously high, and their statement that some precautions had to be taken; the experts' obvious difficulties in formulating simple information on complicated matters and statistical risks; and the media thriving on the disagreements between the experts.

Still, the confidence in information from experts remained high. Nuclear radiation specialists in Norway probably profited by being seen as neutral experts, since the absence of nuclear power plants in Norway means that there have been few professional and political controversies over nuclear power. The latter circumstance, however, may partly explain the low level of personal and public preparedness. It is a rare phenomenon in Norway that interviewees use the extreme values on response scales as they did in this study. Ninety-seven percent admitted they were poorly prepared, 80% expressed discontent with the guidance that was provided by the authorities, and 63% did not trust the official information.

The frequency with which fears of radiation injury were expressed, contrasted sharply with the absence of manifest illness or injury, and the low statistical risk of developing cancer. The threat to physical health by the nuclear material had some characteristics that made it particularly frightening. Individuals lacked personal control over the events. There were no danger signals to monitor; everyone was dependent on outside information but actual data were scarce and ambiguous. Radiation exposure from the Chernobyl disaster was frightening because it was involuntary, caused by another country, and carried the risk of cancer.

It is difficult to judge the clinical importance of the psychological reactions to the Chernobyl disaster. Reactions were more frequent in people with a history of mental health problems. The posttraumatic stress reactions and the frequency of pronounced sadness or depression indicated that perhaps only 1%–3% of the subjects developed a clinically significant reaction numbing hypothesis. One explanation for this finding may be based on psychological defences: Robert Lifton's psychic numbing hypothesis. This was seen as the result of a split between cognitive and emotional functions, much like denial and apathy combined, with hopelessness underlying these feelings.

Studies show that, when asked how they perceive nuclear disasters, people respond by reporting abstract and material destructions. They do not primarily see dead and dying people. The lack of concrete, and widespread, evidence of the destructiveness of the Chernobyl disaster in human costs, may reinforce such defensive perceptions.

Another hypothesis is that of nuclear normalcy. This perspective, derived from optimism and previous experience of mankind's survival, stresses that nuclear threats are like any other threat, greater in magnitude but on a continuum. This tendency of human psychology was clearly exploited by the Soviet authorities, but is probably employed by many individuals in their attempt to cope with the chronic stress imposed by the Chernobyl fallout. The increased sense of vulnerability and awareness of environmental risks that appear to have resulted from the Chernobyl experience indicate that the fear, worry, and sadness may also have initiated some preventive measures.

People over 60 years old reported less worry of being hurt by the radiation; a realistic judgement. Older people also reported stronger threat and emotional reactions than did the younger subjects. Those who were more highly educated, worried more about the destruction of the food and water supplies, an accurate understanding of a real risk of the disaster.

The most striking finding in the study was the greater negative emotional reactions reported by women. This finding was also seen in the two other Scandinavian countries. Multiple regression analysis indicated the sex of the subject was the best predictor of emotional reaction and threat perception. Women reported more emotional reactions, while men reported more intellectual responses to the Chernobyl threat. Women, however, took action, e.g. changing their food habits, more frequently than men (8% versus 3%). The findings may indicate directions for education: men needing to develop their ability to relate to the emotional aspects of severe threat, and women to the cognitive aspects.

In Norway, there were no differences between the sexes in the perception of threat to physical safety. However, women below 45 years of age were significantly more worried about chronic radiation injuries than were older women. Regardless of age, Norwegian and Swedish women worried more about the safety of people close to them than did men. These findings may indicate that the greater concern reported by women may be related to the traditional female role as caretaker, and the fear of harm to future children.

Similar results were reported after the Three Mile Island accident. Women respondents may feel 'closer to life' in the sense that they give birth to children and usually have more responsibility for their care and feeding. The possibility of genetic alterations due to the radiation exposure, and the increased risk to children were highly emotionally charged issues during the information crisis. Through her own body, a mother might poison or damage her fetus, a terribly frightening and unacceptable possibility. The extensive changes in food and drinking habits reported by the women further convey their experience of this risk.

The human consequences of the Chernobyl disaster in the Soviet Union

Thirty people in the Soviet Union died from acute radiation sickness as a result of the Chernobyl accident or its immediate consequences. Perhaps over a half million people received high doses of radiation. Some of those who suffered from radiation sickness initially presented with primarily psychiatric symptoms. Others suffered loss of consciousness, fatigue, nausea, and vomiting. A number of individuals with anxiety reactions were examined to rule out radiation illness. From what is known today, one must assume that a number of the radiation sickness cases were not counted in the official statistics. The official number of deaths in the Soviet Union has risen to 250.

The start of the Chernobyl disaster was similar to many classical industrial disasters: mismanagement leading to a crisis that could not be handled; an explosion that killed people and caused massive destruction. One aspect of this disaster was different from the more common toxic disasters: the lack of clear boundaries of the disaster. The contaminated areas in the USSR alone had a population of 4 million, more than 800 000 of whom lived in regions where the contamination level was above 5 Ci/km². In the Spring and Summer of 1986, 116 000 people were evacuated from the danger zone. As described in a report to the UN general assembly, three stages of the postdisaster period can be distinguished. The first stage, April to May 1986, involved: making initial estimates of the scale of the disaster and the radiation situation; taking action to prevent a spontaneous chain reaction and radioactive emissions from the damaged reactor, identifying areas exposed to radioactive contamination; and evacuating the population and farm animals from a 30 kilometer zone. The May 1 outdoor celebrations in Kiev, however, were arranged as usual; no disturbing information was issued. The following week thousands were evacuated.

The second period, from the summer of 1986 to 1987, involved: mapping out the contaminated areas; construction of the 'encasement' ('Sarcopha-gus'); decontamination of the working area of the nuclear power plant; restarting the No. 1, No. 2 and No. 3 reactors; protecting water resources from radioactivity; decontaminating settlements; scientific investigations; and taking special measures for the agricultural land. Like many technolo-gical disasters, the accident at the Chernobyl nuclear power plant was not an acute, time limited event. Rather, the nuclear plant accident started a sequence of events that continued to unfold over several years, creating a situation of chronic stress for many people.

A World Health Organization working group on the Psychological Effects of Nuclear Accidents (Report of June 21, 1990) emphasized that, whereas a great deal of scientific knowledge exists on the physical effects of radiation, much less is known about the psychological damage and how this can best be handled by the responsible authorities, by the individual health care workers, and by those affected. In the summer of 1990, the working group visited an area with a contamination level of 5–15 Ci/km^2. The members of the group were struck by the degree of anxiety present in individuals who evacuated the area out of fear. The exodus of so many caused considerable social disruption and a shortage of labor.

Very serious worries are now being experienced by the population in the affected areas, worries that appear to be increasing with time. Among the dimensions that need to be understood are the following: changes in illness behavior of the population and of diagnoses made by the doctors; the sociocultural effects of the displacement and social disruption of communi-ties; the psychological aspects of the perception of risk from radiation, and the role of policies on release of information; the socioeconomic dimensions including the return to nonnuclear sources of energy; and, finally, pathoge-nic factors, relating physiological stress reactions and changes in lifestyle, e.g. dietary habits and the consumption of alcohol.

Concern for one's health status has increased enormously since the disaster, and anxiety and its concomitant physiological reactions are spread far beyond the heavily contaminated areas. Shortly after the disaster, subjective and objective symptoms were attributed to radiation exposure. Except for independent sources, the media had little credibility. The public's and the local medical communities' knowledge of the consequences of radiation exposure were limited. Dissatisfaction with medical and administration management was considerable. 'In order to cope with general anxiety and uncertainty about the possible health effects of exposure to radiation, people focus on the more tangible aspects of their physical state of health, seeking out the health care system and requesting explanations. In the absence of reliable data about the health effects of the accident, the medical profession lacks adequate explanations and responds predictably with more extensive and intensive diagnostic screening of populations and individual patients. As a result, hitherto unobserved morbidity patterns and individual variations emerge which are without explanation and which confuse the situation further' (WHO, 1990).

Five years after the Chernobyl accident there are substantial psychosocial problems in its aftermath, particularly in the Soviet Union. The interpretations of these problems differ. One extreme position defines the whole problem as irrational: 'The Chernobyl psychiatric disaster.' The psychiatric label 'radiophobia' was coined to describe the human response. One should be cautious in using psychiatric labels when characterizing such responses, particularly when a large proportion of the population appear to share the response. How fear driven is the response, how irrational is the fear? Could it be understood as a protest, or reflect a distrust in people? After all, people were misinformed about the fallout for a long time, and it is not a new observation that when credibility is lost it may never be won back. The other extreme position holds that the psychosocial responses reflect real and objective factors.

Recently, the International Atomic Energy Bureau proclaimed that the radiation level was far less than feared and, although most radiation experts exercise some caution in long-term predictions, an optimistic forecast has been presented regarding health damage. According to recent reports (end of 1991), half of the population living in contaminated areas experienced psychological stress symptoms. Eventually, these stress reactions will produce psychosomatic and somatic illness in some.

The problems encountered should come as no surprise. For a long time, it was predicted that an information crisis would occur after such an accident. Even in the area of the accident, the major responsibility of the health services should have been to inform and calm the many thousands of scared persons, and not merely treat the acute radiation exposure cases. No country had foreseen the magnitude of the problems involved in handling such an information issue.

Conclusions

Modern technology has a Janus face. On the one side, technology spares lives in natural disasters through better preparedness, prevention and mitigation of the effects of the disaster. On the other side, although technology is becoming relatively safer, there are simply more things that can go wrong. The classical technological disaster is sudden, without warning, tremendously powerful and extremely destructive within a confined area. Usually, it leaves the surrounding environment intact. However, man's increasing interference with nature has not only blurred the distinction between natural and manmade disasters, but also broken down the geographical boundaries of the traditional technological disaster by toxic dispersion. In manmade disasters, failed technology implies a loss of control by those responsible, which contributes to the psychological trauma experienced by the population.

Technological disasters generally cause more severe mental health problems than natural disasters when they are of roughly the same magnitude. This is probably related to the greater unpredictability, uncontrollability and culpability in technological disasters. Compared to peacetime victims of severe violence, however, technological trauma causes less psychiatric morbidity in its victims. Some evidence indicates that the disaster behaviors, the natural responses of manmade disaster victims, such as fight/flight, may be less adaptive than in a natural environment.

Optimal disaster behavior appears to be strongly related to an individual's level of training and experience in handling physical danger situations. In the particular industrial disaster presented here, the later occurrence of PTSD was substantially related to the immediate failure to cope. Thus, a high level of training may be the best preventive of later PTSD. Stress inoculation of employees in high risk occupations has also been shown to increase resilience. The explosion itself in this industrial disaster was severe enough to produce acute PTSD in previously healthy subjects, mainly in somewhat vulnerable personalities.

Finally, the helplessness and anxiety of individuals and the general population when confronted with the invisible danger of a toxic disaster, such as Chernobyl, are substantial. Dissatisfaction with medical advice and the public administration, as well as confusion about the real health effects, lead to substantial psychosocial problems.

References

Baum, A. (1986). Toxins, technology, disasters. In G. R. Vanden Bos & B. K. Bryant (eds.) *Cataclysms, crisis, and catastrophes: psychology in action.* Washington DC: American Psychological Association, pp. 9–53.

Berz, G. (1989). List of major natural disasters, 1960–1987. *Earthquakes and Volcanoes*, **20**, 226–8.

Couch, S. R. & Kroll-Smith, J. S. (1990). Slow burn. *The Sciences*, May–June 1990, 5–7.

Dixon, N. F. (1987). *Our last enemy*. London: Jonathan Cape.

Ekeberg, Ö., Seeberg, I. & Ellertsen, B. B. (1988). The prevalence of flight anxiety in Norwegian airline passengers. *Scand. T. Behav. There*, **17**, 213–22.

Ekeberg, Ö., Seeberg, I. & Ellertsen, B. B. (1989). The prevalence of flight anxiety in Norway. *Nord Psykiatr Tidsskr.*, **43**, 443–8.

Ekeberg, Ö., Seeberg, I. & Ellertsen, B. B. (1990). A cognitive/behavioral treatment program for flight phobia, with 6 months' and 2 years' follow-up. *Nord Psykiatr Tidsskr*, **44**, 365–74.

Erikson, K. T. (1976). Loss of communality at Buffalo Creek. *American Journal of Psychiatry*, **133**, 302–4.

Frederick, C. J. (1986). Psychic trauma in victims of crime and terrorism. In G. R. Vanden Bos & B. K. Bryant (eds.) *Cataclysms, crisis and catastrophes: psychology in action*. Washington DC: American Psychological Association, pp. 59–108.

Gleser, G. C., Green, B. L. & Winget, C. N. (1981). *Prolonged psychosocial effects of disaster: a study of Buffalo Creek*. New York: Academic Press.

Green, B. L. (1982). Assessing levels of psychosocial impairment following disaster: consideration of actual and methodological dimensions. *Journal of Nervous Mental Disease*, **170**, 544–52.

Green, B. L., Grace, M. C., Lindy, J. D., Titchener, J. L. & Lindy, J. G. (1983). Levels of functional impairment following a civilian disaster: the Beverly Hills Supper Club fire. *Journal of Consulting and Clinical Psychology*, **51**, 573–80.

Green, B. L., Lindy, J. D., Grace, M. C., Gleser, G. C., Leonard, A. C., Korol, M. & Winget, C. (1990). Buffalo Creek survivors in the second decade: stability of stress symptoms. *American Journal of Orthopsychiatry*, **1**, 43–54.

Holen, A. (1990). *A long-term outcome study of survivors from a disaster*. PHD Thesis, Medical Faculty, University of Oslo, Oslo.

Hytten, K., Jensen, A. & Skauli, G. (1990). Stress inoculation training for smoke divers and free fall lifeboat passengers. *Aviation Space and Environmental Medicine*, 983–8.

Janis, I. L. & Mann, L. (1977). *Decision making: a psychological analysis of conflict, choice and commitment*. New York: The Free Press.

Lopez-Ibor, J. J., Soria, J., Canas, F. & Rodriguez-Gamazo, M. (1985). Psychopathological aspects of the toxic oil syndrome catastrophe. *British Journal of Psychiatry*, **147**, 352–65.

Luchterhand, E. G. (1971). Sociological approaches to massive stress in natural and man-made disasters. In H. Krystal & W. G. Niederland (eds.) *Psychiatric traumatization: after effects in individuals and communities*. Boston: Little, Brown & Company, pp. 29–51.

Ploger, A. (1977). A 10-year follow up of miners trapped for 2 weeks under threatening circumstances. In C. D. Spielberger & I. G. Sarason (eds.) *Stress and Anxiety*. New York: Wiley & Sons, pp. 23–8.

Raphael, B. (1986). *When disaster strikes: how individuals and communities cope with catastrophe*. New York: Basic Books.

Sethi, B. B., Sharma, M., Singh, T. & Singh, H. (1987). Psychiatric morbidity of patients attending clinics in gas affected areas in Bhopal. *Indian Journal of Medical Research*, 45–50.

Stierlin, E. (1909). Über psychoneuropathische Folgezustende bei den Überlebenden der Katastrophe von Courreère am 10 (Doctoral dissertation, University of Zurich, Marz 1906).

Stierlin, E. (1911). Nervöse und psychische Störungen nach Katastrophen. *Deutsches Medizinisches Wochenschrift*, **37**, 2028–35.

Sund, A., Holen, A. & Weisaeth, L. (1983). *The Alexander Kielland oil rig disaster, March 27, 1980*. Report to Ministry of Health. Division of Disaster Psychiatry, University of Oslo.

Weisaeth, L. (1984). *Stress reactions to an industrial disaster*. Phd Thesis, Medical Faculty, University of Oslo, Oslo.

Weisaeth, L. (1985). Post-traumatic stress disorder after an industrial disaster: point prevalences, etiological and prognostic factors. In P. Pichot, P. Berner, R. Wolf & K. Thau (eds.) *Psychiatry – the state of the art*. New York: Plenum Press.

Weisaeth, L. (1989a). The stressors and the post-traumatic stress syndrome after an industrial disaster. *Acta Psychiatrica Scandinavica Supplementum*, **80**(355), 25–37.

Weisaeth, L. (1989b). A study of behavioral responses to an industrial disaster. *Acta Psychiatrica Scandinavica Supplementum*, **80**(355), 13–24.

Weisaeth, L. (1989c). Torture of a Norwegian ship's crew. *Acta Psychiatrica Scandinavica Supplementum*, **80**(355), 63–72.

Weisaeth, L. (1990). Reactions in Norway to fallout from the Chernobyl disaster. In T. Brustad, F. Langmark & J. B. Teitan (eds.) *Radiation and cancer risk*. New York: Hemisphere, pp. 149–55.

Weisaeth, L. (1991a). The information and support center. In T. Scrensen, P. Abrahamsen & S. Torgersen (eds.) *Psychiatric Disorders in the Social Domain*. Oslo: Norwegian University Press, pp. 50–8.

Weisaeth, L. (1991b). The psychiatrist's role in preventing psychopathological effects of disaster trauma. In A. Seva (ed.) *The European handbook of psychiatry and mental health*. Barcelona. Editorial Anthropos, pp. 2342–58.

Weisaeth, L. (1991c). Psychosocial reactions in Norway to nuclear fallout from the Chernobyl disaster. In S. R. Couch & J. S. Kroll-Smith (eds.) *Communities at risk. Collective responses to technological hazards*. New York: Peter Lang Publishing, pp. 53–80.

Weisaeth, L. (1993). Disasters: psychological and psychiatric aspects. In L. Goldberger & S. Breznitz (eds.) *Handbook of Stress*. New York: The Free Press, pp. 591–616.

World Health Organization (1988). *Resolution on the international decade for natural disaster reduction*. WHO, Geneva: A/44/832/Add. 1.

World Health Organization (1990, June). *Working Group on Psychological Effects of Nuclear Accidents*. [Summary]. EUR/ICP, the WHO Regional Office for Europe.

World Health Organization (1991). *Psychosocial guidelines for preparedness and intervention in disaster*. WHO, Geneva: MNH/PSF/91.3, 1991.

5

Traumatic effects of accidents

ULRIK FREDRIK MALT

Empirical research indicates that the presence of physical injuries and suffering increases the prevalence and incidence of psychological and psychiatric problems after disasters and accidents (Gleser, Green & Winget, 1981; Malt, Blikra & Høivik, 1989a; Malt & Ugland 1989; Patterson et al., 1990; Raphael, 1986; Smith et al., 1990; Ursano et al., 1990). In a three-year retrospective study of 551 patients who were admitted to a surgical ward of a general hospital due to accidental injury, reduced physical function was significantly correlated with worse bodily health, and worse psychological health (correlation 0.299 and 0.498 respectively) (Malt et al., 1989a). Only one study reported no association between the severity of injury and psychological distress (Curran et al., 1990).

A number of war casualty studies also have shown that the frequency of psychiatric problems increases with the presence of physical injury (Chemtob et al., 1990; Crocq et al., 1990; Palinkas & Coben, 1987; Pitman, Altman & Macklin, 1989; Rundell et al., 1989; White & Faustman, 1989). Findings of the epidemiologic catchment area survey showed that about 3.5% of the nonwounded Vietnam veterans had a history of posttraumatic stress disorder compared to 20% in veterans wounded in Vietnam (Helzer, Robins & McEvoy, 1987). This difference was not explained by differences in combat intensity among the groups. Thus optimal planning and treatment of disaster and accident victims must include adequate knowledge and attention to the psychological and psychiatric aspects of physical injuries. This chapter is, to our knowledge, the first comprehensive effort to address this problem for a general readership.

Table 5.1. *Type, severity and frequency of injuries sustained according to the abbreviated injury scale (AIS) in a cohort of adults (15–69 years of age) discharged alive from a surgical department of a general hospital (n = 683). Minor injury AIS = 1; extremely severe injury AIS = 5*

	AIS-score						
Body area injured	1	2	3	4	5	Total	%
General (external)	3	11	1	1	1	17	2.5
Head (face, ear, eye)[a]	25	189	35	7	9	265	38.8
Neck (cervical spine, throat)	4	3	6	3	0	16	2.3
Chest (thoracic organs/spine)	12	26	33	5	0	76	11.1
Abdomen (incl. pelvic organs, lumbar spine)	9	18	12	7	2	48	7.0
Pelvis (bony structures only)	1	6	7	0	0	14	2.0
Extremities[b]	23	127	228	7	0	385	56.4
Total number of AIS-ratings						821	

Notes:
[a] 181/683 (25.5%) had sustained head injury only.
[b] 232/683 (34.0%) had sustained injury to an extremity only.
Source: Malt et al. (1989*a*).

Type and frequency of physical injury in accidents and disasters

Different types of physical injuries may be associated with rather specific psychological and psychiatric problems (e.g. burn injuries and affective problems related to permanent change of the body image; severe head injuries and disruptive behavior caused by cognitive impairment). The most common cause of traumatic injury is accidents. Accidents affect millions of individuals each year. In the United States of America, the annual incidence of nonfatally injured persons is estimated to be more than 8 million individuals (Munoz, 1984). In Britain alone, more than 13 000 hospital beds are occupied every day by accident victims. About half of the persons brought to general hospitals for injuries have sustained injury to the extremities and more than one-third had injuries to the head (Table 5.1).

The Abbreviated Injury Scale (AIS) is the method used most often to assess the severity of injuries. An Abbreviated Injury Scale (AIS) score of 1 denotes a minimal injury (e.g. bruises of the skin only). An uncomplicated head concussion is given an AIS score of 2. An uncomplicated ankle fracture is given a score of 3. A single AIS rating of 4 or 5 reflects a severe injury. Table 5.1 shows that injuries to the chest, abdomen and neck are less frequent in civilian accidents but often are more serious (e.g. gunshot, crush injuries) than the more frequently seen types of injuries.

The Injury Severity Score (ISS) is the sum of the squares of each of the three highest single AIS ratings for a patient and a very well accepted index for severity of physical trauma (Greenspan, McLellan & Greig, 1985). An ISS score above 10 usually defines patients with multiple injuries or more severe single injuries. In random hospital samples of injured patients, only 10–15% of the patients have sustained severe injuries, according to the ISS or overall clinical evaluation (Malt, 1988; Malt et al., 1989a). Rape is often associated with injuries (bruises, fractures, wounds in the genital area). Current research suggests that injuries increase the likelihood of post-traumatic psychiatric consequences (Steketee & Foa, 1987).

The type and severity of injuries seen in disasters vary depending on the type of disaster and the climate. Natural disasters, like earthquakes and tornadoes, most often cause crush injuries due to falling buildings or flying objects. Avalanches may also cause crush injuries and fractures, but suffocation is the biggest danger. Exposure to blasts causes internal injuries, e.g. pneumothorax without external evidence of injury. Severe bleeding and/or choking may be the result of such injuries. Air transport disasters, e.g. air plane crashes, cause fractures and burn injuries. Ground transportation disasters, e.g. train and bus accidents, are frequently associated with fractures of the limbs and injuries to the head (concussion, contusion). Shipwreck disasters are associated with cooling down (hypothermia) and electrolyte disturbances due to exposure of the lungs to sea water. Fires and explosions on ships and oil rigs cause burn and other types of injuries (fractures, crushes).

Disasters also can create smoke inhalation casualties, conjunctival irritation, shortness of breath, retrosternal pain and expectoration of bloodstained sputum. Suffocation occurs in some instances. Accidents and disasters associated with the inhalation of toxic gases other than smoke may cause pulmonary edema or shock lung. Disasters and accidents in a cold climate are often complicated by cold injuries; most often affecting the feet (i.e. damage to the peripheral nerves and vasculature with symptoms of paraesthesia and loss of sensation, swollen and painful feet). In the most severe cases, gangrene and subsequent amputation may be the sad end result. Time spent on thorough planning of how to organize physical and psychosocial care of all possible types of injuries is crucial to reducing the frequency and severity of the negative short- and long-term effects of physical trauma.

Psychiatric problems following traumatic injury

Acute phase

The period after traumatic injury is often called the emotional shock, denial numbness phase or the outcry phase. It may last from minutes to hours or even longer. The behavioral and emotional responses seen at this time result from both the emotional impact of the accident/disaster and the impact of the injury. Gross behavioral disturbance or emotional distress is infrequent. These responses can be thought of as the human expression of phylogenetically determined responses to acute danger and injury: fight (aggression), flight (panic) or freeze (apathy, lack of affect).

At the accident/disaster site or in the emergency room, aggression, bewildered and aimless running away, or apathy causing lack of appropriate lifesaving activities, are the major clinical problem from a psychiatric point of view. In fact, the word panic derives from the idea of running away from the forest god, Pan. In civilian accidents, aggressive behavior in the injured person is the single most frequent behavioral disturbance, occurring in about 5% of individuals in our own research. Aggressive behavior is associated more often with substance use (intoxication) and preexisting personality disorder than with the psychological impact of the accident or the injury. In such cases, the presence of undetected brain damage or hypoxia must be ruled out. Clear-cut individual panic reactions ('blind flight') or complete lack of psychomotor and affective responses (freeze response) occur in less than 1% of the injured. In disaster situations, the two latter responses occur more often. Aggressive reactions are less frequent among injured disaster victims compared to injured victims of civilian accidents and more often they are provoked by the emotional impact of the accident or trauma per se.

Being aware of the acute emotional response to injury may be important to the proper handling of patients in the acute phase even if the behavior of the patient is calmer. Physical injury may color the emotional responses. Thus patients report things in a way that may endanger an accurate medical understanding of the type and severity of the injury.

Strong anxiety, without loss of behavioral control, is very common and seen in about 10–20% of injured patients. The anxiety often reflects vivid fantasies of having sustained severe injuries, with a concomitant increased activation of the nervous system (e.g. increased pulse rate and blood pressure). Sometimes these patients claim severe pain as a reflection of the anxiety, and provide misleading information to the rescue/medical personnel.

Clinical case A 20 year-old woman was in a front-to-front vehicle collision. During the impact period, she experienced the situation as dreamlike ('derealization'; an acute dissociative response of short duration (seconds) seen in about 10% of accident victims). She felt pain in her abdomen due to the sudden pressure of the safety belt, which prevented any serious injury. She thought her abdominal wall was ruptured and that her 'guts' were falling out under her dress. She screamed in intense fear. The rescue personnel thought she was badly injured, gave her morphine IV, and brought her to a hospital in an ambulance at high speed. No severe injury was found.

In rare instances, emotions may be so strong that the patient suffers from psychological amnesia. 'I cannot remember anything. It was just horrible!' Other patients may be overtly confused (acute confusional psychosis), but such reactions are very rare. If amnesia occurs, it is most often determined by psychological factors. The psychological impact of the event has overwhelmed cognitive processes. However, physical injury may also manifest itself as amnesia or as confusion (i.e. a head concussion with organic amnesia; contusio cerebri with confusion upon awakening). This problem of medical diagnosis emphasizes the need to have an experienced trauma psychiatrist at the disaster site and in the trauma center.

Severe injuries are at times completely denied in the first minutes after a disaster/trauma. Quite often, a full understanding of the extent of the injury occurs over the following days to weeks. In the acute phase, this means there are often few lifesaving activities undertaken by the patient (e.g. does not move away from a dangerous area). Some patients deny the need for medical help despite obvious injuries.

Clinical case A 17 year-old boy climbed the roof of a train and touched a 17 000 volt electricity line. He fell to the ground with visible burns to the left leg and the right arm, which later had to be amputated. He refused help, 'I have not been injured'. An ambulance was called, disregarding his protests.

Clinical case The clothes of a 32 year-old woman caught fire in a tent explosion when she was camping. After escaping the burning tent, she stood passively watching the fire not noticing that her clothes were on fire. Bystanders had to tell her to jump into the nearby swimming pool in order to extinguish the fire.

Despite these dramatic examples, it should be remembered that the majority of traumatized persons respond in a controlled and unremarkable way. Nevertheless, a substantial number, about 40% in our research, are very emotionally upset despite their lack of deviant behavior or obvious emotional response. The inner turmoil reduces the cognitive capacity of the victim. The most significant clinical sign of this inner turmoil is shivering or shaking. The presence of a head concussion increases cognitive impairment. For these reasons, information to victims must be repeated often. As a rule, any important information given during the acute phase should be repeated later.

Except for head injuries associated with impaired cognitive function and injuries that significantly interfere with ventilation and cardiovascular function (e.g. leading to agitation due to hypoxia or apathy due to cardiovascular hypotension), the type and location of the injury plays a minor role in the acute response. The real threat to life, i.e. the circumstances and psychological meaning of the accident or disaster, or the injury, are the most important variables for predicting acute responses. In the subacute phase, injury and treatment related variables become more important for the emotional and behavioral responses seen.

Subacute phase

The subacute phase occurs within hours or less frequently (days) and lasts from several days to several weeks. In this phase, behavioral dysfunction and observable emotional reactions occur most frequently. Carefully conducted longitudinal studies in Norway by our group suggest that about 45% of injured adults have periods of marked emotional and behavioral change during this phase. These reactions do not warrant a psychiatric diagnosis in about two-thirds of the cases.

The subacute phase is crucial to the outcome: restoration of the psychological health of the individual or the development of a psychiatric disorder. In the hospital, the main clinical problems are organic brain dysfunction (delirium), deviant social behavior, somatization and affective responses (anxiety, depression). These may interfere with the treatment and healing of wounds and injuries and thus lead to surgical and long-term complications of the injury.

Most surgical departments cope with these problems without asking for help from the psychiatrist or mental health team, even in hospitals with a Consultation–Liaison (C/L) service. Quite severe emotional reactions, however, may be overlooked by the surgical staff as long as they are not associated with deviant behavior. These emotional reactions may precede the development of a psychiatric disorder. Accordingly, early detection and intervention is needed.

Psychologically, the subacute phase is characterized by intrusion and repetition of the trauma (Horowitz, 1986) and has personal implications and meaning for the individual. The clinical picture is influenced by the physiological and psychological effects of the physical injury, and the psychosocial effects of treatment. As time passes, the so-called secondary events (e.g. family attitudes, police and insurance investigations, press activities) become more important to the clinical picture.

Delirium Delirium is an acute organic brain disorder characterized by a reduced ability to maintain attention to external stimuli and to appropriately shift attention to new external stimuli. Patients show signs of disorganized thinking, a reduced level of consciousness and perceptual disturbances. Psychiatric symptoms such as panic, aggression and hallucinations are common, and may be the only signs of a delirium.

A substantial number of patients with delirium show no increased psychomotor activity. Accordingly, in hospital wards 'silent delirium' may remain undiagnosed. The risk of overlooking a delirium is increased if the patient is on certain types of drugs (e.g. beta-blockers). During the delirium, the patient may have vivid dreams and nightmares which may merge with hallucinations and cause postdelirium psychiatric disorders (Blank & Perry, 1984).

Often, high risk delirium patients have a history of difficulty tolerating passivity and acknowledging their dependency needs. They prefer to be active and dominant. After their sensoria clear, they feel humiliated for having 'gone crazy' and having revealed their weaknesses and potential insanity. Relatives may detect the changed consciousness of the patient, but abstain from discussing this with the staff for fear of labeling their relative as 'crazy'. If the delirium remains undetected by the staff, the 'secret' may be a tremendous source of distress and anxiety to both the patient and the relatives.

Delirium after physical injury is most common among elderly persons, individuals with a preexisting cognitive impairment (e.g. due to substance abuse) and among those with severe physical injuries. As a rule of thumb, all patients put on artificial ventilation and may have experienced periods of delirium, particularly those with very severe injuries (e.g. more than 30% of the body surface burned).

Clinical case   A 62 year-old man was severely burned (40% of body area with second and third degree burns) in an industrial explosion. During the hospital stay, the nurses reported that he appeared reasonable, calm and collected, and behaved in a controlled manner. But they also noted periods of sudden movements of his arms and legs when he was 'sleeping'. After a few days, the patient's wife became increasingly depressed and irritable. Because her behavior interfered with the nursing activities, a C/L psychiatrist was called. She told the psychiatrist that she thought her husband had 'gone crazy'. She feared that he would have to be transferred to a state mental hospital after discharge from the general hospital. An examination of the husband demonstrated a typical delirium which had been undetected by the nurses and treating physicians. At times, the patient thought he was at home, while at other times, he thought he was driving a car. Intensive care equipment was misinterpreted as traffic lights. His sudden movements had been efforts to push the brakes and change the direction of the car in order to avoid a collision.

Behavioral dysfunction

Severe behavioral dysfunction interfering with the medical care of injuries is infrequent following civilian accidents (less than 5% in a random sample of injured patients in our own research). If such reactions occur, they are usually due to preexisting psychopathology. About one-third of adults admitted to a hospital owing to a traumatic injury suffer from an Axis I, DSM-III-R psychiatric disorder at the time of the accident. About one-fifth suffer from a developmental condition (personality disorder, Axis II, DSM-III-R) (Malt et al., 1987). Substance abuse and dependence, and antisocial personality disorders are most frequently seen.

Clinical case   A 22 year-old male patient with fractures of the long bones became increasingly disruptive after admittance to the hospital. He appeared anxious with symptoms of increased sympathetic activity. Clinical examination by a C/L psychiatrist revealed longstanding cocaine and alcohol abuse in a person with a borderline personality disorder. The current behavioral dysfunction was due to both abstinence and fear of being crippled.

Clinical case   A 19 year-old male patient was hospitalized with a spinal cord injury after being shot during a burglary. During the hospital stay, he was extremely difficult to handle. He did not cooperate. He complained about his treatment and shouted at and offended the nurses, interfering with the nursing care of his roommates. Clinical examination revealed an individual with an antisocial personality disorder who was feeling extremely threatened by the enforced passivity due to his severe injuries. He felt both despair and worthlessness as he thought of facing a future in a wheelchair.

In rare instances, guilt over an accident provokes hypomanic, and even manic, behavior as a defense against overwhelming guilt and depression. Disruptive behavior (i.e. quarreling, suspiciousness, irritability, aggression) can occur frequently. This reaction can be seen in persons without a previous personality disorder. These patients may demonstrate the same characteristics as the patients at risk for postdelirium psychiatric disorders. They feel threatened by their loss of autonomy and independence and feel shame and anxiety as part of feeling humiliated at being a victim and being weak. Disruptive, manic or rude behavior in middle aged or older persons should always raise a suspicion of an underlying organic mental disorder.

Clinical case   A 56 year-old man, with no preexisting psychiatric disorder, ate a nice dinner at home with his wife. They shared half a bottle of wine. Later, they quarreled when the wife refused to have sex with her husband. In anger, he left the bedroom with his bedsheet. Outside the bedroom door, he stumbled on the bedsheet and fell down a very steep staircase. He was found unconscious by his wife. Upon arrival at the hospital, he was awake but with retro- and antegrade amnesia. He was aggressive and somewhat verbally abusive with the staff. There were no clearcut neurological findings on admittance. The doctor made a diagnosis of uncomplicated head concussion. Due to the smell of alcohol on his breath, the doctor on duty considered the patient's deviant behavior to be due to alcohol intoxication. He also stated in the medical records that the fall was due to alcohol intoxication. He did not question the wife to confirm this assumption, and she did not tell him what had really happened due to her guilt feelings about the incident. After discharge from the hospital, it was established that the man had sustained a severe head concussion (contusio cerebri) with posttraumatic dementia. One hundred percent disability was the final result. Initially, the insurance company refused to pay disability insurance because the medical notes stated that the injury was due to self-induced alcohol intoxication.

Severe organic mental disorder should also be suspected if the patient does not recognize the seriousness of his/her accident or injury, or denies any emotions despite having sustained serious physical injuries involving the head. In some cases, these behavioral responses ('denial–elation response') are the only hints of a brain dysfunction. The surgeons and ward staff may overlook the organic basis of these signs and symptoms.

Clinical case In a disaster at an industrial plant, a 63 year-old man fell four meters hitting the concrete floor with his head. After a short period of unconsciousness, he awoke. At the hospital, no neurological damage was found. The patient claimed to feel well and angrily refused to stay in the hospital. At follow-up, there was evidence of a severe head injury with permanent cognitive impairment and symptoms of anxiety.

Somatization and psychological factors affecting the injury

Some patients report little emotional disturbance but do report strong pain, reduced appetite and poor sleep. However, the clinician may observe marked anxiety even though the patient denies such emotions. The majority of these patients describe an immediate psychophysiological response (shivering, shaking) to the accident.

This subacute response is typical of males with obsessive–compulsive personality traits and little premorbid psychopathology. These individuals are threatened by passivity and the perceived lack of control associated with their injury and treatment. This situation increases neurophysiological activation and is associated with changes in levels of hormones, peptides, transmitters and function of the immune system (Eysenck, 1987). These persons run a high risk of developing surgical complications like embolus, infections, delayed healing of wounds and fractures (Line & Malt, unpublished observations). In a few cases, persisting complications may be the only sign of current psychosocial conflicts.

Clinical case A 26 year-old male was admitted to a surgical ward after 20% of his body surface was burned in an industrial accident. The wounds did not heal but no biological explanation could be found. Factitious disorder was ruled out by 24-hour nursing observation. The psychiatric interview revealed that when the patient was discharged from the hospital, he would have to serve a jail sentence unrelated to his accident. When a 6-month postponement of the sentence was obtained, the wounds healed within a short time.

Anxiety

During the subacute phase, anxiety is a common clinical feature of physical injury after accidents and disasters. The most frequent symptoms of anxiety are worrying, compulsive thoughts about the accident or the injury, inner

Table 5.2. *A 3-year biopsychosocial follow-up study of accidentally injured adults. The frequency of symptoms reported to be bothering and present the last 6 months before follow-up.*

Symptom	Persons with one or several negative consequences (%) ($N = 298$)	Persons with no negative consequences (%) ($N = 232$)	$\times 2^b$ (df = 1)
Fatigue	49.3	28.9	21.93
Pain in the body	43.9	17.7	39.96
Decreased performance	43.2	8.6	75.78
Traumatophobia	41.0	17.7	32.55
Emotional lability	36.7	22.0	13.03
Irritability	36.7	19.4	18.44
Sweating	33.1	20.3	10.51
Restless	32.7	19.4	11.50
Sleep disturbances	31.7	19.4	9.86
Startle reaction	30.6	16.4	13.93
Tense	29.1	16.8	10.68
Lack of initiative	29.1	13.4	18.36
Vertigo	29.1	12.1	21.92
Memory impairment	27.0	6.0	38.51
Trouble concentrating	25.9	12.1	15.35
Headache	23.7	41.4[a]	18.15
Depressed mood	21.9	10.8	11.25
Weakness	21.6	4.3	31.86
Fearful/anxious	20.1	9.5	11.10
Isolation	19.8	6.0	20.44
Digestive problems	18.7	15.1	1.17
Bitterness	14.7	3.4	18.59
Breathlessness	9.0	5.2	2.74
Nightmares	6.8	5.2	0.61

Notes:
[a] Highest frequency reported in the nonconsequence group.
[b] All symptoms significant at $p < .001$ except digestive problems, breathlessness, and nightmares.

tension, startle reactions, and concentration difficulties. Sleep problems also may be present and related to physical pain and treatment procedures. Contrary to what one might think from reading the literature about war and PTSD, nightmares are not common in a general population of accident victims (Malt, 1988; see also Table 5.2). If present, nightmares usually occur several days after the accident. Persistent nightmares, which over time do not show any signs of mastery in the dream content, are highly significant for the development of posttraumatic stress disorders.

Anxiety is most often related to the accident or the injury situation including real or imagined fear of body damage. Anxiety may also be related to fear of police or press investigation. This is particularly so if the patient feels he or she has broken rules or is responsible for the damages.

Clinical case A 43 year-old male, with obsessive–compulsive personality traits, was slightly injured in a traffic accident which involved four cars and injured seven other persons. The patient was the driver of one of the cars. His passengers, his daughter and her girlfriend, were among the injured. He felt responsible for the accident. During the hospital stay, he was observed walking restlessly in the corridors with a worried appearance. Upon examination, he reported strong anxiety and poor sleep, reexperiencing the accident in his dreams.

Clinical case A 35 year-old woman ran across the street, fell over a road block, and sustained a minor injury to her abdomen. She was admitted to the trauma unit for observation because of pain. Physical examination was negative. In the following days, she complained of an increasingly strong pain. Finally, her abdominal wall was 'as hard as a wooden plate'. An exploratory operation was performed in order to rule out an intraabdominal pathology. Nothing was found. On psychiatric evaluation, the woman reported that her husband had died one year ago of a heart attack. Hours before he died, he had been examined by a doctor who said 'nothing was wrong'. Before her admittance to the hospital, the admitting doctor had told her that observation was necessary to rule out inner bleeding from the liver or rupture of the intestine. This was, in fact, ruled out by the hospital staff but she was not explicitly told this. Her anxiety increased the pain she was feeling and she began to think she would die because of undetected pathology, as had happened to her husband. The surgeons and nurses did not ask about her vivid fantasies and their nonspecific statement, 'nothing is wrong', increased her anxiety, reminding her of the fate of her husband.

Depression

Depressed mood during the first days to weeks following an accident may be due to guilt, shame, or grief due to real or imagined losses. However, premorbid causes of depression, such as bereavement and the presence of a mood disorder at the time of the accident, must be kept in mind (Malt et al., 1987). A loss that interferes with cognitive processes is more devastating for the patient whose career, recreation, self-esteem, and defensive and coping mechanisms are based on intellectual functioning (Krueger, 1986). The patient whose self-esteem, work, coping interests, and lifestyle are centered around physical activities has a more marked reaction and greater difficulty adjusting when a true or imagined physical disability occurs.

Clinical case A 23 year-old salesman suffered a moderate injury to his knee (rupture of a tendon). Postoperatively he became very depressed. He lost his appetite, could not concentrate, thought of dying and showed little interest in social interaction with other patients. Clinical examination revealed that he had been a very active baseball player, devoting much of his leisure time to this activity. This activity had been crucial to his feelings of wellbeing and worth. Now he felt his whole life had been ruined by his injury.

Severe injuries may cause a permanent loss of physical function or a permanent change in appearance. Severe burns and spinal cord injuries, in particular, create such losses. Depression is frequently seen following such injuries (Craig et al., 1990; Judd et al., 1989; Malt, 1980; White, 1982). In part, this may reflect mourning over the lost functions or body image. The stronger the personal investment in the lost function or body part, the greater the depressive reaction.

Accidents and disasters may be associated with acts involving aggressive and sexual themes. These 'current concepts' may be incongruent with the patient's 'enduring concepts' of social morality and self-image (Horowitz, 1986). Guilt, shame and depressed mood may be the result. In the majority of cases, this response is transient and dealt with by the ward staff. In severe cases, however, the depression may be more persistent. Such persistent depression may cause a sustained neuropsychological activation and have detrimental effects (Baker, 1987).

Family responses

Sometimes, the reaction of the family to the trauma is crucial. A patient with a head concussion may react with more emotion if the family has emphasized intellectual functioning as necessary for future success, glory and pride. (For further discussion, see Peterson & O'Shanick, 1986; Livingston, 1987).

Clinical case A 15 year-old boy was injured in a traffic accident, sustaining a minor head concussion and several fractures to the long bones. During his hospital stay, he did not worry much about the fractures but showed marked distress about the clinically insignificant head concussion, with depressive and anxious symptoms. The boy was the oldest son of a Jewish couple. During the war, all the property of their wealthy grandparents was stolen by the Nazis, and several of the relatives were killed in the Holocaust. Since then, his parents felt that money and wealth could always be lost. However, cognitive abilities and high intellectual achievement were one's life insurance. Now the parents felt extremely threatened by the boy's head concussion. They reported vivid fantasies about cognitive deterioration and had conveyed these to the patient.

Staff problems

In addition to these individual problems, physical injuries increase the stress upon health care personnel and social support systems. In situations where the victims are injured far from home, the psychosocial needs of the injured victims may be enormous. The increased demand for basic human contact and social support may exceed the capacity of the hospitals and health care systems. It is our clinical experience that this burden is easily overlooked by surgeons and medical staff. In disaster situations, the hospital may have dozens of injured patients admitted within hours. Without specific actions to counteract the increased stress on the staff in such instances, the treatment and nursing capacity of the staff may be exhausted within a week. Increased psychiatric and behavioral disturbances among the patients, and sick leave due to burnout of the staff, may be the result.

Long-term reactions

Incidence of long-term psychiatric problems

In a random sample of accidentally injured adults (where less than half of the patients were injured in traffic accidents or shooting incidents), the incidence of nonorganic psychiatric disorders was 17% during the first year and 9% after about 2 years (Malt, 1988). Approximately one-third of these patients suffered from organic mental disorders two years after the trauma. In addition, 6% suffered from an organic mental disorder only. Other studies suggest a somewhat higher prevalence of psychiatric disorders after physical injuries, but these studies are based on nonrandom samples and only use self-report instruments (Feinstein & Dolan, 1991; Landsman et al., 1990). These factors tend to increase prevalence rates over studies which use comprehensive clinical interviews and consider information about the premorbid status of the patients (Malt, Blikra & Hoivik, 1989*b*).

The incidence of psychiatric problems after physical injuries associated with disasters per se is probably somewhat higher (Helzer et al., 1987; Raphael, 1986). However, we lack studies that report the frequency of psychiatric problems after disasters separately for victims with and without physical injury. Several studies have demonstrated that severe injuries are associated with more psychiatric problems than less severe injuries. This is most obvious among patients with head injuries (for a review, see Lishman, 1988), but it is also true for other types of injuries. In a follow-up study of burn injured patients (n = 70), 44% of the more severely injured patients suffered from psychiatric problems compared to 16% of the less severely injured patients (Malt & Ugland, 1989). Similar findings have been reported in other studies of burn injured adults (Patterson et al., 1990).

The relationship between the severity of the injury sustained in civilian accidents and posttraumatic psychiatric problems may partly be explained by the fact that individuals with psychopathology more often sustain severe injuries (Kuhn et al., 1989; Malt et al., 1987; Rockwell et al., 1988). However, this finding does not fully explain the observed relationship. Similar relationships between the severity of the injury and the prevalence of psychiatric disorders have been observed after disasters and warfare (Raphael, 1986), but empirical studies are few.

Despite this association, measures of the severity of injury alone are by no means a sufficient predictor of outcome. All available information suggests that sociodemographic and psychosocial variables are crucial for the psychosocial and functional outcome of accidental injuries (Krueger, 1984; Landsman et al., 1990; Malt, 1988; Mossey et al., 1989; Roessler & Bolton 1978; Ward et al., 1987).

The majority of injured persons involved in accidents sustain minor injuries (Malt, 1988). In the general population, the personal meaning of the accident or injury, and the secondary events of the accident have greater predictive power of psychiatric outcome than the severity of the physical injury per se. Accordingly, an Injury Severity Score (Greenspan et al., 1985) above 10, which includes about 20% of the most severely injured patients, will identify only a quarter of those who develop long-term psychiatric consequences. Even the behavioral and functional sequelae of brain injury are only modestly predicted by the severity of brain damage.

A strong emotional response to the accident or injury during the first weeks after the event usually predicts about half of the patients who will develop long-term psychiatric syndromes. Nevertheless, several patients who developed long-term psychiatric syndromes after accidents or traumatic injury, did not show any deviant behavior or adjustment reactions during their hospital stay. But the assessment of the most likely sources of distress will, in most cases, reveal important keys to the understanding of the posttraumatic psychiatric syndrome (for details, see Malt, 1991).

Injuries that cause brain damage and cognitive impairment are regularly associated with a high frequency of long-term psychiatric problems. Enduring personality changes may appear. Brain injury and its sequalae may also lead to behavioral disturbances and violence, causing major problems for spouses and relatives (Rosenbaum & Hoge, 1989).

Some types of nonbrain injury notoriously cause more psychiatric problems than others: injuries associated with significant visual disfigurement (e.g. severe burn injuries) (Bernstein, 1976; Wallace & Lees, 1988) and loss of body parts (e.g. traumatic amputation) or physical function (e.g. spinal cord injury) (Roessler & Bolton, 1978). Major injuries to the neck, pelvis or genital areas are also clinically associated with an increased frequency of problems (Campbell, La Clave & Brack, 1987; Malt, 1991) although such injuries are rather infrequent. Psychiatric symptoms after minor soft tissue injuries due to a whiplash movement of the neck are controversial. This issue is discussed under the somatoform disorders.

Psychiatric disorders

In a retrospective study of 551 adults 3 years after having been hospitalized for accidental injuries, 530 completed a 24-item symptom checklist (Malt et al., 1989b). Each person was asked to check all symptoms which bothered them during the last 6 months prior to the follow-up. They were not asked to consider the cause of the symptoms. A comparison between persons who reported at least one negative consequence after the injury (physical or psychosocial) and those who denied any negative late effects, showed that decreased performance, bodily aches and pain, reduced memory impairment, fear of a situation similar to that in which the accident/injury took place (traumatophobia), and weakness were the symptoms that showed the greatest difference among persons with and without self-reported sequelae. In a factor analysis of the 24 items, only traumatophobia loaded on the anxiety factor (Malt et al., 1989b). It is also of interest to note that nightmares were one of the three symptoms that were not reported significantly more often among those with sequelae (Table 5.2).

The most commonly seen psychiatric disorders after physical injury are listed in Table 5.3. Depression is the single most frequent type of disorder seen. This corresponds well to the fact that symptoms loading high on the depressive factor were most frequently reported (Table 5.2). Other types of anxiety and somatoform disorders are also prevalent (Malt, 1988; Holen, 1991).

Table 5.3. *Most frequently seen long-term psychiatric disorders after physical injury*

Mood disorders
Major depression
Dysthymic disorder
Recurrent brief depressive disorder

Anxiety disorders
Posttraumatic stress disorder
Simple phobia
Social phobia
Somatoform disorders

Somatoform autonomic dysfunction
e.g. hyperventilation syndrome,
    cardiac neurosis
Somatoform pain disorder
Neurasthenia

Psychological factors affecting physical conditions
e.g. tension headache, myalgia

Organic mental disorders
Amnestic syndromes
Posttraumatic dementia
Enduring personality change

Depressive disorders

The long-standing depressive disorders are most often of moderate severity, fulfilling the diagnostic criteria of major depression or dysthymia (DSM-III-R), or recurrent brief depression (ICD-10). Depressive disorders are particularly common in elderly persons (Mossey et al., 1989). They occur more often among persons with loss of physical function or body parts, and among those who expect to perceive reinforcement as contingent upon one's own behavior (internal locus of control). Psychological assessment will identify injuries which may affect highly significant personal physical attributes (i.e. high narcissistic investment in one particular function or body part).

Clinical case A 62 year-old active, hardworking man sustained a head concussion and fracture to one arm and hip in a bicycle accident. During the hospital stay, he was very dysphoric and periodically aggressive, feeling severely threatened by the fact that he might have postdischarge disability problems. He rejected suggestions that he have a psychiatric assessment. On follow-up 3 years later, he reported having to quit some of his more strenuous leisure activities and had some trouble running. Although he had no major physical disability, subjectively, he felt crippled. He was still depressed. He suffered from insomnia, low energy, poor concentration and feelings of low self-esteem and hopelessness. He was bitter about his fate. He remarked, 'It's not fair. I've always been such an active, healthy and hardworking man.' Psychologically, it was obvious that his injury presented a major narcissistic blow.

The risk of having a depressive disorder is increased if people close to the injured person were killed (survivor guilt) or severely crippled during the accident or disaster. The presence of a simultaneous organic mental disorder should always be considered.

Clinical case A 55 year-old male was treated for a fracture to the femur after a traffic accident in which another person was killed. At follow-up in the department of surgery he appeared depressed and suffered from impotence. He was referred for outpatient follow-up. The clinical interview suggested cognitive impairment; the patient was not able to copy a single drawing of a clock and a box. Additional neuroradiological examinations revealed gross posttraumatic atrophy of the brain.

Anxiety disorders

Posttraumatic stress disorder is the most frequent anxiety disorder seen after physical injury. The recurrent and intrusive distressing recollections are most often related to the accident or disaster situation, and not the injury per se. Disaster victims may reexperience the explosion and the immediate chaos of the situation rather than their resulting leg fracture. However, occasionally, aspects of the injury or treatment may represent the main content of the intrusive symptoms. Nightmares, experienced during confusional states when being artificially ventilated, may be relived in later dreams. Torture victims, for example, may reexperience strong anxiety when they are exposed to police inquiry in a friendly country if they were once tortured by police. They also will reexperience anxiety if they are hospitalized and see people with injuries like the ones inflicted upon themselves during torture.

The avoidance reactions of posttraumatic stress disorder are most often related to any stimuli associated with the accident or disaster situation per se or the injury. The person may avoid seeing war movies, or watching surgical operations on television. Symptoms of increased arousal, such as irritability, outbursts of anger, hypervigilance and exaggerated startle response are seen in about 15% of people (Malt, 1988).

Recent research has demonstrated a stimulus-specific autonomic reactivity in PTSD (Giller, 1990; Pitman et al., 1987). This reactivity suggests a role of classic conditioning in the etiology of PTSD. The findings that PTSD is more frequent after frightening experiences which include a physical injury (Helzer et al., 1987; Malt & Ugland, 1989) may suggest that physical injury in disaster may function as an important classic conditioner. Often the symptoms of posttraumatic disorder may be mixed with symptoms of organic mental disorders (postconcussion syndrome), emphasizing the need to consider both organic and nonorganic aspects in all cases of posttraumatic disorder. In the Norwegian studies (Malt, 1988), three out of four persons with a posttraumatic syndrome following civilian accidents had concomitant signs and symptoms of posttraumatic cognitive dysfunction (atypical organic brain syndrome).

Clinical case Due to a communication error not involving the patient, a 20 year-old commando soldier, who was holding onto a rope swinging under a military helicopter, was lifted 30 meters into the air and then fell off. While falling, he managed to keep his body in a 'flight position' and steer towards a pine. He remembered hitting the pine and parts of the period afterwards while lying on the ground. He sustained a number of fractures, including the spine and thorax, and a head concussion. He did not suffer any major neurological damage. During the first year after the event, he had trouble moving freely and had to quit his training as a commando. He developed posttraumatic stress disorder and was referred to the psychiatric stress and disaster team of the Joint Medical Services of the Armed Forces. The referring surgeon stated that the fractures were healed and that his impaired performance could not fully be explained by physical findings. On psychiatric examination, posttraumatic cognitive impairment was detected. This was verified by neuropsychological testing. A rehabilitation program was very successful.

Simple phobia may occur after physical injuries. Most often such reactions are related to the accident or disaster situation (e.g. fear of driving) more than the injury per se. Definite fear associated with exposure to situations that symbolized or resembled the traumatic event was found in 29% of the Norwegian sample of injured adults (Malt, 1988). In some patients, the fear was associated temporarily with avoidance behavior or a compelling desire for avoidance. However, the fear did not constrict normal activities in any of these individuals. Thus, significant phobic behavior appears to be rather infrequent.

Some persons may suffer from social phobia after a physical injury. This occurs most frequently as a consequence of injuries causing visible scars or disfigurement. Burn injury is the most frequent type of injury causing this disorder. In a follow-up study of a consecutive sample of 70 burned adults admitted to a general hospital, 4 (6%) suffered from social phobia (Malt & Ugland, 1989) compared to none of 107 randomly selected injured adults (Malt, 1988) of which only 1% had sustained burn injuries. Sometimes the phobic reactions may be reinforced by society's reaction to visible disfigurement (e.g. public indoor swimming pools may refuse persons with scars and sequelae to injuries that may look like skin diseases.)

Clinical case A 20 year-old woman was seen several years after being severely burned in an airplane crash in which more than 90% of the passengers and all the crew were killed. She had major facial disfigurement despite extensive plastic surgery. To most people, her face looked grotesque. During recent years, she stayed at home with her family most of the time, reading magazines and watching TV. When she began to go out in public after discharge from the hospital, people turned away in order to avoid the frightening sight of her disfigured face. She gradually developed a persistent fear of situations that exposed her to scrutiny by others, and felt anxious when in public places. She also suffered from periods of recurrent, brief, depressive episodes. She had developed a pattern of going out only after dark.

Clinical case A 22 year-old male had sustained partial thickness burns to his thorax in a fire. The injuries left visible thorax scars. He reported suffering from a social phobia after the accident, especially around women and swimming. He was afraid of dating due to the possible exposure of his naked thorax. He also avoided going to beaches and other places where his scars might be exposed to women. This condition led to a rather persistent feeling of depression (dysthymia) for which he had not sought treatment.

Somatoform disorders

Somatoform disorders and psychological factors affecting physical condition is the third major group of nonorganic psychiatric disorders seen after physical injury. Such disorders appear to be rather infrequent, occurring in about 3% of those injured in civilian accidents (Malt, 1988). This figure contrasts with the frequency seen in patients in the process of litigation or compensation (Krute & Burdette, 1978; Mendelson, 1984, Tarsh & Royston, 1985).

Somatoform pain disorder is probably the single most frequent type of somatoform disorder seen after physical injury. It has been suggested that such disorders are more common after occupational injuries due to the compensation issues, however, empirical evidence is lacking. Neither do we know the exact frequency of somatoform pain in different samples of injured populations. Somatoform pain after physical injury is most often related to current psychosocial problems or conflicts (Ford, 1983; Malt, 1991).

The diagnosis of somatoform pain disorder is often understood by the patient as an offense, suggesting that he or she does not suffer from 'real' pain ('hysterics', 'malingering'). Accordingly, patients may vigorously deny any current psychosocial problems and secondary gain, increasing the likelihood of bringing the case to court. This development is reinforced by the simple fact that the diagnosis 'somatoform pain disorder' after physical injury, to a large extent, is based on clinical judgement with limited 'objective' evidence. The DSM-III-R criteria states that this diagnosis may be made 'when there is related organic pathology, [if] the complaint of pain or resulting social or occupational impairment is grossly in excess of what would be expected from the physical findings' (American Psychiatric Association, 1987).

These diagnostic and legal problems are highlighted when looking at injuries caused by a whiplash movement of the neck. Such injuries have been reported to be the cause of chronic pain problems, but the etiology is controversial and in most cases no clear-cut neurological finding can be demonstrated (Malt, 1991; Trimble, 1981). Maimaris, Barnes, and Allen (1988) found that 35 out of 102 patients with such injuries exhibited symptoms after 2 years; pain being the most prominent symptom. Balla and Karnaghan (1987) found that 25% of the people in their study developed chronic disability, mostly headaches. Gargan and Bannister (1990) reported that only 12% of 43 patients with such injuries recovered after a mean of 10.8 years. Some authors claim that these complaints cannot be explained by reference to psychopathology or personality traits (Radanov, Dvorak & Valach, 1989). In contrast to these clinical studies, neuropsychological and neurophysiological studies have not identified any significant signs of cognitive impairment in most of these patients (Jacome, 1987; Olsnes, 1989). More research is needed to settle this issue.

Whatever the cause of this disorder, it is a well established clinical fact that depression is quite often associated with pain, and may be the underlying condition. Many patients still consider depression to represent a weakness and not a stress provoked medical disorder with concomitant biological dysfunction. Thus, patients may often be unwilling to reveal symptoms of depression and accept that a diagnosis of depressive disorder should replace their 'real pain'. Such attitudes may call for a skilled intervention in the early phase in order to avoid chronicity and somatization as a way of life (Ford, 1983).

Clinical case   A 48 year-old woman sustained a minor head concussion and hip fracture in a traffic accident. During the follow-up period, she consistently complained of hip pain which impaired her working capacity as a receptionist and interfered with her quality of life. A careful physical examination found no organic pathology that could explain her pain. She was not suffering from any symptoms or signs of impaired cognitive dysfunction due to her minor head injury. She denied symptoms of depression but felt distressed by her pain. She accepted the idea of seeing a 'stress specialist' as part of a comprehensive assessment of her complaints. It turned out that she had lost her closest friend a fortnight after the accident and was having major interpersonal conflicts at work following this event. The pain had developed during this period. The company doctor put her on sick leave, reinforcing her avoidance tendencies. The secondary gain also reinforced her pain (operant conditioning).

Phantom limb pain is a particular form of pain seen in some patients after traumatic amputation. The etiology is debated but clinically is closely related to feelings of depression. Symptoms like fatigue, weakness, pain and aches, decreased performance, and concentration difficulties are often reported after accidental injury (Malt et al., 1989*b*). Sometimes multiple symptoms without any reasonable organic explanation may be found, suggesting a diagnosis of 'undifferentiated somatoform disorder' (DSM-III-R). In most of these cases, a previous history of 'somatization' when stressed may be identified. Quite rarely, injured patients may complain of a changed visual appearance despite no observable change (body dysmorphic disorder). A strong narcissistic investment in the body area affected by the injury most often underlies this reaction.

Psychotic disorders

While acute, brief reactive psychosis may occur after very upsetting accident situations, the psychological impact of an injury does not increase the frequency of more chronic psychotic disorders like manic depressive illness (bipolar disorder, recurrent unipolar depression with psychotic features) or schizophrenia. This has been most convincingly demonstrated in the long-term follow-up studies of survivors of concentration camps in Nazi Germany (Eitinger & Strøm 1973, 1981; Strøm, 1986). Despite extreme psychological stress and repeated physical trauma from torture and battering, this extreme stress was a causal factor for serious and chronic psychoses only in relatively few cases. However, the presence of severe head injury with brain damage may increase the frequency of schizophrenia.

Organic mental disorders

Organic mental disorders are the most common disorder after physical injury (Malt, 1988). In a general sample of civilian accidents, about 10% will suffer from such disorders. In most cases, the consequences are mild with emphasis on symptoms of memory disturbance and headache (i.e. postconcussional syndrome) (Boll & Barth, 1983; Lishmann, 1988). In samples of patients from lower social economic classes living in societies with insufficient public health services, the consequences (i.e. employment) may be more severe (Rimel et al., 1981). Among child and adult patients with head injuries, there is a clearcut relationship between severe injuries and psychiatric problems, as might be expected (Bornstein, Miller & van Schoor, 1989; Fletchner et al., 1990). Severe posttraumatic encephalopathy (dementia) is an infrequent, but very serious, consequence. Some long-term studies of World War II soldiers suggest that damage to the anterior area of the right hemisphere of the brain may be associated with greater maladjustment (Tellier et al., 1990).

Psychological factors affecting a physical condition

Sometimes current problems and conflicts have a significant negative influence on physical functioning and distress, warranting a DSM-III-R diagnosis of 'psychological factors affecting a physical condition'. These patients seldom report psychological problems. As a rule, the influence of psychological and social factors upon the course of physical injury should be assumed (Ford, 1983).

Quality of life

So far, I have focused only on the psychiatric consequences of trauma. This rather narrow approach does not account for the whole dimension of pain and suffering after physical trauma. A comprehensive picture of the suffering associated with injuries must include reduced quality of life of the patients. This is evident if we compare the frequency of self-reported complaints after physical injury with the frequency of psychiatric diagnosis. About 50% of injured adults will report some kind of permanent distressing symptoms or complaints 2–3 years after their injury (Malt et al., 1989*b*). A psychiatric disorder, however, including mild organic dysfunction is present in less than 20% (Malt, 1988). For the majority of the 30% difference, reduced quality of life is the main problem (Malt et al., 1989*a*).

Mortality

Eitinger and Strom (1973) conducted a retrospective investigation of mortality and morbidity up to the end of 1966 among 5706 male and 487 female concentration camp survivors. The mortality study was based on a comparison between the observed number of deaths and the expected number, based on the mortality of the Norwegian population. Compared with that, the mortality of the ex-prisoners, who had been subject to both extreme psychological and physical stress (beating, torture, hunger, infections), was much higher. Among the most severely physically maltreated persons (Nacht- und Nebel prisoners), the excess mortality was not only due to infections but also to coronary heart disease, lung cancer and violent death due to accident and homicide. The findings correspond well with later studies showing an increased mortality of coronary heart disease and cancer among patients with anxiety disorders (Coryell, Noyes & Clancy, 1982; Eysenck 1987) and increased violent death in Vietnam veterans, particularly those with PTSD. We do not know the figures for persons injured in less traumatic civilian accidents and disasters.

Effects on relatives

The implications of accidents and traumatic injuries for the families of the affected persons must be added to these numbers in order to grasp the tremendous toll put on individuals and the society by accidents and injuries. This is particularly so after brain injuries with personality changes (Livingston, 1987; Rosenbaum & Najenson, 1976) and severe burn injuries (Bernstein, 1976; Blakeney, Portman & Rutan, 1990).

After civilian accidental injuries, the suffering of the victims' relatives may be remarkably high. In a 3-year follow-up study of adults injured in traffic accidents with some type of physical sequelae, a quarter of the 55 close relatives interviewed reported impaired psychological health in themselves as a consequence of the injury to their loved ones (Malt, Blikra & Høivik, 1982).

Economic costs of physical injuries

The economic costs of physical injuries are tremendous. In the United States, the total economic cost of physical trauma was estimated to be $61 billion in fiscal year 1982. These figures do not sufficiently consider the psychosocial implications for the victim and his significant others. Norwegian studies suggest that up to 10% of the relatives of the injured may be on sick leave for a short period of time after the injury (Malt, unpublished data). Psychological stress reactions and the injured's need for care are the main reasons.

Another widely unrecognized problem is the cost associated with longer stays in the hospital. Studies have shown that the length of stay of surgical patients with psychiatric comorbidity is significantly longer than that of other patients (Fulop et al., 1987). Similar observations have been made in trauma patients although evidence from empirical studies is lacking. In the Norwegian 3-year follow-up study of traffic accidents, about 15% of the relatives of injured patients with some kind of physical sequelae reported they had poorer physical health. Seven percent reported a reduced capacity for work and 8% reported taking sick leave due to their injured relative.

Legal aspects of physical injury

In cases of physical injury, compensation often becomes a major issue. In most cases, the issue is settled by agreement without the case coming to court. If not, it is common to have a psychiatric consultation on the case. A proper evaluation must include access to information about previous disabilities, sick leave and psychopathology. Several patients may claim that their mental distress and occupational dysfunction are due to the injury despite positive evidence for similar problems before the accident.

The use of a questionnaire like the Late Effect of Accidental Injury Questionnaire (LEAIQ) may be of value in evaluating the patients' own opinion about late effects of the injury (Malt et al., 1989b). This may be combined with a self-report scale of intrusive and avoidance symptoms like the Impact of Event Scale (IES) (Horowitz, Wilner & Alvarez, 1979). All claims about physical or mental disabilities or handicaps must be supported by positive evidence of a medical investigation. Patients with psychopathology tend to attribute dysfunction and distress to their injury. Such patients may even report intrusion and avoidance symptoms to some degree after trauma which, in fact, were present before the traumatic injury occurred. In the prospective Norwegian study, 75% of the patients claiming insufficient medical treatment for their injuries had, in fact, been given appropriate treatment. The complaints reflected, to a large extent, neglect of psychosocial needs by the helpers.

These findings also underlie the limitations of relying solely on self-report scales (as done by several authors) when assessing the negative long-term effects of traumatic injury (Feinstein & Dolan, 1991; Landsman et al., 1990). Structured interview based measures are of value (Keane, Wolfe & Taylor, 1987; Malt, 1988) as well as psychophysiological methods in assessing PTSD after physical injury (Pitman et al., 1987).

Before accepting any causal relationship between an injury and psychiatric problems, other sources of life stress must be explored (Frank & Elliott, 1987; Malt, 1988). It is also crucial to assess the presence of preaccident personality disorders. In civilian accidents, about one-fifth of the patients suffer from rather severe personality disorders. Persons with psychopathology are more often injured as a result of current psychological distress; they sustain more severe injuries and are injured more often as a result of violence. More often, they have also received social benefits due to accidental injuries.

True posttraumatic stress disorders after usual civilian traumas appear to be infrequent (less than 1%). The studies suggesting higher percentages are based on selected samples with higher levels of trauma or injury and/or rely heavily on scales which do not assess premorbid psychopathology. As a rule of thumb, civilian accidents causing physical injury to a person rarely cause a PTSD reaction unless there is concomitant brain damage and/or premorbid psychopathology, including character traits, predisposing for anxiety and depression (neuroticism) (Hirschfeld et al., 1989). Earlier observations from Ebaugh and Brosin (1943), and Adler (1943) that patients with head concussions and amnesia for the accident situation do not develop injury related posttraumatic stress disorders have been confirmed in a more recent study (Malt, 1988).

Psychological reactions associated with physical illness among rural communities where there is no provision for compensation, differ very little from the reactions described among those injured in compensable accidents (Mendelson, 1984). The assumption that, after the compensation issue is settled, nearly all the cases recover completely without treatment has not been supported in European studies (Foerster, 1983; Mendelson, 1984; Sprehe, 1984). Thus, in cases of chronic disturbances after physical injury, malingering is an unlikely explanation (White, 1982). Most often, major psychiatric disorders are identified explaining the complaints as a 'way of life' (Ford, 1983).

Whatever the status of the patients, the compensation issue should be settled as soon as possible. The American system which provides the lawyers with percentages of the compensation is, from a psychiatric point of view, disastrous. It delays settlements and increases illness behavior while reinforcing psychiatric dysfunctions.

The insanity defense used with dissociative reactions as part of a PTSD syndrome is not easily accepted. Injuries associated with disasters or civilian accidents rarely, if ever, cause major dissociative reactions in persons without premorbid, severe psychopathology according to comprehensive studies of various injured populations in Norway (Malt & Weisaeth, 1989). If such reactions occur after accidental injury, the presence of a severe personality disorder or an organic brain disorder (e.g. temporal lobe epilepsy) should be suspected. There are case reports suggesting that severe anxiety after accidents with minor injury may lead to violent acts (Parker, 1980). There is no support from the research data for this connection between criminal activity and postinjury mental disorders.

Implications for planning and treatment of traumatic injury

Considering the frequency of traumatic injury and the magnitude of the long-term problems, any effort to reduce the occurrence of psychiatric problems after injuries should be welcomed. Clinical experience and studies of the long-term psychiatric effects of traumatic injuries all indicate that intervention should take place during the first days to weeks after the injury to prevent negative effects (Malt, 1991). This is best done by the nursing staff under supervision of a Consultation/Liaison psychiatrist. The helpers should be active and direct in their approach. The key to successful intervention is emotional abreaction and a close collaboration with the families involved (Halmosh & Israeli, 1982; Lenehan, 1986).

Psychiatric interventions may be indicated in select patients (for elaboration, see Malt, 1991). In civilian accidents, disruptive behavior is the most frequent acute problem secondary to the high number of patients with substance abuse and personality disorders among accidentally injured adults. Treatment must be based on the assessment of the cause of the disturbed behavior. Firm, but kind, limits for acceptable behavior should be given. The staff should be taught not to perceive the disturbed behavior as a personal assault. Care must be taken to avoid the development of a ward setting which reinforces disruptive behavior, i.e. the more fuss and disturbed behavior, the more attention by the staff. The best way to achieve this is by allocating a Consultation/Liaison psychiatrist to the emergency and surgical departments (Huyse, 1991).

In disaster situations, several injured persons may arrive at the same time, in addition to the dead. Within hours, many relatives will show up. This may create tremendous problems if the hospital management has made no special arrangements for such events. Relatives of the injured will need different information and support than the relatives of the dead. Accordingly, they should be briefed separately. The hospital disaster plan must include this situation.

In Norway, the leading general University hospital has prepared for such situations by putting a Consultation/Liaison psychiatrist on the disaster steering committee. The committee consists of the chief surgeon, chief anesthesiologist, director of the hospital, the head nurse and the psychiatrist in charge of the Consultation/Liaison Department. The task of the Consultation/Liaison psychiatrist is to evaluate the need for psychiatric interventions and organize the disaster psychiatric service including management of the relatives' needs (for further details, see Weisaeth, 1991). According to the hospital disaster handbook, the psychiatrist is responsible for continuously monitoring the stress reactions of the nursing staff and other medical personnel during disaster situations and, if needed, organizing interventions to prevent burnout and excessive mental distress. Close collaboration with the head nurse and the pastoral service is part of the plan.

In addition to these activities, another Consultation/Liaison psychiatrist is allocated the emergency reception to help the surgeons and anesthesiologist evaluate and treat severe, acute psychiatric reactions. This arrangement has proven very efficient and useful and prevents the problems that may arise if the psychosocial needs of the injured, their relatives, and the staff are neglected. The psychiatrist may also function as a liaison person between crisis centers erected outside the hospital for noninjured disaster victims and the hospital.

The treatment options must include careful assessment of the source of dysphoric emotions, and provision for support and practical help when necessary. In cases where the health service receives several injured persons living far away from home, this need is dramatically increased. Thus, a close collaboration with the social workers of the hospital is needed and must be planned beforehand.

With regard to long-term assessments, the administration of a self-report questionnaire that measures symptoms of intrusion and avoidance (Impact of Event Scale, Horowitz et al., 1979) together with a questionnaire for general distress (e.g. Goldberg's General Health Questionnaire) and specific postinjury problems (Late Effect of Accidental Injury Questionnaire) may be useful as screening instruments (Malt et al., 1989*b*). Repetitive application of such scales increases the positive predictive power (Malt, 1989).

Conclusions

The psychiatric aspects of physical trauma represent a major clinical challenge for the medical profession and health care authorities. Despite the magnitude of injuries and associated problems, this area has been largely neglected until recently. Optimal handling of these problems calls for good planning that takes the special psychosocial implications of traumatic injuries into consideration. The positive experience of having a Consultation/Liaison psychiatrist in the disaster planning and steering committees in Norway suggests that this approach may be useful in other countries in the western world where high quality care of all aspects of human suffering is the optimal goal of the health care system.

References

Adler, A. (1943). Neuropsychiatric complications in victims of Boston's Coconut Grove disaster. *Journal of the American Medical Association*, **123**, 1098–101.
American Psychiatric Association (1987). Somatoform disorders. In *Diagnostical and statistical manual of mental disorders* (3rd edn., rev.) (p. 266). Washington DC: Author.
Baker, G. H. B. (1987). Psychological factors and immunity. *Journal of Psychosomatic Research*, **31**, 1–10.
Balla, J. & Karnaghan, J. (1987). Whiplash headache. *Clinical and Experimental Neurology*, **23**, 179–82.
Bernstein, N. R. (1976). *Emotional care of the facially burned and disfigured*. Boston: Little, Brown, and Company.
Blakeney, P., Portman, S. & Rutan, R. (1990). Familial values as factors influencing long-term psychological adjustment of children after severe burn injury. *Journal of Burn and Care Rehabilitation*, **11**, 472–5.
Blank, K. & Perry, S. (1984). Relationship of psychological processes during delirium on outcome. *American Journal of Psychiatry*, **141**, 843–7.
Boll, T. J. & Barth, J. (1983). Mild head injury. *Psychiatric Developments*, **3**, 263–75.
Bornstein, R. A., Miller, H. B. & van Schoor, J. T. (1989). Neuropsychological deficit and emotional disturbance in head-injured patients. *Journal of Neurosurgery*, **70**, 509–13.
Campbell, J. L., La Clave, L. J. & Brack, G. (1987). Clinical depression in pediatric burn patients. *Burns*, **13**, 213–17.
Chemtob, C. M., Bauer, G. B., Neller, G., Hamada, R., Glisson, C. & Stevens, V. (1990). Post-traumatic stress disorder among special forces Vietnam veterans. *Military Medicine*, **155**, 16–20.
Coryell, W., Noyes, R. & Clancy, J. (1982). Excess mortality in panic disorders: a comparison with primary unipolar depression. *Archives of General Psychiatry*, **39**, 701–3.

Craig, A. R., Hancock, K. M., Dickson, H., Martin, J. & Chang, E. (1990). Psychological consequences of spinal injury: a review of the literature. *Australian and New Zealand Journal of Psychiatry*, **24**, 418–25.

Crocq, M., Macher, J., Duval, F., Barros-Beck, J. & van Valkenburg, C. (1990). The residual effect of cranial injury on post-traumatic stress symptoms over 40 years later. *Biological Psychiatry*, **27**, 54A.

Curran, P. S., Bell, P., Murray, A., Loughrey, G., Roddy, R. & Rocke, L. G. (1990). Psychological consequences of the Enniskillen bombing. *British Journal of Psychiatry*, **156**, 479–82.

Ebaugh, F. G. & Brosin, H. W. (1943). Traumatic psychoses. *Annals of Internal Medicine*, **18**, 666–96.

Eitinger, L. & Strøm, A. (1973). *Mortality and morbidity after excessive stress.* New York: Humanities Press.

Eitinger, L. & Strøm, A. (1981). New investigations on the mortality and morbidity of Norwegian ex-concentration camp survivors. *Israel Journal of Psychiatry and Related Sciences*, **18**, 173–95.

Eysenck, H. J. (1987). Anxiety, learned helplessness, and cancer: a causal theory. *Journal of Anxiety Disorder*, **1**, 87–104.

Feinstein, A. & Dolan, R. (1991). Predictors of post-traumatic stress disorder following physical trauma: an examination of the stressor criterion. *Psychological Medicine*, **21**, 85–91.

Fletchner, J. M., Ewing-Cobbs, L., Miner, M. E., Levin, H. S. & Eisenberg, H. M. (1990). Behavioral changes after closed injury in children. *Journal of Consulting and Clinical Psychology*, **58**, 93–8.

Foerster, K. (1983). Psychodynamic and social development of neurotic patients applying for disability compensation: a catamnestic study. *International Journal of Law and Psychiatry*, **6**, 225–33.

Ford, C. V. (1983). *The somatizing disorders.* New York: Elsevier.

Frank, R. G. & Elliott, T. R. (1987). Life stress and psychologic adjustment following spinal cord injury. *Archives of Physical Medicine and Rehabilitation*, **68**, 344–7.

Fulop, G., Strain, J. J., Vita, J., Lyons, J. S. & Hammer, J. S. (1987). Impact of psychiatric comorbidity on length of hospital stay for medical/surgical patients: a preliminary report. *American Journal of Psychiatry*, **144**, 878–82.

Gargan, M. F. & Bannister, G. O. (1990). Long-term prognosis of soft-tissue injuries of the neck. *Journal of Bone and Joint Surgery*, **72**, 901–3.

Giller, E. L. (ed.) (1990). *Biological assessment and treatment of post-traumatic stress disorder.* Washington DC: American Psychiatric Press.

Gleser, G. C., Green, B. L. & Winget, C. (1981). *Prolonged psychosocial effects of disaster: a study of Buffalo Creek.* New York: Academic Press.

Greenspan, L., McLellan, B. A. & Greig, H. (1985). Abbreviated injury scale and injury severity score: a scoring chart. *Journal of Trauma*, **25**, 60–4.

Halmosh, A. F. & Israeli, R. (1982). Family interaction as modulator in the post-traumatic process. *Medicina del Lavoro*, **1**, 124–34.

Helzer, J. E., Robins, L. N. & McEvoy, L. (1987). Post-traumatic stress disorder in the general population: findings of the epidemiologic catchment area survey. *New England Journal of Medicine*, **317**, 1630–4.

Hirschfeld, R. M. A., Klerman, G. L., Lavori, P., Keller, M. B., Griffith, P. & Coryell, W. (1989). Premorbid personality assessments of first onset of major depression. *Archives of General Psychiatry*, **46**, 345–50.

Holen, A. (1991). A longitudinal study of the occurrence and persistence of posttraumatic health problems in disaster survivors. *Stress Medicine*, **7**, 11–17.

Horowitz, M. (1986). *Stress response syndromes* (2nd edn.). New York: Aronson.

Horowitz, M., Wilner, N. & Alvarez, W. (1979). Impact of event scale: a measure of subjective stress. *Psychosomatic Medicine*, **41**, 209–18.

Huyse, F. (1991). Consultation/Liaison psychiatry: the state of the art and future developments. *Nord Psykiatr Tidsskr*, **45**, 405–22.

Jacome, D. E. (1987). EEG in whiplash: a reappraisal. *Clinical Electroencephalography*, **18**, 41–5.

Judd, F. K., Stone, J., Webber, J. E., Brown, D.J. & Burrows, G. D. (1989). Depression following spinal cord injury: a prospective in-patient study. *British Journal of Psychiatry*, **154**, 668–71.

Keane, T. M., Wolfe, J. & Taylor, K. L. (1987). Post-traumatic stress disorder: evidence for diagnostic validity and methods of psychological assessment. *Journal of Clinical Psychology*, **43**, 32–43.

Krueger, D. W. (1986). Psychological adjustment to physical trauma and disability. In R. Roessler & N. Decker (eds.) *Emotional disorders in physically ill patients*. New York: Human Sciences Press, pp. 250–63.

Krueger, M. (ed.) (1984). *Handbook of rehabilitation psychology*. New York: Brunner/Mazel.

Krute, A. & Burdette, M. E. (1978). 1972 survey of disabled and non-disabled adults: chronic disease, injury and work disability. *Social Security Bulletin*, **41**, 3–17.

Kuhn, W. F., Bell, R. A., Netscher, R. E., Seligson, D. & Kuhn, S. J. (1989). Psychiatric assessment of leg fracture patients: a pilot study. *International Journal of Psychiatry in Medicine*, **19**, 145–54.

Landsman, I. S., Baum, C. G., Arnkoff, D. B., Craig, M. J., Lynch, I., Copes, W. S. & Champion, H. R. (1990). The psychosocial consequences of traumatic injury. *Journal of Behavioral Medicine*, **13**, 561–80.

Lenehan, G. P. (1986). Emotional impact of trauma. *Nursing Clinics of North America*, **21**, 729–40.

Lishman, W. A. (1988). *Organic psychiatry: the psychological consequences of cerebral disorder* (2nd edn.). Oxford: Blackwell.

Livingston, M. G. (1987). Head injury: the relatives' response. *Brain Injury*, **1**, 8–14.

Maimaris, C., Barnes, M. R. & Allen, M. J. (1988). Whiplash injuries of the neck: a retrospective study. *Injury*, **19**, 393–6.

Malt, U. F. (1980). Long-term psychosocial follow-up studies of burned adults: review of the literature. *Burns*, **6**, 190–7.

Malt, U, F. (1988). The long-term psychiatric consequences of accidental injury. *British Journal of Psychiatry*, **153**, 810–18.

Malt, U. F. (1989). The validity of the General Health Questionnaire in a sample of accidentally injured adults. *Acta Psychiatrica Scandinavica*, **80**(355), 103–12.

Malt, U. F. (1991). Psychiatric aspects of accidents and traumatic injuries. In A. Seva (ed.) *The European handbook of psychiatry and mental health. (Volume II)*. Zaragoza: Prensas Universitarias de Zaragoza, pp. 1349–61.

Malt, U. F., Blikra, G. & Høivik, B. (1982). *Bedre føre var: En studie av trafikkskader og deres følger* [A study of traffic injuries and their consequences]. Nordbyhagen: Sentralsykehuset i Akershus. (Only available in Norwegian).

Malt, U. F., Blikra, G. & Høivik, B. (1989a). The three-year biopsychosocial outcome of 551 hospitalized accidentally injured adults. *Acta Psychiatrica Scandinavica*, **80**(355), 84–93.

Malt, U. F., Blikra, G. & Høivik, B. (1989*b*). The late effect of accidental injury questionnaire (LEAIQ). *Acta Psychiatrica Scandinavica*, **80**(355), 113–30.

Malt, U. F., Myhrer, T., Blikra, G. & Høivik, B. (1987). Psychopathology and accidental injuries. *Acta Psychiatrica Scandinavica*, **76**, 261–71.

Malt, U. F. & Ugland, O. M. (1989). A long-term psychosocial follow-up study of burned adults. *Acta Psychiatrica Scandinavica*, **80**(355), 94–102.

Malt, U. F. & Weisaeth, L. (1989). Traumatic stress: empirical studies from Norway. *Acta Psychiatrica Scandinavica*, **80**(355), 1–137.

Mendelson, G. (1984). Follow-up studies of personal injury litigants. *Internal Journal of Law and Psychiatry*, **7**, 179–88.

Mossey, J. M., Mutran, E., Knott, K. & Craik, R. (1989). Determinants of recovery 12 months after hip fracture: the importance of psychosocial factors. *American Journal of Public Health*, **79**, 279–86.

Munoz, E. (1984). Economical costs of trauma, United States 1982. *Journal of Trauma*, **24**, 237–44.

Olsnes, B. T. (1989). Neurobehavioral findings in whiplash patients with long-lasting symptoms. *Acta Neurologica Scandinavica*, **80**, 584–8.

Palinkas, L. A. & Coben, P. (1987). Psychiatric disorders among United States Marines wounded in action in Vietnam. *Journal of Nervous and Mental Disease*, **175**, 291–300.

Parker, N. (1980). Personality change following accidents: the report of a double murder. *British Journal of Psychiatry*, **137**, 401–9.

Patterson, D. R., Carrigan, L., Questad, K. A. & Robinson, R. (1990). Post-traumatic stress disorder in hospitalized patients with burn injuries. *Journal of Burn and Care Rehabilitation*, **11**, 181–4.

Peterson, L. G. & O'Shanick, G. J. (eds.) (1986). *Advances in psychosomatic medicine (Psychiatric aspects of trauma) vol. 16*. Basel: Karger.

Pitman, R. K., Altman, B. & Macklin, M. L. (1989). Prevalence of post-traumatic stress disorder in wounded Vietnam veterans. *American Journal of Psychiatry*, **146**, 667–9.

Pitman, R. K., Orr, S. P., Forgue, D. F., de Jong, J. B. & Claiborn, J. M. (1987). Psychophysiologic assessment of post-traumatic stress disorders imagery in Vietnam combat veterans. *Archives of General Psychiatry*, **44**, 970–5.

Radanov, B. P., Dvorak, J. & Valach, L. (1989). Psychological changes following whiplash injury of the cervical vertebrae [In German] *Schweiz Med Wochenschr*, **119**, 536–43.

Raphael, B. (1986). *When disaster strikes*. London: Hutchinson.

Rimel, R. W., Giordani, B., Barth, J. T., Boll, T. J. & Jane, J. A. (1981). Disability caused by minor head injury. *Neurosurgery*, **9**, 221–8.

Rockwell, E., Dimsdale, J. E., Carroll, W. & Hansbrough, J. (1988). Preexisting psychiatric disorders in burn patients. *Journal of Burn and Care Rehabilitation*, **9**, 83–6.

Roessler, R. & Bolton, B. (1978). *Psychosocial adjustment to disability*. Baltimore: University Park Press.

Rosenbaum, A. & Hoge, S. K. (1989). Head injury and marital aggression. *American Journal of Psychiatry*, **146**, 1048–51.

Rosenbaum, M. & Najenson, T. (1976). Changes in life pattern and symptoms of low mood as reported by wives of severely brain-injured soldiers. *Journal of Consulting and Clinical Psychology*, **44**, 881–8.

Rundell, J. R., Ursano, R. J., Holloway, H. C. & Silberman, E. K. (1989).

Psychiatric responses to trauma. *Hospital and Community Psychiatry*, **40**, 68–74.

Smith, A. M., Scott, S. G., O'Fallon, W. M. & Young, M. L. (1990). Emotional responses of athletes to injury. *Mayo Clinic Proceedings*, **65**, 38–50.

Sprehe, D. J. (1984). Worker's compensation: a psychiatric follow-up study. *International Journal of Law and Psychiatry*, **7**, 165–78.

Steketee, G. & Foa, E. B. (1987). Rape victims: post-traumatic stress responses and their treatment. A review of the literature. *Journal of Anxiety Disorder*, **1**, 69–86.

Strøm, A. (ed.) (1986). *Norwegian concentration camp survivors*. New York: Humanities Press.

Tarsh, M. J. & Royston, C. (1985). A follow-up study of accident neurosis. *British Journal of Psychiatry*, **146**, 18–25.

Tellier, A., Dams, K. M., Walker, A. E. & Rourke, B. P. (1990). Long-term effects of severe penetrating head injury on psychosocial adjustment. *Journal of Consulting and Clinical Psychology*, **58**, 531–7.

Trimble, M. R. (1981). *Post-traumatic neurosis*. Chichester: John Wiley.

Ursano, R. J., Fullerton, C. S., Wright, K. M. & McCarroll, J. E. (eds.) (1990). *Trauma, disasters and recovery*. Bethesda, MD: Uniformed Services University of the Health Sciences.

Wallace, L. M. & Lees, J. (1988). A psychological follow-up study of adult patients discharged from a British burn unit. *Burns*, **14**, 39–45.

Ward, H. W., Moss, R. L., Darko, D. F. et al. (1987). Prevalence of postburn depression following burn injury. *Journal of Burn and Care Rehabilitation*, **8**, 294–8.

White, A. C. (1982). Psychiatric study of patients with severe burn injuries. *British Medical Journal*, **284**, 465–7.

White, P. & Faustman, W. (1989). Coexisting physical conditions among inpatients with post-traumatic stress disorder. *Military Medicine*, **154**, 60–71.

Weisaeth, L. (1991). The psychiatrist's role in preventing psychopathological effects of disaster traumas. In A. Seva (ed.) *The European handbook of psychiatry and mental health Volume II*. Zaragoza: Prensas Universitarias de Zaragoza, pp. 2342–58.

6

The human experience of earthquakes

BRIAN G. McCAUGHEY, KENNETH J. HOFFMAN
and CRAIG H. LLEWELLYN

Destructive earthquakes occur frequently and affect the economic, social, medical, and psychological wellbeing of large numbers of people. World-wide there are 100 000 (Beinin, 1985) to 1 000 000 earthquakes per year (Nichols, 1974); 5 000 000 per year if microearthquakes and tremors are included (Nichols, 1974). Most of these earthquakes go unnoticed, too small to even detect.

Although most earthquakes are harmless to man, either because they are too weak to damage property, or because they occur in nonpopulated areas, many cause considerable destruction, injury, and death (see Table 6.1).

Some of the most destructive earthquakes have occurred in China (Jackson, 1981; Sood, Stockdale & Rogers, 1987). Confirmation of specific details is often difficult to obtain. In China, in 1976, an earthquake reportedly killed 800 000 people (Sood et al. 1987). The amount of destruction was difficult to verify at the time because the information released by the Chinese government was quite limited. Another extremely serious earth-quake, but also difficult to verify, occurred in AD 526 in Antioch; 260 000 died (Miln, 1890). The number of deaths that are caused by an earthquake may be very high, but even more people may be physically injured. The February 4, 1976 earthquake in Guatemala, caused 24 340 deaths, but 90 000 people were injured (Beinin, 1985). Acute and chronic psychological distress are characteristic of earthquakes (Leivesley, 1984). This chapter will discuss the psychological impact of earthquakes. In the process we will review: (1) a commonly used system to classify disasters into manmade or natural, (2) the psychological effects of the threat of an earthquake, and (3) observations on the psychological consequences of the Loma Prieta Earthquake which struck on October 17, 1989 and measured 7.1 on the Richter Scale. Loma Prieta means 'dark hill' and refers to a geographical area near the epicenter of the quake, 60 miles south of San Francisco,

Table 6.1. *Deaths caused by earthquakes*

Number killed	Location	Year
260 000	Antioch	526
800 000	China	1556
300 000	Calcutta	1737
200 000	China	1920
93 000	Japan	1923
25 000	Guatemala	1976
800 000	China	1976
700	San Francisco	1906
10 000	Mexico City	1985
40 000	Iran	1989

California. The resulting destruction was widespread and covered a large area, including San Francisco, Oakland, and Santa Cruz.

Classification of disasters: natural versus manmade

Disasters are often classified as either natural or manmade (Berren, Beigel & Barker, 1982; Dohrenwend & Dohrenwend, 1987) based on their perceived cause. Natural disasters include earthquakes, floods, hurricanes, etc. They are caused by nature or God, but not by man. What we call a natural disaster today has not always been thought of as 'natural'. In Western cultures prior to the eighteenth century, natural disasters were seen as retribution for man's misdeeds; particularly sexual misdeeds (Gilbert & Barkun, 1981). These ideas are still found today. Some religious Iranians said that the June 21, 1990, earthquake in northwestern Iran was God's punishment for religious misdeeds.

Manmade disasters are so called, because the cause is due to some action(s) taken or not taken by man. This classification can be misleading. The Buffalo Creek, West Virginia, flood of 1972, is called a manmade disaster (Chamberlin, 1980), and the 1989 Loma Prieta earthquake is called a natural disaster. It may seem that there is a clear distinction between them, but it is blurred when one considers the following. In *both* cases the etiologic agent was 'natural': rain for the Buffalo Creek flood and earth movement for the Loma Prieta earthquake. In both cases, man made decisions prior to the disasters that strongly influenced the outcome (e.g. death, injuries, and property damage). In the case of the Buffalo Creek flood, it was man's decision: to build a dam in the first place, to build it in its particular location, and to maintain it in the manner that was done. In the case of the Loma Prieta earthquake, it can be argued that the number of dead and injured and the amount of destruction were influenced by man's decisions, just as in the case of the Buffalo Creek flood disaster. The housing codes in the Marina District of San Francisco allowed occupancy in older, unreinforced buildings that were built on unstable land. The ground in the Marina District is filled-in swamp which predisposes it to be unstable during earthquakes. Another example is the elevated $1\frac{1}{4}$ mile section of the Interstate 880 (I-880) freeway in Oakland, which collapsed during the earthquake. It was known to be at risk because of its older design. Thus, the outcome of the 1989 Loma Prieta earthquake, was greatly influenced by man's decisions.

Man's and nature's influence on the outcome of events overlap considerably. Even earthquakes which are almost always thought of as being exclusively caused by nature, can be manmade. For example, nuclear explosions, the construction of manmade lakes, and underground fluid injection can all lead to an earthquake (Nichols, 1974). While a disaster may seem to be due to either nature or to acts of man (including acts of omission), in many cases the results are a combination of the 'natural' etiologic agent and predisaster actions or inactions taken by man. This causative interaction is termed the man–nature etiological dyad.

Considering this confusion of causes, why are disasters classified this way? Why are they classified at all? What effect does it have to classify them this way? Is there a better way to classify disasters? Classifying disasters, like any other problem, implies differentiation through examination. Such study can lead to the identification of unique characteristics that can provide a basis for intervention and management. Even when this is not possible, however, classification systems serve another purpose: they identify the unmanageable or unknown. The act of classifying itself, gives hope, comfort, and a sense of control, even though in the end, this control may be illusive.

This classification system also highlights the aspect of blame. There is a strong belief in western cultures that most events are, or should be, under man's control and that if something goes wrong, it is because of some action or inaction by man. Lawyers frequently like to use the phrase '. . . . knew, or should have known . . .' to comprehensively assign blame. So following a disaster, one of the first questions is, who is at fault? Was it caused by man or nature? If man is the cause of the disaster, frequently other cultural events, such as litigation, victimization, stigmatization, and scapegoating will ensue. At its worst, this system may unfairly find blame, or, unfairly not find blame.

Table 6.2. *Human experience of different types of disasters in the US*

Example	Known to be a potential danger	Potential for warning	Able to take precaution	Can the event be prevented?
Hurricane Hugo	+ + + +	+ + + +	+ + +	− − − −
Mt St Helens	− − −	+	− −	− − − −
Kentucky floods	+ + +	+ + +	+ +	− −
Loma Prieta earthquake	+ + +	− −	− −	− − − −
Three Mile Island	+ +	+ +	+ +	+ + + +
Buffalo Creek	+ +	− −	− −	+ + + +
Hyatt Regency sky walk	− − − −	− − − −	− − − −	+ + + +

The distinction between manmade and natural disasters changes over time and is related to technological advances. Surviving families of fishermen killed at sea during a storm successfully sued the weather service. It was argued that even though the deaths were due to a storm, they were preventable. The weather service did not maintain a data collection buoy correctly, and thus did not issue a timely warning. This legal outcome would have been impossible 100 years ago.

The manmade versus natural disaster classification system has short-comings, but it is so culturally entrenched that it must be taken into account.

While not meant to be exhaustive, Table 6.2 compares the human experience of earthquakes with other kinds of disasters. Many aspects of natural and manmade disasters are quite similar. All disaster victims face some common experiences.

In Table 6.2, disasters are compared on the following characteristics: 1) Was the threat known to exist? In the case of the collapse of the Hyatt Regency sky walk there was no suspicion that a disaster would occur. This added to the shock when it suddenly collapsed. 2) Was there an opportunity to warn potential victims ahead of time, so that they could take pre-cautions? Of the disasters considered, some people were warned. For Hurricane Hugo this meant a reduction of injury and loss of life. When there is no chance of bracing for the shock, such as with an earthquake, there is the potential for feelings of helplessness and feeling overwhelmed. 3) Were the potential victims able to take precautions after the warning? Similar to the potential for warning, only those disasters where the velocity of the destructive evolution was low, such as Hurricane Hugo, was there enough time to take preventive or life saving measures. 4) Can the event be

Table 6.3. *Characteristics of earthquakes*

Unpredictable – unknown when one will occur
Instantaneous – sudden death, injury and destruction
Concentrated – high velocity destructive evolution
Uncontrollable – its acute effects can not be modified
Powerful – causes a wide area of destruction
Elusive – cause is unseen; only the effects are seen
Total involvement – encompassing all senses
Unexpected continuation – aftershocks cause vigilance

---

prevented? This returns us to a manmade versus natural cause, which must be considered. Victims want to know where to direct their anger. Man was blamed for failures at the Three Mile Island nuclear plant, Buffalo Creek flood, and the Hyatt Regency sky walk collapse.

Characteristics of earthquakes and their psychological impact

Earthquakes are greatly feared, probably more than most other kinds of disaster (Table 6.3). Earthquakes occur unpredictably. Even scientific methods do not help. Predictions of time, location and intensity are limited to the crudest estimates which leads to feelings of helplessness. This results in attempts to predict earthquake occurrence by any means, including observations of animal behavior (Medici, Frey & Frey, 1985), and psychic exploration (Kautz, 1982). In contrast, satellites can track hurricanes and provide lifesaving information.

Earthquakes also occur instantaneously. There is no warning; not a few minutes or even a few seconds. Victims experience a complete and sudden change from the calm of their normal routine, to the full force of mass destruction. The earthquake's full destructive force occurs in a brief period of time, usually less than a minute: earthquakes have high velocity destructive evolution. A hurricane's destructive force lasts for hours or days. Even though in the end, both are quite damaging, the velocity of the evolution of an earthquake adds additional destructive force and psychological trauma. Measures to prevent injury or death during an earthquake are quite limited. Hurricane victims may feel better because they can take some action to help themselves, such as evacuating to another area, erecting sand bags, etc.

Earthquakes are also uncontrollable; nothing can control their progression, (Jackson, 1981). They are extremely powerful, causing buildings to collapse, landslides, etc. The New Madrid, Missouri, earthquake of 1811, changed the course of the Mississippi River. Earthquakes can affect an extremely large area. Some earthquakes have been felt over as much as a 1.5 million square mile area (Nichols, 1974), causing considerable psychological distress to a large number of people. During the 1811 earthquake in New Madrid, earth movement was felt as far away as the East Coast of the United States and Canada. Bells rang in Virginia and clocks stopped in Boston (Nichols, 1974). An earthquake in Chile on May 22, 1960 caused a tsunami (tidal wave) that spread across the Pacific Ocean at 500 miles per hour (Keys, 1963). Sixty-one people were killed and 282 injured thousands of miles away in Hawaii (Cox & Mink, 1963). The wave reflected off the coast of several countries, including, Japan, Russia, New Zealand, Australia (Seivers, Villegas & Barros, 1963).

The fear associated with earthquakes is also due to their elusiveness. You cannot see the cause of an earthquake, only its effects (Jackson, 1981). During a hurricane you can see, hear, and feel the etiologic agent; the storm clouds, the wind, and the rain. Everything near the epicenter is involved in an earthquake. There is no island of safety. Buildings move and may break apart; the ground shakes. Aftershocks occur following the main seismic event and create a repetition of the original psychological trauma producing a forced and unrelenting vigilance. This diminishes the individuals ability to relax, and focus on rebuilding the community, delaying the resolution of psychological distress.

There are many psychological effects of earthquakes. Each of them, if taken individually, causes considerable psychological distress, however, the terror of an earthquake is that they all occur at the same time.

Phases of an earthquake disaster

The time periods, phases, of disasters are classified in various ways (Chamberlin, 1980; Boyd, 1981). One way is preimpact, impact, and postimpact. In this chapter, corresponding terminology will be used: pre-, during, and postearthquake. The postearthquake period can be subdivided into early and late.

The preearthquake period

Threat

Most psychological studies examine victims who are recovering during the postearthquake period. Very few studies consider the psychological aspects of the preearthquake period. It is a psychologically active period in parts of the world where earthquake threat is well known, such as the Pacific seismic belt, including Japan and parts of North America. This region accounts for 80% of all of the world's earthquakes (Jackson & Mukerjee, 1974).

Many people living in this area know they are at significant risk of death, injury, and destruction. Some authors have suggested that people should not be allowed to live in these high risk areas (Nichols, 1974), however, many do (Ayres & Sandilya, 1986). In Turkey, rebuilding continues along a fault where there have been 11 earthquakes in 30 years (Nichols, 1974).

Why do some people continue to live in these high risk areas when they could live somewhere else? Some are unaware of the destructive threat. Others are aware of the threat but are more concerned about the more visible, here and now problems. Residents ($N = 302$) of Los Angeles, Vancouver, and Anchorage were asked what they thought were the disadvantages of living in their city. Only 1.7% cited earthquake hazard as a disadvantage, compared to air pollution, crowding, traffic, climate, noise, and crime (Jackson, 1981).

Others continue to live with the threat because the social, economic, and cultural advantages outweigh the disadvantages (Sood et al., 1987). After Hurricane Hugo, homeowners rebuilt their houses near the water, stating that they realized that the same thing would likely happen again, but that the pleasure they got from living near the ocean was worth the cost of rebuilding. The costs of rebuilding in an area known to be at high risk for a disaster is termed the 'Eden overhead'; the cost of rebuilding when the Garden of Eden is destroyed.

Preparation

Governments are aware that people continue to live in high risk areas, so they develop emergency plans (Edwards, 1976) and training programs (de Bruycker et al., 1983) to prepare for disasters. Governments use this information to instruct their citizens on how to prepare. It might be expected that residents who live in a seismically active area and hear warnings, would want to increase their individual preparedness. Sometimes this is the case, but often it is not. In Japan, the news media quite vigorously disseminated information based on a prediction made by scientists in August 1976, that an earthquake would occur in the Shizuoka Prefecture. The population was strongly advised to prepare (Hirose & Ishizuka, 1983). Follow-up surveys found that initial warnings had a positive effect on preparedness, but eventually motivation diminished (Hirose & Ishizuka, 1983). In another survey on preparedness, residents were given a considerable amount of information about earthquake risk through the mass media. This initially increased preparedness, but later it plateaued, because the population had 'learned to live with the threat ...' (Hirose, 1986).

University of California administrators publicized a report that predicted which campus buildings would be damaged, and how severely, if there was an earthquake with a magnitude of 7 or greater. Two groups of students were asked about their perceptions about future earthquakes (Lehman & Taylor, 1987). The students ($n = 51$) living in structures identified as seismically 'very poor' were more likely to deny that the threat was serious, than the other students ($n = 50$) who lived in seismically 'good' structures. But neither group was knowledgeable about basic earthquake safety information, and no one took preparatory safety measures.

In a study of 123 residents of San Francisco, most (96%) thought there would be an earthquake in the future, but few thought that they would have property damage (Jackson, 1981). They either did nothing to prepare for an earthquake (36.7%) or thought they would rely on emergency services (42.5%) if one occurred. Very few had insurance (7.5%) or housing modifications to improve earthquake protection (7.5%). A problem of possible bias (78% questionnaire refusal rate) was cited as limiting the study's usefulness. Even this, however, may be important information because the fact that so few participated may indicate strong denial.

It would seem to be a simple matter to educate people about earthquake risk, and that they would react appropriately and in accordance with the facts. This may be true in some cases. The studies cited above suggest that the amount of preparation is related to how much publicity the problem is given. But, there are other reasons. To make decisions you need to be able to know the risks, understand probabilities and assess uncertainty. Multiple risk assessments are difficult for the average person to make. Even when there are effective warnings that raise appropriate public concern, there may be limitations to how prepared a population can be (Slovic, Kunreuther & White, 1974). Also, no one is aware of all the possibilities for preparation for an earthquake. Therefore, the choices as seen or used are narrowed. In addition, people prefer to respond to the most urgent demand in the present rather than one in the future.

The most prominent psychological aspect of the preearthquake period is denial. For many this is a strong defense. As noted by Wolfenstein, 'even when the denial of a threatened danger occurring .... yields to contrary evidence, the belief remains: it can't affect me. The pre-disaster conviction seems to be: it can't happen, but if it does, I will remain immune' (Wolfenstein, 1957).

During the earthquake

Injuries, deaths and a variety of psychological reactions occur during an earthquake. Experiencing an earthquake is terrifying, and while the main seismic shock most often lasts less than a minute (usually several seconds) the perception is that it lasts much longer (Nichols, 1974). Following an earthquake in New York State on October 19, 1985, 246 people were asked to estimate its duration. According to scientific measurements, it lasted about 30 seconds; for the subjects it seemed to last more than twice as long. The mean estimate was 61 seconds, with a range of 1 to 300 seconds (Buckhout, Fox & Rabinowitz, 1989).

Psychotherapy patients who experienced the February 9, 1971 earthquake in Los Angeles reported their reactions to their psychotherapists. They ranged from fright and fear, to seeming indifference (Greenson & Mintz, 1972). Another report described individuals vacillating between the extremes of denial and fantasy, but usually settling on reality (Wolfenstein, 1957).

While many people may do worse during an earthquake, some who have psychological problems actually improve, at least temporarily. Some psychotic patients were more rational for a short period of time, following the destruction of the Los Angeles County Olive View Medical Center on February 9, 1971. One patient, who was more disturbed than the others, was able to help dress a blind patient and then lead him to safety. This more rational state among the patients lasted from one hour to two weeks (Koegler & Hicks, 1972).

There are also immediate psychophysiologic reactions to earthquakes. The February 9, 1971 earthquake in Los Angeles caused 'over eight heart attacks brought on by fright' (Greenson & Mintz, 1972). In addition, earthquakes may cause considerable anxiety and subsequent cardiac arrhythmias. Several cardiac patients were wearing Holter monitors during the February 24, 1981 earthquake in Athens, Greece (Voridis, Mallios & Papantonis, 1983). An analysis of the data showed that a number of the patients had a disturbance of cardiac rhythm during the earthquake. This was attributed to increased vagal or sympathetic activity.

The feeling of terror that occurs during an earthquake can be overwhelming. The 1989 Loma Prieta earthquake in the San Francisco region was a moderate one. The amount of damage and number of deaths was much less than it could have been. Even so, many people reacted strongly to the event. The following are the experiences of three residents of the Marina District of San Francisco.

Miss L.: Miss L, an 11 year-old girl, was at home with her father during the earthquake. Although previously in good health she became 'paralyzed', during the earthquake, and unable to leave her home. She was carried out by her father. Part of her fear was caused by the inability to see, because of the thick dust from collapsing buildings.

Mr S.: At the time of the earthquake, Mr S saw and heard buildings collapsing around him. He braced himself, working to remain upright as the ground shook. Over the years he had tried to prepare himself psychologically for an earthquake. But he did not anticipate that suddenly and unexplainably, a thick dark material came up through the cracks in the ground near where he was standing (he found out later this was silt mixed with water being forced out of the ground). He also heard the sounds of distressed people and a cloud of dust disoriented him. Because of all of this, there was nothing that he could see, hear or feel, to reassure himself. He thought he was experiencing what it would be like to be in hell.

Ms B.: Ms B, a Marina District resident was on the fourth floor of an apartment building when the earthquake struck. Within a few minutes, the first three levels of the building collapsed, accordion style. The fourth floor remained intact, but was now at ground level. She climbed out the fourth floor apartment through the window, onto the street, physically uninjured.

These cases convey the extremely stressful nature of an earthquake. In a sense, the earthquake is a metaphor for what takes place in a person; a sudden upheaval of emotions and fear where there had been calm. An earthquake is terrifying because there is no way to escape; 'It is as if the entire world were trembling and falling apart ...' (Greenson & Mintz, 1972).

Postearthquake period

After an earthquake, many groups intervene, if they still exist. Initially, this includes locally based medical personnel, rescue units, government agencies, engineers, news media, etc. Later, they may be supported by groups outside the community. Each have their own tasks, their difficulties trying to complete their jobs, and their associated psychological stresses. The decisions they make and their performance affect their own psychological wellbeing and that of the community at large. They must overcome a variety of problems.

Rescue workers' success, that is, whether victims live or die, often depends on how soon after an earthquake they can complete their rescue (de Bruycker et al. 1983). This often depends on what local capabilities were in place before the earthquake and how effectively they can be used. Physical barriers, such as impassable roads are a significant problem. This was a major problem in Guatemala in 1976 (Spencer et al. 1977) and Peru in 1970 (Rennie, 1970). Medical personnel may be forced to combine old, inelegant techniques like amputation (Bialik et al., 1989; Ishmukhametov, l'Initskaia & Tsepliaeva, 1989; Kliukvin & Zolotukhina, 1989; Yuan, 1989) with newer ones. Hemodialysis for acute renal failure secondary to crush injuries or dehydration, was provided locally for some patients following the 1988 Armenian earthquake (Tattersall et al., 1990).

Government officials must cope with a number of problems, including some that cannot be anticipated. Following the Mexico City earthquake, homeless people living outside the damaged area surprised rescue workers by coming into the damaged area. They thought the assistance they could get would be an improvement over their usual living standards (Gavalya, 1987). Government policies and decisions, some of which are influenced by political considerations, affect large populations (Spencer et al., 1977), may be unpopular and may cause anger (Gavalya, 1987; Edwards, 1976).

The news media is a very important factor during the postearthquake period. During this time communications can be dramatically impaired (Spencer et al., 1977). The news media can pass important information even though their means may be limited (Sood et al., 1987). After the September 19, 1985, Mexico City earthquake telephone service was disrupted; radio and television stations used their facilities to help dispatch rescue equipment. At other times, the news media have been viewed unfavorably. The same television stations in Mexico City replayed death and injury scenes, which unnecessarily upset the population (Palacios et al., 1986).

Disaster victims manifest a wide range of psychiatric symptoms. Historically, symptoms resolve quickly with simple humane treatment; providing rest, food, drink, clothing, and a chance to talk (Edwards, 1976). Some earthquake victims' reactions fit the definition of posttraumatic stress disorder. As a stressor, an earthquake universally evokes fear. After an earthquake, many people report intrusive thoughts with alternating periods of emotional numbing and hypervigilance. There can be long-term effects on sleep and dreaming (Hefez, Metz & Lavie, 1987). There are also rare but true psychiatric emergencies, which require immediate intervention and a disposition plan for long-term chronic care (Baldwin, 1978).

Loma Prieta earthquake (1989)

The Loma Prieta earthquake caused immediate destruction, death, and injury, much of it along the 1¼ mile collapsed Interstate 880 (I-880) overpass in Oakland, Claifornia. Rescuing survivors and recovering bodies started almost immediately. Several groups were involved: construction workers, engineers, coroner personnel, police, firefighters, Navy corpsmen, and Air Force Pararescue. They worked long hours in a dangerous situation, on a gruesome task. Some psychological stress was attributable to the tragic circumstances of the victims' death. One victim was crushed by a cross beam from the second level of the interstate highway. Because the car's emergency break was set, rescuers thought that the victim mistakenly chose where he stopped. Probably the victim thought he would be safer under a cross beam. In fact, this decision may have caused his death; some motorists who stopped away from cross beams survived. This twist of fate added to the impact of the tragedy on the rescue workers. In another situation, rescuers recovered a body with an electronic pager that was still receiving messages being sent by worried family members.

After the Loma Prieta Earthquake, officials were concerned about the psychological impact of the tragedy on the rescue workers. Many of the military personnel were young, inexperienced in the medical field, and used to working with patients, but not recovering bodies. They and the construction workers were strongly encouraged to talk about their experience after each shift. A debriefing tent was established for that purpose. The Alameda County Coroner's office established a policy that required its employees to work less than their normal shifts to limit their exposure to the body recovery and identification process.

In contrast to the meager amount of resources that are available in some countries, those available to the communities affected by the Loma Prieta earthquake were plentiful. So numerous were the fire appliances at the I-880 site, that one observer said it looked like a sales lot for used fire trucks. There were so many fire trucks that only a small percentage could be used at any time. A large amount of donated food was distributed by numerous disaster workers. One fast food chain brought a truck with cooks to the disaster site to make free hamburgers and french fries. Two masseuses also donated their services. Within three days after the earthquake it was decided to add an extra lane to the highway leading to the San Mateo Bridge to alleviate the increased commuter traffic due to another bridge having to be closed. The additional lane was built in part of a day. Leading a line of construction equipment was a grader, followed by a truck laying gravel, then another grader, then trucks with blacktop, etc. At the end of the line was a machine putting stripes on the road. The effect of this resource rich environment on the psychological recovery is unknown, but anecdotal accounts suggest that it was helpful.

Local governments faced a number of difficult problems during the postearthquake period. In Oakland, how to dismantle the I-880 overpass was a problem. If it was dismantled slowly, it would take a long time, be expensive and risk additional injury or death, especially if strong after-shocks occurred. A much less expensive, safer, and quicker way to dismantle the bridge was to blow it up. But this risked further emotional shock to the community and governmental embarrassment if additional bodies were found under these distasteful circumstances. It was decided to slowly dismantle it. This illustrates the complexity of the issues that officials must deal with, the extremely stressful nature of their work and how their decisions can influence the psychological wellbeing of the community.

Officials in the Marina District also faced difficult choices. Buildings collapsed on their own during the first week after the earthquake; it was dangerous just to walk down some streets. But residents wanted to enter their homes and recover things they needed for basic living: medications, financial papers, etc. Engineers, who had been identified as part of the areas disaster plan, determined which buildings were safe. While some residents complained that it took too long to get into their homes, it was clear that, for most, the disaster plan was carried out well and contributed to the recovery process.

The news media actively gathered information in the Marina District following the Loma Prieta earthquake. Some residents were irritated by their aggressiveness. Others were even more distressed when they saw media personnel crossing police lines into the District although the residents were prohibited from entering. The residents were also irritated by the curious, those who came to see the destruction. They felt violated when they saw these people looking into their houses and taking broken parts of buildings as souvenirs.

Marina District residents were affected by the disaster in many different ways. Some of the homeless, who were quite used to living on the street, improved their situation by moving into shelters. Several of them presented with chronic, severe mental illness, which placed additional demands on shelter managers. Many of the wealthier residents moved into motels. Some moved in with friends. The ones who seemed most adversely affected were the near homeless; the ones living in inexpensive single occupancy rooms. They could not afford a hotel and did not have friends or relatives to stay with. Many had to move to a shelter.

A few days after the earthquake, some Marina District residents were allowed to reenter the area. Very early on, some talked about their future and how the earthquake affected them.

Mr K.: Mr K was a single businessman in his late 20s. He had lived in an apartment for the last few years. He said that even before the earthquake he never intended to live there for any length of time, but that because of the damage and possible future threat of another earthquake he wanted to move out as soon as possible. Not only was he thoroughly convinced that he wanted to leave, but he couldn't understand why anyone would want to stay. They were crazy. 'Their favorite food must be jello', he said. He complained that the government moved too slowly to resolve issues that would allow residents to reclaim their necessary possessions: business papers, etc. He was also angry with the rich owners of the local apartment buildings that lived in the suburbs, and were spared earthquake damage.

Mr T.: Mr T and his wife were allowed to occupy their house in the Marina District a few days after the earthquake. They were alone because most other nearby houses remained unoccupied. Mr. T. was not sure that his house was undamaged, but he was confident that if something wrong was found, it could be repaired and he could continue to live there. He liked his house, a three-storey dwelling that was owned first by his grandfather, and then by his father who passed it on to him. Within a week prior to the earthquake he received an unsolicited offer from a real estate agent to sell the house for at least $700,000. He rejected the offer, as he had similar offers in the past. He was a little concerned about continuing to live in San Francisco because of the threat of another earthquake. But he reasoned that his grandfather survived the 1906 earthquake, his father never experienced one, and because previous generations never experienced more than one, and he had one in his lifetime, he did not expect another.

He was very concerned about how the neighborhood would change. He thought that several apartment houses would have to be destroyed. This would force out the elderly residents who lived in the relatively inexpensive apartments. In their place would come new, more expensive apartment buildings and the young urban professionals that could afford the higher rents. For him, the community would change in an unpleasant way.

These reactions demonstrate several points. Both individuals lived within a few blocks of each other in the Marina District and both considered the future risk. Their plans for the future were, however, quite different, and were related to their emotional investment in the community. Mr T was well established in the community and saw his life as part of it. He viewed the earthquake as a problem, but one that he could overcome, based at least in part on his family's experience. For him, there was a generational effect; denial was prominent. He had already started to deal with the loss of his community as he knew it. In contrast, Mr K's ties to the community were weaker. He had more ease of mobility; he lived in a rented apartment and had lived there for only a short time. He was quite willing to move and change his job if needed; something seen in other disaster situations (Crabbs & Black, 1984).

Mental health programs were established in various locations soon after the earthquake. Counsellors were available in several shelters. Over time, counsellors and others reported the ways in which people cope with the regions earthquake threat. Anecdotal reports from the San Francisco Bay area indicated that some drivers unbuckled their seat belts while stopping for a red light when they were underneath a freeway. This was to facilitate a rapid exit from the car if an earthquake occurred. The concern about the ease of escape following an earthquake was also seen among children following the July 26, 1963 earthquake in Skopje (Popovic & Petrovic, 1964). After evacuation from the damaged area, some children took the locks off the doors of their homes so they would not be trapped.

Other ways of coping have also been observed. In the Los Angeles area, seismological offices continually receive a variety of calls from concerned citizens. They notice that the number of calls increases following news about any earthquake. Some people call repeatedly asking for predictions about when the 'big one' will occur. One person called ten times a day for a month. This led the seismographic office staff of one office to use of the term 'seismophobia' to describe the over concern among some people. Others call the offices to suggest theories about how to predict earthquakes.

There is a recurring three part rumor in some communities in Los Angeles. Part one is that a seismographic office in Southern California has predicted the date and location of a major earthquake and secretly called out the National Guard. The second part is that, if you call the seismographic office to confirm this information, you will be told that no prediction was made. According to the rumor, this is to prevent panic. In the third part of the rumor, citizens call the seismographic office and are told that no prediction was made, which confirms in their minds that the rumor is true.

Conclusions

Earthquakes are important because they affect individuals, families, communities, and government organizations. Their negative effects cause change and demands for readjustment, which are quite stressful. Dealing with earthquakes can be difficult at every phase. During the preearthquake phase, denial of risk makes it difficult for governments to design and implement effective prevention and rescue programs. During the period of earthquake activity and the postearthquake period many problems present. Inadequate preparation can highlight these problems. But even with adequate preparation, improbable or illogical things occur, such as the unanticipated flow of the homeless into the earthquake damaged areas of Mexico City.

The Loma Prieta earthquake in San Francisco and the surrounding communities can be viewed in several different ways. From one perspective, it was a small earthquake that provided valuable training for massive, future earthquakes. The psychological experience was a beneficial inoculation (Norris & Murrell, 1988). From another perspective, citizens witnessed a massive, efficient rescue effort, which will reinforce the belief that future earthquakes will be handled with as much ease. This might mistakenly suggest to some that there is no need for preparation.

It is important to understand the basic concepts of how earthquakes affect individuals and communities in order to use this information for training individuals and organizations. Individual preparation should include first aid training, maintaining a small stockpile of basic necessities, fundamental aspects of rescue work and how to avoid hazards. Government, and nongovernment organizations need to plan, educate, and especially, practise disaster response. They also need to prepare for the social, economic, and psychological impact on survivors and rescue personnel, and establish programs to address these issues.

Acknowledgements

The authors thank the following individuals for contributing to this chapter: Joshua Vayer, Linda Curtis, Robert Finn, and Dr Thomas Heaton.

References

Ayres, R. U. & Sandilya, M. S. (1986). Catastrophe avoidance and risk aversion: implications of formal utility maximization. *Theory and Decision*, **20**(1), 63–78.

Baldwin, B. A. (1978). A paradigm for the classification of emotional crisis; implications for crisis intervention. *American Journal of Orthopsychiatry*, **48**(3), 538–51.

Beinin, L. (1985). *Medical consequences of natural Disasters*. Berlin Springer-Verlag.

Berren, M. R., Beigel, A. & Barker, G. (1982). A typology for the classification of disasters: implications for intervention. *Community Mental Health Journal*, **18**(2), 120–34.

Bialik, I. F., Borovkova, T. F., Vasina, T. A. et al. (1989). Treatment of open injuries in the victims of the earthquake in Armenian USSR. *Soviet Medicine*, **10**, 18–21.

Boyd, S. T. (1981). Psychological reactions of disaster victims. *South African Medical Journal*, **60**(2), 744–8.

Buckhout, R., Fox, P. & Rabinowitz, M. (1989). Estimating the duration of an earthquake: some shaky field observations. *Bulletin of the Psychonomic Society*, **27**(4), 375–8.

Chamberlin, B. C. (1980). The psychological aftermath of disaster. *Journal of Clinical Psychiatry*, **41**(7), 238–44.

Cox, D. C. & Mink, J. F. (1963). The tsunami of 23 May 1960, in the Hawaiian Islands. *Bulletin of the Seismological Society of America*, **53**(6), 1191–209.

Crabbs, M. A. & Black, K. U. (1984). Job change following a natural disaster. *Vocational Guidance Quarterly*, **32**(4), 232–9.

de Bruycker, M., Greco, D., Annino, I. et al. (1983). The 1980 earthquake in southern Italy: rescue of trapped victims and mortality. *Bulletin World Health Organization*, **61**(6), 1021–5.

Dohrenwend, B. S. & Dohrenwend, B. P. (1987). Some issues in research in stressful life events. *Journal of Nervous and Mental Diseases*, **166**(1), 7–15.

Edwards J. G. (1976). Psychiatric aspects of civilian disasters. *British Medical Journal*. **1**, 944–7.

Gavalya, A. S. (1987). Reactions to the 1985 Mexican earthquake: case vignettes. *Hospital and Community Psychiatry*, **38**(12), 1327–30.

Gilbert, A. N. & Barkun, M. (1981). Disaster and sexuality. *Journal of Sex Research*, **17**(3), 288–99.

Greenson, R. R. & Mintz, T. (1972). California earthquake 1971: Some psychoanalytic observations. *International Journal of Psychoanalytic Psychotherapy*, **1**(2), 7–23.

Hefez, A., Metz, L. & Lavie, P. (1987). Long-term effects of extreme situational stress on sleep and dreaming. *American Journal of Psychiatry*, **144**(3), 344–7.

Hirose, H. (1986). The pschological impact of the Tokai Earthquake predication: individual's responses and the mass media's coverage. *Japanese Psychological Research*, **28**(2), 64–76.

Hirose, H. & Ishizuka, T. (1983). Causal analysis of earthquake concern and preparing behavior in the North Izu Peninsula. *Japanese Pscyhological Research*, **25**(2), 103–11.

Ishmukhametov, A. I., I'Initskaia, T. I. & Tsepliaeva, G. I. (1989). Functional methods of examination of the victims of the earthquake with crush syndrome in the Armenian USSR. *Soviet Medicine* **10**, 12–14.

Jackson, E. L. & Mukerjee, T. (1974). Human adjustment to the earthquake hazard of San Francisco, California. In G. F. White (ed.) *Natural hazards: local, national, global*. New York: Oxford University Press, pp. 160–6.

Jackson, E. L. (1981). Response to earthquake hazard: the west coast of North America. *Environment and Behavior* **13**(4), 387–416.

Kautz, W.H. (1982, September). Earthquake triggering: a psychic exploration. *PSI Research*, **1**(3), 117–25.

Keys, J. G. (1963). The tsunami of 22 May 1960, in the Samoa and Cook Islands. *Bulletin of the Seismological Society of America*, **53**(6), 1211–27.

Kliukvin, I. & Zolotukhina, I.G. (1989). Formation of functional stumps of the extremities in severe mechanical trauma. *Soviet Medicine*, **10**, 14–17.

Koegler, R. R. & Hicks S. M. (1972). The destruction of a medical center by earthquake. *California Medicine*, **116**(3), 63–7.

Lehman, D. R. & Taylor, S. E. (1987). Date with an earthquake: Coping with a probable, unpredictable disaster. *Personality and Social Psychology Bulletin*, **13**(4), 546–55.

Leivsley, S. (1984). Psychological response to disaster. In J. Seaman, S. Livesley & C. Hogg (eds.) *Epidemiology of Natural Disasters*. New York: Karger, pp. 109–17.

Medici, R. G., Frey, A. H. & Frey, D. (1985). Response facilitation: implications for perceptual theory, psychotherapy, neurophysiology, and earthquake prediction. *International Journal of Neuroscience*, **26**(1–2), 47–52.

Miln, J. (1890). *Impact of earthquakes on man.* Nauka Zhisn, pp. 243–4.

Nichols, T. C. (1974). Global summary of human response to natural hazards: earthquakes. In G. F. White (ed.) *Natural hazards: local, national, global.* New York: Oxford University Press, pp. 274–84.

Norris, F. H. & Murrell, S. A. (1988). Prior experience as a moderator of disaster impact on anxiety symptoms in older adults. *American Journal of Community Psychology*, **16**(5), 665–83.

Palacios, A., Cueli, J., Camacho, J., Clergia, R., Cuevas, P., Ayala, J. & Cossoff, L. (1986). The traumatic effect of mass communication in the Mexico City earthquake: crisis intervention and preventive measures. *International Review of Psychoanalysis*, **13**(3), 279–93.

Popovic, M. & Petrovic, D. (1964). After the earthquake. *Lancet*, 1169–71.

Rennie, D. (1970, January). After the earthquake. *Lancet* 704–7.

Seivers, H. A., Villegas, G. & Barros, G. (1963). The seismic sea wave of 22 May 1960 along the Chilean coast. *Bulletin of the Seismological Society of America*, **53**(6), 1125–90.

Slovic, P., Kunreuther, H. & White, G. F. (1974). Decision process, rationality, and adjustment to natural hazards. In G. F. White (ed.) *Natural hazards: local, national, global.* New York: Oxford University Press, pp. 187–205.

Sood, R., Stockdale, G. & Rogers, E. M. (1987). How the news media operate in national disasters. *Journal of Communication*, **37**(3), 27–41.

Spencer, H. C., Campbell, C. C., Romero, A. et al. (1977, July). Disease-surveillance and decision-making after the 1976 Guatemala earthquake. *Lancet*, 181–4.

Tattersall, J. E., Richards, N. T., McCann, M. et al. (1990). Acute haemodialysis during the Armenian earthquake disaster. *Injury*. **21**(1), 25–33.

Voridis, E. M., Mallios, K. D. & Papantonis, T. M. (1983, June). Holter monitoring during 1981 Athens earthquakes [letter to the editor]. *Lancet*, 1281–2.

Wolfenstein, M. (1957). *Disaster.* New York: Macmillan.

Yuan, S. Y. (1989). Superficial blood flow (SBF) in 193 patients with traumatic paraplegia. *Chung Hua I Hsueh Tsa Chih* **69**(9), 482–5.

7

Psychological effects of toxic contamination

BONNIE L. GREEN, JACOB D. LINDY and MARY C. GRACE

In recent years, increased attention has been directed to the short- and long-term psychological effects of exposure to certain toxins in the environment, such as dioxin and radioactivity. The accident at Three Mile Island, the toxic chemical spills at Love Canal and Times Beach (and the more immediately devastating nuclear meltdown at Chernobyl), reminded all of us that we are at the mercy of technological catastrophes. Silent and invisible pathogens may contaminate our homes and bodies, and risks such as cancer and infertility may not be known for years. Because toxic threat cannot be seen, heard or smelled, it is tempting for authorities to deny or minimize its effects. This new type of 'disaster' is unlike its more acute, traditional predecessors, such as floods, fires, explosions, where the physical effects on property and persons are immediate and obvious. Because of the different nature of this type of threat, it is certainly possible (indeed evidence is accumulating) that the nature of the psychological response is somewhat different from that which follows more traditional events.

The purpose of this chapter is to describe, clinically and empirically, the nature of the symptom picture that emerged following residents' receipt of information about their exposure to radioactive contamination from a nuclear weapons plant in Fernald, Ohio. The data from 50 individuals who were active participants in a class action lawsuit were used for these purposes. Because the subjects were highly selected, they are not seen as necessarily representative of all individuals so exposed, particularly with regard to their extent of psychopathology. Rather, we will focus on the types of symptoms which were relatively prominent, and which of these decreased over time and which remained more chronic.

Characteristics of contamination stressors

Baum and his colleagues have written extensively about 'technological catastrophe' (Baum, Fleming & Davidson, 1983; Davidson, Fleming &

154

Baum, 1986). Based on their work at Three Mile Island, they contrasted such events (generally what others called 'manmade' disasters) with natural disasters along several critical dimensions. Natural disasters remind us that there are certain forces over which we have no control, although some, like hurricanes, may be somewhat predictable. Technological catastrophes, on the other hand, represent a *loss* of control of systems over which we presume to control. Further, disasters such as Three Mile Island have no clear 'low-point', i.e. a point where clearly the 'worst is over'. Exposed residents may expect that the consequences of the event will be development of disease in themselves and their children years after the exposure, providing an ongoing, chronic stressor. Confidence in future controllability of technology is also likely to be eroded (Baum, Fleming & Davidson, 1983).

Bromet (1989) separates chronic technological events like Three Mile Island, Chernobyl and Bhopal from more acute other 'manmade' events like train crashes. Actually, these three events were both acute (onset) and chronic (continued impact). Other nuclear or toxic disasters may unfold more slowly, less dramatically, and residents may not be aware of their exposure until the process has been going on for quite some time. Bertazzi (1989) referred to this latter type of industrial disaster as a 'diluted disaster' which becomes apparent only because human targets happen to be in the way of toxic releases, or because, over time, environmental evidence crops up that something is wrong.

A further characteristic of these slowly unfolding technological disasters is that fears may be elevated by agencies that seem to be unresponsive or concealing facts, so that people come to believe that there is a hidden, but serious, threat (Hallman & Wandersman, 1989). Also, the announcement of the discovery of the contamination is frequently the first awareness residents have that a disaster occurred (Edelstein & Wandersman, 1987).

Bertazzi (1989) suggested that all industrial accidents (including more 'overt' events) have the following characteristics: 1) uncertainty (fear of unknown health damage along with a strong feeling of lack of protection); 2) insecurity about housing and jobs (e.g. fear of contamination of homes); 3) social rejection (discrimination based on perceived contamination); 4) media siege; and 5) cultural pressure (public pressures on how to behave, political issues such as whether exposed women should have abortions, etc).

Psychological responses to contamination stressors

What kind of psychological effects accompany this unique type of stressor? Bromet (1989) described four sets of studies that were conducted by a variety of research groups following the Three Mile Island radiation leak. Homogeneous samples were studied as well as specific groups, such as workers at the plant, mothers of small children, psychiatric patients, and children. The mothers seemed to be the most affected group of all, showing higher levels of depression, anxiety, hostility, and somatization than controls. When the reactor was restarted, this group showed distress scores elevated over all previous levels (Dew et al., 1987). Neither workers nor children showed elevated symptom rates. Bromet (1989) concluded that:

1) contrary to early findings of the President's commission (Bromet, 1989 for a summary), long-term studies have revealed persistent elevations in psychological distress, but 2) the levels are by and large at the high end of the normal range, and functioning ... appears not to have been impaired. ... (p. 130)

Baum and his colleagues (Baum, Gatchel & Schaeffer, 1983; Davidson et al., 1986) followed Three Mile Island residents over time. While their work was summarized by Bromet (1989), it will be discussed separately because it provides specific information regarding symptoms and their course. These studies showed that at about $1\frac{1}{2}$ years postaccident, subjects had elevated scores on the following SCL-90 scales relative to controls: anxiety, alienation, and somatic distress (Baum, Gatchel & Schaeffer, 1983). The highest scores for the Three Mile Island subjects were in the areas of somatization and obsessive–compulsive thoughts (labeled 'concentration' by the study group), which covers repeated unpleasant thoughts that won't leave your mind, trouble concentrating, etc.

By 5 years postevent (Davidson et al., 1986), most of these scores actually increased, with obsessive thoughts remaining high relative to other scales, but with hostility and suspiciousness showing particularly dramatic increases (scores were among the highest). Long-term effects were also evident in a task of concentration (proofreading) and in physiological measures. Also, Three Mile Island residents showed higher levels of norepinephrine and cortisol than controls.

This group also studied residents within a one-mile radius of a toxic waste landfill in a Mid-Atlantic state about a year after the announcement that the site was among 10 of the most potentially hazardous in the country (Davidson et al., 1986). Subjects in this group had depression, anxiety, fear and suspiciousness symptom levels elevated over those of the Three Mile Island residents at 5 years. They also were more distressed than nonexposed controls. Both the TMI and the toxic landfill groups showed elevated scores on the Impact of Event scale, particularly on intrusive symptoms (e.g. 'I thought about it when I didn't mean to'; 'I had dreams about it'). Intrusive symptoms were more prominent than avoidance symptoms (e.g. 'I tried to remove it from memory'; 'I stayed away from reminders of it') in these samples.

A study of residents exposed to dioxin and floods at Times Beach, Missouri, focused primarily on diagnosis (Smith et al., 1986). This study found poorer psychological health in residents exposed directly to the disasters than in indirectly or nonexposed samples. Furthermore, flood and dioxin exposure together caused more problems than either disaster alone. The most common diagnostically related symptoms for the residents directly exposed to dioxin were somatization and depression. With regard to 'new' (since disaster) symptoms, somatization and depression far surpassed other types of symptoms in terms of their frequency.

Coping with radioactive contamination

In terms of individuals' attempts to *cope* with this type of event, Baum, Fleming, and Singer (1983) examined the types of coping styles that were used by residents of Three Mile Island. High use of emotion focused coping was associated with significantly lower levels of stress (distress), while problem focused coping was associated with higher levels of distress. The authors hypothesized that these paradoxical relationships held because there was little that individuals could do to alter the situation. Thus, regulation of one's emotional response might be a realistic way of exerting some control in a basically uncontrollable situation. Further, self-blame was associated with less stress, and it was also associated with the subject's perception of control over things that happened to them.

The Fernald disaster

The revelations about possible contamination following exposure to radioactive leaks into the air and groundwater at the Fernald, Ohio Feed Materials Production Center (FMPC) followed the pattern noted by several investigators cited above. Although some information was released earlier, in October of 1984, the media focused on information that the facility was negligent in the disposal and storage of toxic waste. Many residents learned about the danger from the plant for the first time at this point. During congressional hearings in 1985, the Environmental Protection Agency (EPA) reported that FMPC was the worse emitter of radioactive materials in the nation (Carpenter, 1986). It was later learned that the government intentionally withheld information about contamination for decades. These revelations were shocking to many residents who had lived in the area for years, or had moved there to build their dream homes because they liked the pastoral nature of the area: hills, trees, cows grazing. Most were not even aware that the 'Feed Materials Processing Plant', with the red and white checked towers, processed *nuclear* feed, rather than animal feed, so the information was doubly distressing. Information about the extent of radioactive leakage from this nuclear weapons production facility was released gradually, often preceded by denials, disclaimers or minimizations about the extent of exposure. In 1987, residents and landowners living within a five mile radius of the plant were named as plaintiffs in a class action against the company that managed the plant. The authors served as expert witnesses in the portion of the case that related to claims of 'emotional distress' and examined a small subset of the class. The data reported upon in this chapter were collected in November of 1987.

As we listened to the residents we were evaluating, we were struck by differences between their stressor experiences and those of survivors we had previously studied from a slag dam collapse, a supper club fire and the Vietnam war (see Table 7.1).

Lack of warning

There was no warning of the increased hazard. Indeed, only retrospectively were residents aware of previously released radioactivity, or that their water well contained dangerous radioactive elements. By and large, there was no odor, sight, or sound which could alert them to hazard. Faced with this situation, the residents became sensitized to those warning systems, accurate or inaccurate, upon which they had to rely: increased dust; the sound of a siren, presumably from the plant at Fernald; an unusual metallic odor; increasingly sophisticated monitoring devices.

Diffuseness of impact

The danger of this type of radioactive contamination is chronic and diffuse, that is, it has already been active, continues to be active, and for the foreseeable future continues to present danger. Residents were being exposed long before they were aware of this. The continued storage of radioactive material and likelihood of its seepage into surrounding land and water created a situation where the exposure might well continue into the future.

Table 7.1. *Contamination
stressors at Fernald*

Lack of warning
Diffuseness of impact
Information as stressor
Chronicity of threat
Economic features
Stigma

Information as stressor

Unlike the vivid picture of a tornado, earthquake or flood, a seemingly normal environment served as the backdrop against which the Fernald resident learned of possible disaster. Only a news report or information from a neighbor identified this situation as a disaster, and the resident as one who had been exposed to it. Information, per se, was the initial stressor. Additional information served as secondary stressors. The residents felt that they had to rely on the authoritative sources of information yet at the same time they feared and distrusted them. The resident was understandably concerned, lest the information be inaccurate out of self-interest.

Chronicity of threat

As noted by Baum et al. (1983), nuclear disasters have no 'low point' where the worst is over; future threat is ongoing. Increased exposure to radioactive materials increases the likelihood of the development, many years later, of a variety of illnesses, including cancers and leukemias, decreases the effectiveness of the immunologic system, and increases the likelihood of radioactive exposure to genes, affecting rates of miscarriages, birth anomalies, and fertility. The medical consequences are described as probabilities, not certainties, and society places the burden of uncertainty on the inhabitant.

Lifton (1967) described this uncertainty in the 'hibakusha' (survivors of the A-bomb in Hiroshima) he interviewed many years after their exposure. While the severity of exposure clearly differs between the two incidents, the quality of the feeling is similar: 'survivors feel themselves involved in an endless chain of potentially lethal impairment, which, if it does not manifest itself in one year – or in one generation – may well make itself felt in the next' (p. 130).

Fernald residents had to cope with the ongoing fear of a contaminated habitat. Some residents reported being careful not to use water from the tap for drinking. Some were cautious about the amount of time they spent outside exposed to the air. They worried about dangers to children and grandchildren, and about the longevity of their ancestral line.

Economic features

The loss in market value of the residents' property is an understandable consequence of the above dangers, and becomes a secondary stressor. The inability to receive a fair price for their homes meant, practically speaking, that many residents felt 'trapped' in this potentially contaminated place.

Fears of radioactive contamination of the crops which grew on residents' properties created a secondary level of problems. Danger existed for those who relied on the sale of small crops to supplement their income. The crops identified as coming from the Fernald region might not be bought. At the same time, if the crops were successfully raised and sold, the resident was left with a gnawing sense of guilt at having potentially exposed others.

Stigma

As noted by Bertazzi (1989), contemporary society is frightened of and, to some extent, unkind towards innocent victims of radioactive contamination. Because we fear the unknown, we tend to stigmatize those who have been contaminated. Again, referring to the 'hibakusha' of Hiroshima, Lifton (1967) argued that outsiders, when observing those who were exposed to contamination, saw the survivors as tainted with death. This perception caused them to experience a threat to their own sense of continuity and immortality, and to 'feel death anxiety and death guilt activated within themselves' (p. 170). In defending against this guilt and anxiety, others may turn upon the exposed residents in an attempt to distance themselves from the threat. For example, residents at Fernald reported, with distress, jokes about their 'glowing in the dark'.

In light of the special characteristics of these stressors and on the basis of exploratory interviews with six Fernald residents, review of the depositions of the nine representatives of the class action, and notes on past interviews with residents at TMI (about 12), we hypothesized a spectrum of symptomatology which would be similar to, yet distinguishable from, posttraumatic stress disorder (PTSD) that would manifest itself in the quantitative measures. Like PTSD, the syndrome we would expect following possible radioactive contamination at Fernald would be set in motion by events which are outside of the range of normal, or expectable, human experience. The pathology would likely arise due to failure of successfully processing the intrusive cognitive problems that were presented by the stressor. Unlike PTSD, however, the stressor in this case was ongoing, future oriented, somatically based, and not confined to a single past event that could be processed by the senses.

Based on the characteristics of the stressor and research by other investigators, we expected several types of responses including obsessive/intrusive thinking related to worries about future illnesses along with attempts to avoid such thoughts. Because of the type of perceived risk, we expected somatic concerns to be high relative to other symptoms, although general anxiety symptoms were expected to be prominent as well. Finally, the way in which residents were informed about the leaks (i.e. the attempts to hide exposure, etc.) was expected to produce symptoms of suspiciousness/mistrust. We were interested in whether a unique cluster of symptoms defining a specific syndrome would emerge from the clinical observations and the research instruments.

Method

Participants

The 57 plaintiffs who had previously filled out questionnaires and interrogatories were identified by their lawyers as the respondent pool for first wave of interviewing. Not all of these 57 people were seeking restitution for *emotional* distress. Their names, addresses, and phone numbers were provided to the Traumatic Stress Study Center (TSSC) at the University of Cincinnati for the purpose of scheduling interviews. Preceding phone calls by interviewers was a letter that was sent by the law firm to each of the 57 plaintiffs informing them of the involvement of the TSSC and explaining the interview that was being requested. Residents were encouraged, but not required, to participate. Each of the six interviewers were given the names of six to eight residents to interview. Interviews were usually conducted in the resident's home and averaged approximately $1\frac{1}{2}$ hours in length.

Interviewers

Four advanced clinical psychology students, the research coordinator for the Traumatic Stress Study Center and an experienced survey research interviewer served as interviewers for this project; four were female, two were male. All but one had worked on previous research studies at the TSSC doing field interviews of a similar sort to the one employed in this investigation. Extensive training in the administration of the interview protocol was completed before the interviewers entered the field. This included: reading the training materials for the use of the Psychiatric Evaluation Form (PEF) (see below); attending two 3-hour meetings to discuss these materials and to practise using the rating scales; rating and discussing two audio training tapes. The training also addressed the administration of the remaining interview materials. Since the PEF requires some judgment on the part of the trained raters, a small reliability study was conducted to assure that raters were using the scales the same way. Six of the residents were seen by two interviewers. One interviewer conducted the interview, making ratings as he/she went along, while the other observed and rated. Considering all 19 scales and the overall severity for the six subjects for two time periods (i.e. 240 pairs of ratings), there were only six pairs of ratings (2.5%) where there was disagreement by more than one point. In 20% of the cases there was a disagreement of one scale point, while in 77.5% of the cases there was perfect agreement. Disagreements did not occur appreciably more often in particular scales, or time periods, or with particular raters. Disagreements were discussed following these preliminary interviews with an attempt to clarify the ratings.

Instruments

Psychiatric evaluation form (PEF)

This rating scale is based on both the observed and reported information obtained during a structured clinical interview (Endicott & Spitzer, 1972). Nineteen dimensions of psychological functioning and a measure of global *Overall Severity* are rated by the interviewer along a six-point scale. The scale ranges from 'no pathology' (1) to 'extreme impairment' (6). Two sets of ratings were obtained: one for the period of one month preceding the interview, and one for the 'worst time' for the resident during the period following their knowledge of events related to the plant. The 'worst time' was determined by the resident and was based on his/her memory of when their distress about the plant was the highest. Because all residents did not receive the same information at the same time, particularly about their own exposure or property values, the actual time frame for 'worst time' varied by subject and covered the entire period from 1952, when one resident was forced to move from his original residence and lost a relative to cancer, to the time the data were collected.

Impact of event scale (IES)

This self-report questionnaire (developed from Horowitz' model of stress response syndromes) consists of 15 statements which the subject is asked to rate in terms of response to a specific stressful life event along a four-point continuum (0, 1, 3, 5) (Horowitz, Wilner & Alvarez, 1979; Zilberg, Weiss & Horowitz, 1982). The statements are scored as pertaining to intrusion and avoidance subscales. The IES is used frequently in trauma research and has demonstrated extensive reliability and validity.

Symptom checklist-90 R (SCL-90 R)

This self-report instrument consists of 90 symptoms which the subject rates as having bothered him or her during the past week on a five-point scale ranging from 'not at all' to 'a great deal' (Derogatis, 1983). It may be reduced to nine subscale scores including anxiety, depression and hostility, and items may be averaged into a Global Severity Index.

Coping strategies inventory (CSI)

The coping strategies inventory (Short Form) is a 40-item self-report questionnaire designed to assess coping thoughts and behaviors in response to a specific stressor, in this case, reminders of the Fernald plant. The CSI contains eight primary scales. These can be combined hierarchically into four secondary scales, and two tertiary scales. (Tobin et al., 1989). Construction of the subscales for the longer form was based on a review of the coping assessment literature. Factor analysis confirmed the structure. The primary subscales consist of specific coping strategies people use in response to stressful events: problem-solving, cognitive-restructuring, social support, express emotion, problem avoidance, wishful thinking, social withdrawal and self criticism.

Stressors

The information about the subjects' stressor experiences was collected via a structured interview format: how the resident first learned about the problems at the Fernald plant; what other information they received, particularly with regard to their own property or selves; changes noted in plants and animals; changes in habits or activities relative to the information; medical problems of self and family that might be attributable to the plant; and content of worries, ruminations and dreams.

Demographic information was also collected.

Results

Demographic description

Fifty residents of Fernald were interviewed for purposes of this report. There were 57 potential interviewees, however, one resident died. Fifty-one of the remaining interviews were completed (a 91% completion rate), however, one person did not fill out the self-report instruments completely enough to be included.

Of the 50 cases, the average age of subjects was 46.78 (range 29–69). Men represented 58% of the sample; while women represented 42%. Ninety percent of the residents were married; they had an average of 2.5 children. With regard to education, 74% completed high school. All but five residents owned their own homes and lived in them for an average of 9.8 years. Occupationally, the majority of subjects, if they worked, were either blue collar workers or in business, and most were working full time. The average family income was $39 000.

Specific stressors

The subjects lived an average of 1.6 miles from the plant, and approximately two-thirds of the sample lived within a one mile radius. Slightly over a quarter of the sample reported some illness. About half reported the illness of an acquaintance or family member that they thought could be related to the contamination. No one thought that they had cancer caused by the plant, but 35% thought that other friends, relatives and acquaintances had contamination related cancer.

Content of worries and dreams

In order to assess the content of mental phenomena, we asked the residents during their interview to address their specific concerns, i.e. what did they worry, ruminate, or dream about that was related to the plant. Of the 40 subjects with completed data on these items, most subjects (95%) named a worry of some type. The most common of these (overlapping) concerns were fear of illness in self (45%) or family (48%), and fears about contamination (43%). Many residents also worried about housing or property devaluation (30%). Less often, residents mentioned distrust of authorities and concerns regarding fertility, ineffective warning systems, and safety of their children.

Regarding dreams, 43% of the sample reported a frightening dream of some sort. These dreams usually involved being endangered in some way and/or being chased, trapped or a family member in danger. Examples include: 'alarm at the plant going off', 'dream about dying', 'the plant blowing up', 'locked in a vault with rising water', 'tragedy in the family', 'wife dying', and 'baby dying'.

Symptom profiles

Fig. 7.1 shows the 'worst time' and 'current' profiles on the Psychiatric Evaluation Form for the fifty residents. Shown for comparison purposes is the group profile for nonexposed residents of the Big Coal River Valley in West Virginia, originally used as a comparison sample for a follow-up study of survivors of the Buffalo Creek dam collapse (Green et al., 1990). This comparison sample consisted of 50 people (48% men) whose average age was 55.6 years, slightly older than the Fernald subjects. All subjects were white; 77% were married; and 64% completed high school. Average family income was $25 500. A second comparison is of ratings from a sample of 325 outpatients that were collected by the authors of the PEF (Endicott & Spitzer, 1972).

For Fig. 7.1 the main points to note are the high points in the Fernald profiles at the two points in time. For 'worst time', elevations were noted in anxiety symptoms, depression, belligerence and daily routine. Highest rated symptoms at the time of the assessment were anxiety, depression, somatic concerns and belligerence. With regard to *changes* over time, significant decreases were found for ratings of anxiety, depression, daily routine impairment, belligerence and agitation. However, elevations *remained* (i.e. changes were *not* significant) for somatic concerns, social isolation and suspiciousness. Alcohol abuse was not elevated to begin with. Levels of ratings for this selected group were somewhat lower than outpatients, but clearly higher than nonexposed, nonpatients. Anxiety and depression ratings were highest for all groups.

Fig. 7.2 shows the subjects' current self-report symptoms on Derogatis' SCL-90 subscales. Derogatis' standardization samples (1983) of outpatients

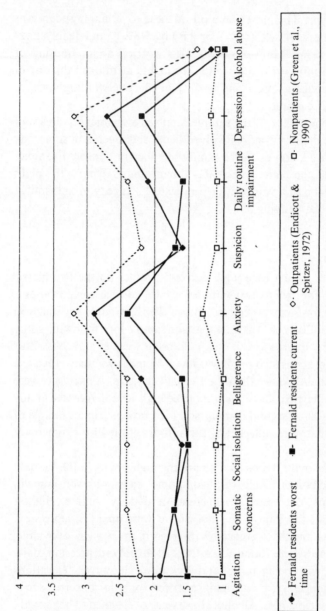

Fig. 7.1. Average clinical ratings on selected scales of the PEF for Fernald residents and comparison samples.

•- Fernald residents worst
   time

■- Fernald residents current

◇· Outpatients (Endicott &
   Spitzer, 1972)

□· Nonpatients (Green et al.,
   1990)

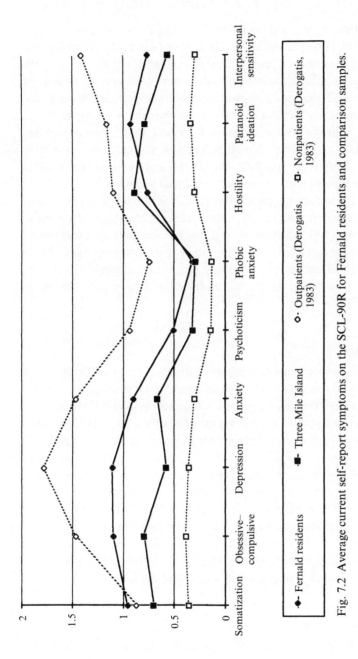

Fig. 7.2 Average current self-report symptoms on the SCL-90R for Fernald residents and comparison samples.

and nonpatient scores are included for comparison purposes, as are Davidson et al. (1986) scores for 53 Three Mile Island subjects which were collected approximately 5 years after the accident there. The two populations exposed to radioactive contamination were quite similar, despite the time difference (3 years vs. 5 years after information about exposure) and other differences (e.g. acuteness of onset) between the two situations. The subjects in both samples were generally worse than normals but less impaired than outpatients. Symptom levels of somatization, obsessive–compulsive symptoms, hostility, paranoid ideation and interpersonal sensitivity (e.g. feeling others cannot be trusted) were elevated.

The pattern of findings on the impact of event scale was particularly interesting. Avoidance scores ($M = 2.0$) were somewhat higher than Intrusion scores ($M = 1.8$), which is a reversal of the usual pattern found among other samples of bereaved or traumatized people (Horowitz, 1986). Mean scores for intrusion were in the same range as a sample of bereaved nonpatients (Horowitz, 1986), but lower than means of a sample of bereaved patients.

Coping strategies

Coping strategies also showed some interesting patterns (see Table 7.2). In general, Fernald residents tended to use *fewer* coping strategies than either patients who were recently diagnosed with cancer or college students who were told to think about a recent stressor. However, they were higher than both groups on 'problem avoidance', which was consistent with their IES scores. They were also similar to patients who were recently told they had a diagnosis of cancer on 'wishful thinking' and 'social withdrawal'. The hierarchical structure of the *Coping strategies inventory* includes four engagement and four disengagement strategies. Each of these general types include both problem focused and emotion focused strategies. Relative to either of the comparison groups, the Fernald residents were relatively low on engagement strategies despite the fact that they were 'active' plaintiffs in the law suit. Overall, disengagement levels were similar.

Prediction of outcome

The range of responses was really too narrow to be able to assess the relationships of these various stressors to outcome. However, there were some trends worth noting. Distance had a low, negative relationship with outcome: those residents who lived closer to the plant tended to have more symptoms. People who lived in their houses *longer* tended to have fewer

Table 7.2. *Coping strategies employed by Fernald residents*

	Fernald residents	Cancer patients	College students
Engagement strategies			
Problem solving	1.9	2.5	2.6
Cognitive restructuring	1.3	2.5	2.1
Express emotions	1.7	2.4	2.5
Social supports	1.7	3.1	2.6
Average engagement	1.7	2.6	2.5
Disengagement strategies			
Problem avoidance	1.1	0.7	0.8
Wishful thinking	2.5	2.5	1.8
Self-criticism	0.2	0.4	1.0
Social withdrawal	1.0	1.1	0.9
Average disengagement	1.2	1.2	1.2

symptoms. Having an illness was the strongest predictor of poor outcome, showing significant correlations with SCLGSI, IES Intrusion, and PEF Overall Severity. Knowledge of the illnesses of others did not predict outcome. However, those who believed more of their neighbors had contamination related illnesses were more symptomatic overall and had more intrusive imagery. Thinking that others had contamination related cancer did not predict outcome except, again, identification of neighbors in this way predicted 'worst time' PEF Overall Severity.

Coping strategies were also related to outcome. The use of disengagement strategies was associated significantly and substantially with all three of the self-report measures of distress. Also, people who used engagement coping strategies had more intrusive thoughts.

Case reports

The following are two case vignettes. They are residents who were seen by one of us (JDL) during the course of evaluating the plaintiffs for the lawsuit. The presentations and concerns are characteristic of the individuals we interviewed.

Mrs K.

Mrs K. was a 35 year-old, married mother of two daughters, ages 9 and 6. She and her husband, both college educated, built their dream house in rural Ohio, within commuting distance of Mr K.'s executive position in a Cincinnati firm. Mrs K. told a friend they were moving to a location that was not far from the 'Ralston grain plant', referring to the checkered tower of the 'feed' processing plant. Three years prior to being seen, she and her husband had learned through the news media that the plant at Fernald processed radioactive material, not grain; that venting of radioactive materials was occurring; and that radioactive waste which had been generated as far back as the Manhattan project in the 1940s, was inadequately stored and seeping into the community water system.

Mrs K. became an active citizen participant with other neighbors in speaking with, and engaging, scientific experts on the extent of the danger. She and her immediate family underwent total body radiation counts. She unsuccessfully sought adequate monitors. The couple invested in an extensive purifying system. They explored selling their house, but learned they would have to inform the buyer of the risks from Fernald. Selling the house under these circumstances would have been a catastrophic financial loss.

During this period she became anxious, irritable, and preoccupied with fears of the possibility of her children developing leukemia. To a lesser extent, she also worried about her husband and herself. Each ache, pain, fever, stirred intense worry which she told herself was irrational, but which she could not contain. Sleep was restless and dreams were ominous but indistinct. She began to repeat tasks, double check the stove, and overprotect her children. Hearing from the school nurse that her child was ill set off a panic attack, and she had an auto accident on the way to pick her up. The 6 year-old daughter began sleeping in the parent's bed after her unsettling experience in the body radiation chamber. Although test results were not abnormal, anxiety worsened after the testing procedure. Abruptly, Mr K. ordered Mrs K. and the rest of the family *not* to seek further information about the plant, because each time they learned something new, everyone got worse. They were not to speak of the Fernald danger any more in the home. She noticed after this that tension grew between the two of them. Further, taking the worries of Fernald on by himself, her husband performed worse at work and for the first time was passed over for a promotion. Mrs K. was now giving up the idea of having more children because of the risk of genetic danger to an unborn child. She felt desperately trapped in the four walls of her dreamhouse; dreading the present and fearful of the future.

Mr J.

Mr J. was a 65 year-old retired assistant manager at the local dry goods store. Mr and Mrs J. lived on 3 acres near Fernald as had their families for generations. Only their children had moved to the city. Mr J. had developed congestive heart failure about 8 years earlier. Along with bronchitis, high blood pressure and rare episodes of alcohol abuse, he was not a picture of perfect health. But, while these ailments made life annoying, he did enjoy his large vegetable garden which supplemented his income, the company of his wife and visits from their grandchildren.

Mr J. grasped only the rudiments of the scientists' explanations regarding radioactive contamination from Fernald. He learned of it directly from the neighbor whose water well was contaminated. He thought this must explain those albino animals, and the poor crops. He remembered when the Fernald plant opened, and never gave a second thought to its safety.

He cried easily as he explained this breach in trust with the Government. While not serving in combat, Mr J. was a veteran and deeply patriotic in his views. His wife articulated even better how betrayed he felt. Joy seemed gone from Mr J.'s life. He no longer knew where he would sell his crops; and worried that the persons who bought them might be contaminated. Neither he nor his wife thought that the grandchildren should visit, fearing contamination, and indeed they had stopped coming. Unbidden thoughts, restless sleep, depression, and alienation characterized his psychic life. Each spot on the skin got inspected nightly for cancerous growth. Each morning as water from the shower struck his skin, he thought about radioactive particles. Each time he drank a glass of water the same thoughts intruded. Mr J. could not remove obsessive thinking of the effects of Fernald from his mind.

Discussion

Being informed that one lives in an area contaminated by radiation is a unique type of stressor experience. Radiation cannot be seen, felt, tasted, or smelled. There is no agreement among experts about what the effects of such exposure are, and authorities often have their own interests in mind when providing information about such effects. By the time one finds out about the exposure, it has already taken place (although it may continue), and it is never quite clear whether or not one was harmed. Fears arising from such exposure may be labeled unreasonable (blaming the person exposed), while at the same time the person may be stigmatized by acquaintances.

From a psychological perspective, any one of these elements is likely to lead to uneasiness or preoccupation at best, because of the vagueness, all pervasiveness, and chronicity of the threat. Erikson (1990) captured the essence of the potential response to this intangible stressor when he distinguished the 'dread' associated with toxic contamination from the fear of natural disasters. The comments of residents he interviewed, living near a toxic dump, were remarkably similar to those at Fernald.

Research designed to assess the psychological effects of contamination is increasing. With few exceptions, however, it has tended to focus on the extent of impairment rather than the particular constellation of symptoms that make up the psychological reaction to this type of event. However, there are data available, particularly from Baum and colleagues' (Baum, Fleming & Davidson, 1983; Baum, Fleming & Singer, 1983; Baum, Gatchel & Schaeffer, 1983) work on Three Mile Island, that addresses this question. In general, the findings from the present report coincide well with findings from TMI even though the two events were dissimilar in several ways, including the acuteness of the onset and the length of exposure.

Limitations of study

As noted earlier, the conclusions that can be drawn from our empirical findings are limited in several ways. First, the subjects participated as part of the process of a lawsuit and there is no reason to believe that the individuals who agreed to make themselves available from the designated class for the study were necessarily typical of class members in general. Secondly, we did not have a control group for this particular study. Thus, the findings presented do not attempt to draw conclusions about the extent of impairment. Rather, we have focused on the constellation of symptoms and the interaction of symptoms and stressors in the particular individuals we did see to suggest hypotheses about the nature of the impact of this particular type of event. Further, subjects provided retrospective data on their psychological condition which is another reason that it needs to be viewed with caution. For all of these reasons, findings which coincided with other studies were given most credence and all of the findings are clearly tentative until replicated on more extensive and general samples. We wish mainly to stimulate thinking about the nature of the reactions to this chronic and vague stressor.

Symptom constellation and duration

Generally speaking, the overall profile of the Fernald group, and the TMI group as well, were not unlike profiles of outpatients (although not as elevated), with relatively (compared to other types of symptoms) high levels of the general symptoms of anxiety, depression and impairment of daily routine. However, individuals with radioactive exposure are also high (relative to their own scores on other measures, and to 'normals') on somatic symptoms and concerns, obsessive thoughts, and suspicion and mistrust of others. It is this latter group of symptoms that may distinguish the reaction to toxic exposure, particularly 'human caused' exposure. As noted earlier, subjects worry about what physical harm may have been done to them, that they can't seem to get thoughts and worries about the exposure out of their minds, are not trusting of others (neighbors/ authorities) and feel alienated from the rest of the world. These symptoms make sense given the diffuse and vague nature of the stressor and the chronic, unknown and future threat.

Further, there is evidence from TMI and our Fernald subjects that these latter symptoms are ongoing over relatively long periods of time. Davidson et al. (1986) showed continued high levels of obsessive thoughts in their TMI subjects between $1\frac{1}{2}$ years and 5 years, with hostility (including feelings of fear of losing control) and suspiciousness becoming especially pronounced. In the Fernald sample, anxiety, depression and impairment of their daily routine improved (decreased) for most subjects between their 'worst' time (in terms of knowledge/revelations about the plant and their symptoms) and the time they were evaluated for the present study. However, similar to the Three Mile Island findings, there were no changes in the areas of somatic concerns, social isolation and suspicion. These areas remained elevated. While neither study was a rigorous longitudinal one, the findings are strikingly similar and clearly suggest that at least some individuals exposed to nuclear radiation continue to be obsessively worried about their health and the future, and are suspicious and untrusting of others. Davidson et al. (1986) noted continued effects on physiology and cognitive capabilities over this period as well.

Fenald residents' attempts to cope with this particular threat were primarily trying to avoid it and to wish it away. Avoidance of thoughts of the events surrounding the plant were particularly high, as expressed on both the Impact of event scale and the coping inventory. This coping activity fit well, both as a response to the high level of intrusion/obsessive thoughts and in terms of the actual situation. No active coping strategy can undo the threat, therefore, not thinking about it may make the most sense. Residents also used other disengagement strategies; social withdrawal (also noted in the other measures) and wishful thinking (e.g. 'I hoped a miracle would happen,' 'I wished that the situation would go away or somehow be over with'). These coping strategies aren't usually associated with healthy functioning.

Syndrome proposed

From a clinical perspective, we would like to propose a name for the syndrome just described, and to note briefly its similarities and differences from other diagnoses, along with its hypothesized dynamics and associated features. This proposal represents an hypothesis based on our beginning clinical work in this selected population, and on our own and others research findings to date. More research is clearly needed to document the existence of this syndrome.

The Informed of Radioactive Contamination Syndrome (IRCS) is both similar to, and distinguishable from, posttraumatic stress disorder and adjustment disorder of adulthood. Like PTSD, the syndrome is set in motion by events which are outside the range of normal, expectable human experience. Like PTSD, pathology arises in the failure to be able to process successfully the intrusive cognitive problems which the stressor presents and which would be stressful to most persons. But unlike PTSD, the stressor is ongoing and future oriented. It is not confined to a single happening which can be processed by the senses and, therefore, the pathology is less likely to include nightmares and reenactments.

Like adjustment reactions of adulthood, which may follow common stressful life experiences like divorce, job loss, etc. IRCS may occur to anyone, regardless of predisposition, and often contains features of depression and anxiety. But, unlike the adjustment reaction, this syndrome is not necessarily self limited; it is not healed by a shift in philosophical perspective. It mimics, in ways that adjustment reactions do not, the features of an obsessive–compulsive disorder.

For persons informed that radioactive contamination of their living space is present, a set of unsatisfactory cycles of mental activity begin to occur. The resident at one phase struggles with the temptation to worry. His first line of defense is to cut the worry off before it begins. He seeks to sequester the problems so that they will not interfere with daily function. For those who live in the backyard of a nuclear waste dump, however, denial has already been pierced by actual findings of increased thorium, uranium, etc. and such denial can no longer be totally effective. Efforts expended in turning away decrease the energy available for pleasurable activity, and are accompanied by a low grade agitation and depression. The presence of any new symptom, any unusual odor or metallic taste, a piece of information from a community meeting or newspaper, all act to catalyze worry.

In another phase of the syndrome, an action oriented phase, residents acknowledge the hazards and decide that they *must* cope. They inform themselves of the nature of the plant, the nature of the contamination so far reported, and the consequences. They attempt to clear their homes of radon, inform themselves about monitors. But how can they truly clear their habitat from contamination? And where can they go to feel safe? The normally successful coping method of confronting difficulties actually increases intrusive symptoms, and as these coping strategies become less effective, residents may become more anxious, depressed, and hopeless. Residents may also become angry and frustrated, particularly with public officials and spokespersons for the site of the contamination. They may become alienated from their neighbors who are attempting to deny or minimize the problems.

Implications for intervention

Treatment implications for residents near contaminated nuclear facilities who show the spectrum of symptoms outlined above are not yet clear. Psychotherapy can neither remove the source of contamination nor the potential effect of contamination already experienced. Residents' primary concern is to find a safe place for their families. As in other ongoing traumatic situations, like spouse abuse, or rape threat when the offender is at large, the first task is to remove or contain the noxious agent. Thus, it may be that social and legal action, and economic activity which permits relocation to a safe environment may be the most reasonable first efforts to prevent further damage. A supportive treatment relationship by mental health professionals may reduce unnecessary distress. Clinicians need to learn more about this syndrome as, sadly, our technological society will likely have much more of it in coming years.

References

Baum, A., Fleming, R. & Davidson, L. M. (1983). Natural disaster and technological catastrophe. *Environment and Behavior*, **15**, 333–54.
Baum, A., Fleming, R. & Singer, J. E. (1983). Coping with victimization by technological disaster. *Journal of Social Issues*, **39**, 117–38.
Baum, A., Gatchel, R. & Schaeffer, M. A. (1983). Emotional, behavioral, and physiological effects of chronic stress at Three Mile Island. *Journal of Consulting and Clinical Psychology*, **15**, 565–72.
Bertazzi, P. (1989). Industrial disasters and epidemiology. *Scandinavian Journal of Work Environmental Health*, **15**, 85–100.
Bromet, E. (1989). The nature and effects of technological failures. In R. Gist & B. Lubin (eds.) *Psychosocial aspects of disaster*. New York: Wiley Press.

Carpenter, T. (1986). *Fernald fact sheet summary.* Government Accountability
    Project: Washington, DC. (Available from Cincinnati Nuclear Weapons
    Freeze Campaign, Cincinnati, OH).
Davidson, L., Fleming, I. & Baum, A. (1986). Post-traumatic stress as a function
    of chronic stress and toxic exposure. In C. Figley (ed.) *Trauma and its wake.*
    vol. II, New York: Brunner/Mazel.
Derogatis, L. R. (1983). *SCL-90 R version: Manual I.* Baltimore, MD: Johns
    Hopkins University.
Dew, M. A., Bromet, E., Schulberg, H. C., Dunn, L. & Parkinson, D. (1987).
    Mental health effects of the Three Mile Island nuclear reactor restart.
    American Journal of Psychiatry, **144,** 1074–7.
Edelstein, M. R. & Wandersman, A. (1987). Community dynamics in coping
    with toxic contaminants. In I. Altman & A. Wandersman (eds.)
    Neighborhood and community environments. New York: Plenum.
Endicott, J. & Spitzer, R. (1972). What! Another rating scale? The Psychiatric
    Evaluation Form. *Journal of Nervous and Mental Disease,* **154,** 88–104.
Erikson, K. (1990). Toxic reckoning: business faces a new kind of fear. *Harvard
    Business Review, January–February,* 118–26.
Green, B. L., Grace, M. C., Lindy , J. D., Gleser, G. C., Leonard, A. C. &
    Kramer, T. L. (1990). Buffalo Creek survivors in the second decade:
    comparison with unexposed and non-litigant groups. *Journal of Applied
    Social Psychology,* **20,** 1033–50.
Hallman, W. & Wandersman, A. (1989). Perception of risk and toxic hazard. In
    D. Peck (ed.) *Psychosocial effects of hazardous waste disposal on community.*
    Springfield, IL: Charles C. Thomas.
Horowitz, M. J. (1986). *Stress response syndromes.* 2nd edn, New York:
    Aronson.
Horowitz, M., Wilner, N. & Alvarez, W. (1979). Impact of event scale: a measure
    of subjective stress. *Psychosomatic Medicine,* **41,** 209–18.
Lifton, R. J. (1967). *Death in life: survivors of Hiroshima.* New York: Random
    House.
Smith, E., Robins, L., Przybeck, T., Goldring, E. & Solomon, S. (1986)
    Psychosocial consequences of disaster. In J. Shore (ed.), *Disaster stress
    studies: new methods and findings.* Washington, DC: American Psychiatric
    Press, pp. 49–76.
Tobin, D. L., Holroyd, K. A., Reynolds, R. V. & Wigal, J. K. (1989). The
    hierarchial factor structure of the Coping Strategies Inventory. *Cognitive
    Therapy and Research,* **13,** 343–61.
Zilberg, N. J., Weiss, D. S. & Horowitz, M. J. (1982). Impact of event scale: a
    cross-validation study and some empirical evidence supporting a conceptual
    model of stress response syndromes. *Journal of Consulting and Clinical
    Psychology,* **50,** 407–14.

Part III

The role of psychosocial context in responses to trauma and disasters

8

Social support and perceived control as moderators of responses to dioxin and flood exposure

SUSAN D. SOLOMON and ELIZABETH M. SMITH

This chapter discusses the impact of exposure to flooding and/or dioxin contamination on rural St. Louis residents experiencing these events in late 1982. Our study was designed to describe the type and extent of psychiatric disturbance that followed these events, and to see if victims' reactions varied for the different types of disasters. We were also interested in learning how social support and family role affected victims' reactions and which victims were most likely to experience psychological problems following exposure. Finally, we wanted to help answer the question of why some people react more negatively to both disaster exposure and the lack of social support than others do. Toward this end, we explored perceived control as a possible explanation of victims' responses to disaster.

Natural and humanmade disasters

While precise estimates are not available, it is clear that an enormous number of people in the United States are exposed to both natural and human-made hazards every year. For example, with regard to natural disasters, in its 1986 reporting year, the American Red Cross responded to 43 658 disaster incidents. In that same year, the Federal Emergency Management Agency (FEMA) responded to 30 presidentially declared disasters and obligated $648 011 810 in funds for disaster relief; the National Institute of Mental Health (NIMH) also responded to nine of these disasters and distributed $1 885 654 of FEMA funds for mental health services to victims. Based on a random national survey of telephone owning households in which people were questioned concerning their disaster experience during the 10-year period 1970–1980, an estimate was made that almost 2 million households per year (24.5 per 1000) experience injuries and/or damages from either household fires or one of the four most common natural hazards (floods, hurricanes and severe tropical storms, tornadoes and severe windstorms, earthquakes and severe tremors) (Rossi et al., 1883).

Further, human-made disasters such as chemical pollution, transportation accidents, explosions, structural failures, terrorism, and the like, pose an ever increasing threat to physical and mental health. Although the extent of exposure to technological disaster is difficult to estimate, a 1980 Senate Subcommittee concerned with only one such hazard (chemical dumps) noted that as many as 30000 sites may be capable of causing significant health problems due to their proximity to public ground water supplies for drinking (Cohn, 1980). The work of Baum and his colleagues (Baum, Fleming & Davidson, 1983) suggests that disasters of human origin may be particularly damaging to the mental health of victims.

The St. Louis disasters

The human made disaster to which the present study sample was exposed is called dioxin. The dioxin in Missouri has been traced back to a plant in Verona, Missouri, which was leased to Northeastern Pharmaceutical and Chemical Company (NEPACCO) in November, 1969, for the production of hexachlorophene, a disinfectant. Hexachlorophene is produced by heating and distilling 2,4,5-T. The desired product, hexachlorophene, rises to the top, leaving a thick, tarry waste sludge called still bottoms. Found in the still bottoms is 2,3,7,8 tetra-chloro-dibenzo-p-dioxin (2,3,7,8-TCDD) (more commonly referred to as dioxin). This is one of a group of 75 poly chloro-dibenzo-p-dioxins, and is considered to be the most toxic. NEPACCO contracted with Independent Petrochemical Company of St. Louis to haul the waste. Independent Petrochemical, in turn, subcontracted with the Bliss Waste Oil Company to dispose of the waste. Every confirmed dioxin site in eastern Missouri has been traced to NEPACCO and the operations of the Bliss Waste Oil Company.

It is believed that, between February 1, 1971, and October 15, 1971 Bliss removed six loads of approximately 3000 gallons apiece of still bottom waste from NEPACCO. Another 4300 gallons of still bottom waste remained at the Verona Plant in a storage tank. When waste from this tank was tested in September, 1974, it contained 343 parts per million (ppm) of dioxin, an extremely high level of contamination. The National Centers for Disease Control (CDC) now estimates that exposure to concentrations of over one part per billion (ppb) may cause adverse health reactions. It can be inferred that the waste Bliss hauled was contaminated in equally high concentrations.

Most of the still bottom waste Bliss hauled was mixed with waste motor oil and stored in tanks. Some of the stored oil was then sold to refineries as salvaged oil. This oil was also used as 'dust suppressant', and sprayed on roads and horse arenas in eastern Missouri. From 1971 through 1975 the CDC, the Missouri Division of Health (DOH), and the Missouri Department of Natural Resources investigated the dioxin problem. At no time during this period were the owners of contaminated areas advised what to do, nor was Bliss advised to cease his dust control operation. Thus while CDC and DOH investigations continued, Bliss continued to spray the waste oil on roads and parking lots throughout Eastern Missouri through 1976. After test results showed dioxin contamination in July 1974, the CDC and DOH began new investigations. Both the DOH and the CDC concluded their investigations in early 1975. In March 1975, CDC recommended that soil around the residential areas in Jefferson County be removed. However, no action was taken on this recommendation until 1982, when further tests were conducted (Smith, 1984).

During the winter of 1982, many rural residents of the St. Louis area experienced a series of traumatic events. These began on December 1, 1982, with the onset of torrential rain, accompanied by violent wind, numerous tornadoes, and intermittent hail. The resulting flood, considered one of the worst in Missouri history, was responsible for five deaths and forced approximately 25 000 people to be evacuated, thousands of whom remained homeless when their houses were destroyed. Although this area had been flooded in the past, this flood was unique both in terms of the extent of its devastation, and its untimely occurrence, coming at a season of year when none of the usual community flood preparations was in place.

One of these flood devastated communities, the town of Times Beach in Jefferson County, experienced additional difficulties. Because of a suspicion that dioxin contamination might be present on the streets of Times Beach, the Environmental Protection Agency (EPA) began tests of that site. Right before Christmas the EPA announced that dioxin levels in Times Beach were 300 times higher than the level identified by the CDC as a potential health risk (one part per billion). Residents were told to abandon flood clean-up attempts and relocate elsewhere. After a protracted period, the federal government bought out the town, forcing residents to scatter widely to various unwelcoming communities.

Although Times Beach was the only community offered a federal buyout, it was not the only Missouri site found to have an unsafe level of dioxin. As of April 1983, the Environmental Defense Fund confirmed 29 dioxin-contaminated sites, the majority in the St. Louis area. The residents of these other contaminated sites were confronted with conflicting reports, from the

EPA and other sources, about the extent of danger dioxin posed to human health. The follow-up survey for this study took place at a time of great uncertainty for the dioxin victims: uncertainty about what government clean-up efforts, if any, would be undertaken; uncertainty about whether it was wiser for residents to remain in their communities, or to sell their homes at a substantial loss and move; and uncertainty about what long-term health problems might result from dioxin exposure the victims had already experienced.

Methods

Sample

By chance, these disasters took place just as Washington University was completing its second wave of interviews in a major epidemiological program designed to assess the psychiatric status of the region (for a description of the entire NIMH Epidemiological Catchment Area (ECA) program, see Eaton & Kessler, 1985). The present investigation took advantage of this coincidence by recontacting 452 ECA respondents, comprised of both individuals in disaster-affected rural areas, and a randomly selected control group of one half of the ECA respondents presumed to be outside the area of impact. Data for the disaster follow-up were collected over an eight month period, beginning approximately 11 months after disaster onset. Because few ECA respondents had been exposed to dioxin, the study targeted an additional sample of 100 individuals residing within one mile of confirmed dioxin sites, including 80 adults from the 800 households formerly comprising Times Beach. In addition, a control group was included, consisting of 100 randomly selected adults from an area flood plain, matched on socioeconomic status to the ECA sample. Like the dioxin sample, this control group had not been previously interviewed for the ECA program. A total of 543 interviews (84% of those targeted) were successfully completed. To our knowledge, our study sample is the first one constituted so as to permit systematic comparisons of the effects of natural and technological disaster, in that it contains victims exposed to either or both of these kinds of events.

All of the respondents in the study were over 19 years old, and most were white. Two-thirds were married and had at least a high school education. Median income for this sample was between $20 000 and $30 000, and 55% of the sample was female. Those exposed to the dioxin tended to be younger that the other respondents. Both flood and disaster victims tended to have

Table 8.1. *Sample demographics by disaster exposure*

	Exposure to disaster			
	Unexposed ($n=325$)	Flood ($n=75$)	Dioxin ($n=28$)	Flood + dioxin ($n=66$)
% Male	43	57	52	39
% Separated/divorced	9	13	10	28[a]
Mean years' education	12.0	10.7[a]	11.6	10.9[a]
Mean age	46	45	36[a]	42

Note:
[a] Significantly different from unexposed.

less education, lower incomes, and higher rates of divorce or separation than the study respondents who did not experience disaster (see Table 8.1). These differences suggested that victims may have been at higher risk for psychological problems than nonvictims, even before they were exposed to dioxin and/or the flood (Smith et al., 1986). Knowing this, we took the precaution of controlling for predisaster psychiatric symptoms in our analyses of this data.

Instrument

The study employed a structured interview, the Diagnostic Interview Schedule/Disaster Supplement (DIS/DS) (Robins & Smith, 1983). The core of the instrument is the Diagnostic Interview Schedule (DIS) (see Robins et al., 1985), a comprehensive instrument originally covering 34 DSM-III psychiatric diagnoses (American Psychiatric Association, 1980), and subsequently enhanced to include questions about generalized anxiety and posttraumatic stress disorder (PTSD). For present purposes, the DIS was further adapted to omit diagnoses of low incidence and/or relevance to disaster exposure (see Table 8.2). (For detailed information about the DIS, including reliability and validity assessments, as well as interviewer training procedures, see Eaton & Kessler, 1985.)

The instrument also included a standardized supplement describing health care services utilization, as well as assessments of family history of psychiatric disorder, health status, social support, life events, and functioning levels in occupational and interpersonal arenas. The newly designed Disaster Supplement added questions about specific disaster exposure,

Table 8.2. *Interview questions: DSM-III disorders*

Affective
Major depression, single and recurrent episodes
Dysthymia

Substance use
Tobacco use
Alcohol abuse/dependence

Anxiety/somatic
Phobias
Panic
Somatization
Generalized anxiety
Posttraumatic stress disorder
Anorexia

Antisocial personality (adult component)

Note:
DSM-III = *Diagnostic and Statistical Manual of
Mental Disorders* (third edition, 1980).

including material losses, extent of harm, attributions of blame for the
events, and help sought and received from formal relief agencies (see Table
8.3).

The findings

Three basic questions guided our analyses. What kind of psychiatric
symptoms result from exposure to dioxin and floods? Which people are
most likely to experience negative effects? And why are some people more
distressed than others by exposure to disaster? Of course, no one study can
hope to comprehensively answer these broad questions, but our study of
the St Louis community was able to uncover findings that shed some light
on each of these issues.

What kinds of psychiatric symptoms result from disaster exposure?

Our earliest analyses were concerned with epidemiological questions: what
kinds of psychiatric symptoms did those exposed to disaster display, and
how do victims of dioxin and flood exposure compare to those who did not
experience disaster?

(Separate analyses were performed on just those respondents who had

Table 8.3. *Interview questions:*
disaster and background related

News coverage
Stigma
Blame/attribution
Residency/quality of housing
Household composition
Exposure, nonhousehold members
Job exposure
Life events
Other's posttraumatic stress
Damage by disaster
Losses/gains
Unemployment
Confidant/social support
Demography/pregnancy
Daily functioning
Health status/functioning
Health services
Barriers to care
Psychoactives
Health problems
School, service, employment, income
Family history
Locus of control

been included in the ECA study and for which we therefore had baseline data. However, since this subsample did not include victims who had been hardest hit by the disasters, these results are not discussed in this chapter. See Robins et al., 1986, for a report on the ECA subsample. The present discussion focuses on those analyses that included the sample as a whole.)

We began by comparing the experience of psychiatric symptoms since the disaster (Smith et al., 1986). A significantly higher proportion of those exposed to disaster had experienced at least one psychiatric symptom in the year following exposure. And among respondents with symptoms, victims of disaster had experienced significantly more symptoms than those who were not exposed. Exposure to all types of disaster (flood only, dioxin only, both flood and dioxin) showed the same pattern, although the flood and dioxin group had the highest proportion of those with symptoms and the highest level of symptoms in the past year.

We next looked at the types of psychiatric symptoms that were experienced during the year following the disasters. Disaster victims significantly exceeded the unexposed group in symptoms of depression, somatization, phobia, generalized anxiety, posttraumatic stress disorder, and alcohol abuse. Each type of disaster exposure contributed to the higher rate of these symptoms. Anorexia, drug abuse, and panic disorder showed no increase with exposure. Although these results seem to suggest a powerful effect as a result of direct exposure to disaster, they do not consider whether these are new symptoms or whether those experiencing disasters might have had these symptoms even before the disasters occurred. In order to assess the degree to which the disasters were responsible for producing new symptoms, we determined for each disorder the proportion of respondents reporting a symptom as occurring for the first time since the disaster. When the data were examined this way, the differences were much less dramatic. Only two significant differences were found. More of the disaster exposed group had new symptoms of depression and posttraumatic stress than did the nonexposure group.

New symptoms might have been a first occurrence of a disorder's symptoms or an increase in preexisting symptoms. To learn which the new depressive and posttraumatic stress symptoms were, we divided each group into those who had had any symptom of each disorder prior to the disasters and those who had not. We found that disasters appeared to exacerbate preexisting depressions rather than to initiate symptoms of the disorder in those previously symptom free. In contrast, for posttraumatic stress there was a strikingly greater increase in symptoms for those with exposure, whether or not they had had prior posttraumatic stress symptoms. Their rate of new symptoms was eight times greater than the no exposure group, both with and without prior symptoms. We concluded that the disasters produced new posttraumatic stress symptoms in respondents both with and without previous experience of these symptoms (see Smith et al., 1986, for an in-depth discussion of these findings).

While the above findings indicated that exposure to disaster resulted in increased symptoms of PTSD, subsequent multivariate analyses which controlled for both lifetime predisaster PTSD symptomatology and other more common stressful events found that disaster exposure in and of itself did not predict PTSD symptomatology, while more common stressful experiences such as experiencing a move, money difficulties, or an illness/injury in the household *did* significantly increase PTSD symptomatology (see Solomon & Canino, 1990). However, two of these more common stressful events (money difficulties, household illness/injury) were related to disaster exposure, and may have resulted from it. In addition, the St. Louis victims did show significantly higher levels of generalized anxiety than nondisaster victims, even after controlling for other negative life events and prior psychiatric symptomatology.

In summary, the findings indicate that psychiatric symptoms of PTSD, generalized anxiety and depression may have resulted from, or been exacerbated by, exposure to disaster. Yet responses in general were not that severe. Many of the symptoms that appeared immediately after the disaster dissipated by the time of the interview one year later (Smith et al., 1986). However, it should be noted that these results reflect the responses of victims taken as a whole. We asked ourselves whether some people may be more at risk than others. That is, do the group averages disguise people who are especially vulnerable when disaster hits?

Which people are most likely to experience psychological distress following disaster exposure?

We wondered if people's responses to disaster varied according to whether or not they had adequate social support systems to see them through the period of crisis. However, we knew from the research of others that social networks can be a mixed blessing in times of trouble (for a review, see Solomon, 1986). Most research models have tended to consider only the positive effects of social interactions, despite the fact that interpersonal encounters may also have negative consequences (Shinn, Lehmann & Wong, 1984). We were interested in not only the effects of social support availability, but also in the effects of a particular aspect of social involvement: support provision. Research on common stressful life events suggests that furnishing support can be costly to the provider (Kessler & McLeod, 1984). Although providing support under normal conditions may benefit the provider as well as the recipient, Shumaker and Brownell (1984) point out that large-scale emergencies force providers to give support at a time when they too need it, thereby making the supportive role in itself a source of stress.

Because other research also indicates that the burden of providing support may weigh more heavily on women than on men (Kessler & McLeod, 1984), we were interested in exploring sex differences in response to disaster as these responses are affected by having access to support, and providing support to others (Solomon et al., 1987).

Effects of providing and receiving support

We first examined the effects of support provision. In contrast to the findings of Kessler and McLeod (1984), we found only a slight (nonsignificant) tendency for women to be greater providers of heavy levels of support following disaster. Further, both sexes found an overload in such demands to be a source of emotional distress. However, especially for male disaster victims, moderate demands for support were generally associated with better outcomes than were low support demands.

Turning then to an examination of the effects of availability of social support, we found that for women, mid-range levels of support availability were associated with the most favorable outcomes. More specifically, access to all four forms of social support measured in this study (advice, trust, support, and/or defense) was associated with significantly higher somatization than was mid-range support availability for our female respondents. These findings suggest that, for females in particular, too much involvement has its cost. Although the study data do not tell us why women might negatively respond to a wide range of available support, other research suggests that it may be because of the obligation to reciprocate implied by accepting informal help (Shumaker & Brownell, 1984; Solomon, 1986). This norm may be more salient to women than to men, in that there tends to be greater reciprocity between two women than between two men, or between a man and a woman (House & Kahn, 1985). Thus even when women are not actually being called upon to provide more support than are men, women may feel more burdened by the obligation implicit in accepting support from others.

Sex differences in response

Our study also found men to be more adversely affected than women by personal exposure to disaster. This finding was of interest to us because of its contrast with findings for other stressors, such as daily hassles and chronic problems, to which women have been shown to be more vulnerable (Kessler & McLeod, 1984; Belle, 1982). We speculated that the reason that major catastrophes appear to have a greater direct effect on men is that disaster disrupts the role of the provider, a role traditionally assigned to men. Past research has shown that men are more emotionally affected than women by financial difficulties (Kessler, 1982). Families personally exposed to disaster are likely to experience financial problems, and perhaps occupational disruption as well. Accompanying these losses is the stigma associated with the need to ask for help from strangers; as a rule, people prefer to turn to their social network in times of trouble, and contact formal assistance agencies only as a last resort (Cowen, 1982; Solomon, 1986). Judging from their relative underutilization of health and mental health resources, this reluctance is particularly characteristic of men (Shapiro et al., 1984). Perhaps for these reasons, then, the combination of stressors uniquely associated with catastrophe has a greater direct effect on men than on women.

In contrast, the results indicated that women cope well with the direct effects of personal disaster exposure (see also Belle, 1982). Only when exposure is accompanied by heavy demands for nurturance – an obligation traditionally associated with the female role – does it have a negative impact on women's mental health (in this case, somatic symptomatology). The victim population in our study was dominated by lower income, married respondents with children (Smith et al., 1986). Women in these circumstances are already contending with a demanding set of role responsibilities, prior to disaster impact. Because women are more often called upon to provide emotional support than are men (Fischer, 1982; Gove & Hughes, 1984), household exposure to disaster may serve to overload the capacity of women to provide the nurturance asked of them. Perhaps it is for this reason that the present study found women with excellent spouse relationships to have worse outcomes following disaster than those with weaker spouse ties. This finding was in direct contrast to that for personally exposed males, whose outcomes positively related to the strength of the spouse relationship. Along these lines, Gleser, Green and Winget (1981) found that married women victims of the Buffalo Creek disaster showed higher psychopathology than women victims who lived alone; further, a spouse's anxiety and/or depression more seriously distressed women than men. Gleser et al.'s findings suggest that women in the present study may have been responding as much or more to their husband's mental health problems as to the disaster that precipitated them.

Effect of family role

The above interpretation of the results in terms of provider/nurturer role disruptions suggested the need for additional analyses, this time focusing directly on family role as a predictor of outcomes following disaster (Solomon, Bravo, Rubio-Stipec & Canino, 1993). We therefore decided to test whether adults occupying different marital and parental statuses were at differential risk for mental health problems in disaster's wake.

Research exploring responses to common undesirable events and role strains have generally found that the unmarried are at higher risk for mental illness following the experience of these events (see Thoits, 1987, for a discussion of this literature). We wondered if the same pattern prevails following exposure to disaster. We hypothesized that, because disaster seems to disproportionately burden providers of support, those victims with greater family responsibilities may find the disaster experience most directly debilitating. Therefore, victims with children were predicted to fare worse than victims without children. Moreover, since research has generally found that the unmarried are at higher risk for mental illness following the experience of undesirable events, and parenting may constitute an additional burden to these vulnerable people, it was predicted that exposure to disaster would have the most negative effect on the mental health of single parents. That is, single parents exposed to disaster were predicted to have highest rates of psychiatric symptomatology, especially exceeding both nonvictims, and married victims without children.

Our findings in St. Louis supported our prediction that worst outcomes would be found for *single parents* exposed to disaster; these respondents showed the highest levels of anxiety and overall total symptomatology of any of those interviewed (although married victims with children and unexposed single parents were almost as high). A possible explanation for this finding is that single parents are already experiencing heavy demands on their time, as well as on their financial and emotional resources; the experience of disaster may serve to make the already difficult dual roles of provider and nurturer overwhelmingly stressful for these individuals. (Results in Puerto Rico differed somewhat; see Solomon et al., 1993).

On the other hand, we reasoned that the presence of moderate levels of social support may alleviate the burden imposed by family or network responsibilities, thus overriding this burden's effects. Since the availability of emotional support has been shown to be an important moderator of stress, it was hypothesized that people with low levels of social support, regardless of their marital or parental status, would show poorer psychological outcomes when hit by a disaster than those with moderate levels of support. As predicted, respondents reporting low levels of available emotional support showed higher levels of depression, posttraumatic stress, anxiety, and total symptomatology than did those with higher levels of perceived support.

Moreover, additional analyses also showed that single parents who were exposed to disaster had substantially reduced levels of emotional support available to them, as compared to unexposed single parents. Thus single parents appear to be at particularly high risk for losing access to emotional support following a disaster, and, as noted above, perceived emotional support was found to be a particularly important moderator of disaster's effect on psychiatric distress. Thus it may be that the loss of social support, rather than simply the family role per se, places single parents at particularly high risk following disaster impact.

Why do some people respond especially negatively to disaster exposure?

If, as our results suggest, disaster disrupts both social support and the ability to perform one's role in the family, we wondered what psychological mechanisms could be used to explain how this disruption can lead to increased psychiatric distress. To assist us in understanding our findings, we turned to literature on perceived control and learned helplessness (Abramson, Seligman & Teasdale, 1978; Dweck & Wortman, 1980; Seligman, 1975; Taylor, 1983). We reasoned that a sudden, extreme event such as disaster can easily undermine an individual's sense of control over his/her life. According to Taylor (1983), an important aspect of successful adjustment to trauma is gaining a sense of control over the emergency event, so as to either manage its effects or prevent its reoccurrence. It is possible that individuals suffering the most psychological disturbance in the wake of disaster are those whose sense of mastery over their lives has been most undermined, and that disruptions in family role and/or social support are deleterious primarily when they are viewed by the disaster victims as evidence of a loss of this kind of mastery or control (see Solomon, 1986, for a more extensive discussion).

Exposure to negative events perceived as uncontrollable and, or unpredictable has been linked to adverse mental and physical outcomes such as depression and death (Seligman, 1975). Wallston et al. (1983) suggest that the way in which social support networks influence health is by enhancing perceptions of control over the environment. For example, Schulz (1976) randomly assigned institutionalized elderly to groups who received either regular visits, visits at random, or no visits from college students, and found that the elderly patients receiving regular visits were rated healthier and required less medication than the elderly in either of the other two groups. This work indicates that it is not merely the occurrence of interpersonal contact but its predictability/ controllability that contributes to recovery.

Theories of perceived control and learned helplessness may also explain the deleterious effects associated with loss of support. Lowenthal's (1964) work indicated that lifelong isolates were no more prone to illness than those with adequate support systems and were less vulnerable to physical and psychological impairment than the recently widowed. Again, these findings suggest that the predictability/controllability of social support may be of greater importance to wellbeing than interpersonal contact per se. In other words, it may not be the *lack* of social support, but rather the *loss* of it that causes so much psychological distress following disaster. And loss of support has been found to be widespread among not only directly affected (primary) victims, but also for secondary victims who experience a disaster in their community (see Norris, Phifer & Kaniasty, this volume).

Role of perceived control

Based on these speculations, we decided to more directly explore the role of perceived control as a moderator of disaster response. We wanted to examine the role of perceived control both in the development of symptoms of mental illness and in decisions to seek different types of formal assistance, following exposure to disaster. We were also interested in examining how the nature of the disaster event (i.e. natural or technological) affected victims' attributions of control and subsequent response (Solomon, Regier & Burke, 1989).

Pioneering work by Baum and his colleagues (Baum et al., 1983*a*,*b*; Collins, Baum & Singer, 1983) suggests that natural and technological disasters importantly differ in control related ways. While neither natural nor technological catastrophe can be controlled, Baum et al. argue that there is a fundamental psychological difference between *lack* of control over natural disasters never perceived as controllable, and *loss* of control over technology, for which expectations of control have been disrupted. For most victims of natural disaster, the consequences of exposure are immediately apparent; the devastation may be severe, yet active problem solving offers the prospect of eventual control over many of the losses sustained. In contrast, technological disaster poses greater uncertainty about physical consequences associated with chronic exposure, as well as the threat of ever increasing catastrophe, given the expansion of waste production and demands for energy (Baum et al., 1983*b*). Our next study examined whether the differing perceptions of control associated with natural and technological hazards differentially affect symptoms of mental illness and help seeking in disaster's wake (Solomon, Regier & Burke, 1989).

Which disasters disrupt control? Based on the work of Baum et al., (1983*b*), we expected that the individuals exposed solely to dioxin, the technological hazard, would display more symptoms of psychological distress than individuals exposed only to the natural hazard (the floods), since technological hazards are theoretically more disruptive to victims' perceptions of control. Those exposed to both kinds of hazards were expected to display the highest symptom levels of any exposure group, and the unexposed control group was predicted to report the fewest symptoms of current psychiatric disturbance. Our findings were in line with these predictions. Victims exposed only to dioxin had more symptoms of anxiety than did the flood only victims. Further, the doubly exposed victims had higher levels of depression, somatization, and anxiety than did either the unexposed respondents, or those exposed only to the floods.

Attributions as modifiers of response We wondered how these disaster effects would be modified by the victims' explanations for the disasters, i.e. their attributions of causality for these different kinds of events. Brickman and his associates (Brickman et al., 1982) have suggested that it is important to draw a distinction between attribution of responsibility for a problem (i.e. who is to blame for a past event), and attribution of responsibility for a solution (i.e. who is in control of future events). Brickman et al. maintain that victims of stressful events may cope most effectively if they do *not* blame themselves for the victimizing event, but believe that it is their responsibility to deal with the consequences of the event now that it has occurred. According to Brickman et al. (1982), this perspective 'allows people to direct their energies outward, working on trying to solve problems or transform their environment without berating themselves for their role in creating these problems' (p. 372).

While we agreed that this attributional pattern is likely to result in the healthiest emotional outcomes, we thought that this would only pertain for those victims involved in events that lend themselves to problem-focused coping. As Baum et al. (1983*b*) work suggests, this is more likely to be the case for flood victims than for dioxin victims. Natural and technological hazards generally present victims with very different kinds of problems. For example, the flood victims were confronted with unambiguous pragmatic difficulties: the situation required that they attempt to salvage their homes, businesses and possessions, or sell them and relocate elsewhere. In other words, effective coping with the flood exposure demanded a problem focused orientation, i.e. coping directed toward ameliorating the external stressor (Lazarus, 1966). We used help seeking from formal relief agencies as an indicator of problem focused coping.

In contrast, solutions to the problems posed by dioxin were unclear, and/ or beyond the control of the victims themselves. Consequently, victims of dioxin who cope effectively may rely more heavily on emotion focused coping in dealing with the effects of disaster exposure. We used visits to a professional for help with an emotional or substance abuse problem as a measure of emotion focused coping.

Fig. 8.1 displays the prediction model for this study, showing how attributions were expected to differentially modify the responses of the flood and dioxin victims. The predictions for the flood victims are shown on the top half of this Figure. We predicted that flood victims who did not blame themselves for the flood damage would have fewer psychiatric symptoms than would flood victims who did hold themselves accountable for the flood's effects. Flood victims who blamed themselves were also predicted to engage in less problem focused coping, as measured by relief agency assistance seeking, and more emotion focused coping (mental health visits) than the nonself blamers.

Attributions were expected to display a different pattern of effects for dioxin victims. Self-blame for dioxin victims was expected to be rare. While some flood victims might realistically blame themselves for locating in an area where floods were known to occur, few, if any, dioxin victims could have known at the time of purchase that their homes would prove to be contaminated with a deadly toxin. Therefore, to the extent that these individuals made any sort of attribution for their exposure, they were likely to chose other human agents, such as business or government, as the cause of their troubles. Further, for reasons noted earlier, problem focused coping was less available to dioxin victims than to flood victims. Dioxin victims with the best outcomes were therefore predicted to be those who demonstrated an effort to manage their internal emotional response to the situation. More specifically, it was predicted that dioxin victims who blamed other human agents for their exposure would have better mental health outcomes then individuals who did not blame others for this event. Other blaming dioxin victims were also expected to report relatively greater rates of mental health visits than dioxin victims who did not blame others for their exposure (see bottom of Fig. 8.1).

Results were generally in line with these predictions. Particularly *high* in somatization were victims who blamed the *flood* damage on themselves. These self-blaming flood victims were also less likely to seek help from relief organizations, and more likely to seek mental health counseling, than were flood victims who did not hold themselves accountable for the flood damage. In contrast, assigning blame (in this case, to others) for the *dioxin* damage related to *lower* anxiety levels in dioxin victims. However, contrary to prediction, few of the dioxin victims sought mental health help, regardless of their attribution.

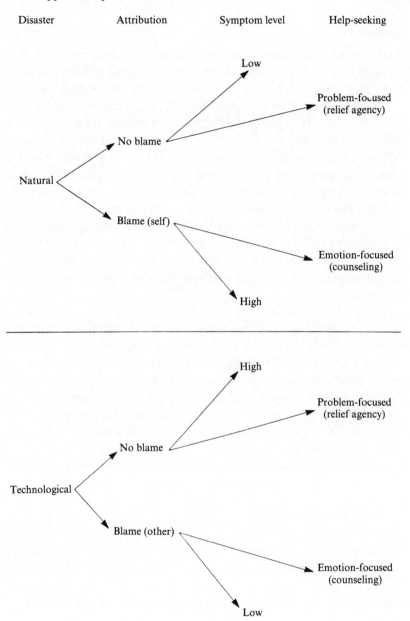

Fig. 8.1. Prediction model: disaster attributions as mediators of psychological symptoms and help seeking.

Discussion

Our results indicate not only that exposure to disaster can result in persisting emotional distress, but also that the degree of distress will vary according to both type of exposure and victims' explanations for their misfortune. These findings suggest that assigning blame (particularly to the self) may impede psychological recovery in natural disaster situations which lend themselves to more active, problem focused responses, such as seeking agency assistance for flood relief. However, in more ambiguous disaster situations, such as exposure to dioxin or other technological hazards, the external environment may not be amenable to individual control. While these situations are likely to produce higher levels of distress overall, some of this distress may be alleviated by blaming others for the exposure. This kind of attribution may serve as a form of emotion focused coping, one which facilitates emotional recovery by imparting a sense of meaning to the event, and with it perhaps the hope that others can and will make restitution.

Our findings are in line with the work of Taylor (1983), who maintains that when direct mastery is a viable alternative, energies diverted into attempts to find meaning in the event (e.g. blaming the self) are more likely to impede than enhance psychological recovery. However, in situations where direct control over consequences is *not* possible, Taylor (1983) agrees that successful adjustment will require the ability to summon cognition which imparts the *illusion* of control. In our study, blaming other human agents for the dioxin damage may have provided such an illusion of control, by fostering the belief that the identified guilty party will be forced to assume the responsibility for finding solutions to dioxin related problems.

Conclusions and implications

Taken as a whole these studies offer some intriguing implications for both victim assistance and further research. Our studies show that for some victims, disaster can have lingering effects. These effects may be more likely to occur in situations characterized by a chronic toxic stressor like dioxin, than by an acute natural stressor such as a flood (see also Baum et al. 1983*b*).

Since disaster tends to disrupt the role of provider, those with the expectation of fulfilling this role may find the disaster experience most directly debilitating. Individuals expecting to fulfil a nurturant role may experience negative psychological effects when disaster intensifies nurturance demands beyond the supporter's capacity to satisfy. Because single parents fulfil both these roles, experiencing a disaster may be most stressful of all for these kind of victims. Our results suggest that although previously unrecognized in the disaster literature, single parents appear to constitute an important high-risk victim group, in need of emotional assistance in disaster's wake. However, these findings also suggest that 'objective' indicators such as demographics may not be sufficient to identify disaster victims in need of counseling, since perceived levels of available emotional support importantly modified the effects of disaster exposure, regardless of family role.

These results suggest that prevention interventions for disaster victims should not only target single parents for special help, but should also routinely assess perceptions of emotional support available to victims in general. When diagnostic indicators suggest the presence of psychiatric problems, victims may need to be encouraged and/or assisted in locating sources of emotional support other than the nuclear family. These might most effectively consist of self-help groups tailored to particular victim subgroups, such as groups for single parents.

Our study brought to light a concern rarely expressed in the disaster mental health literature: that some of the disaster victims with the greatest emotional problems may not be getting the other kinds of formal assistance that they need; i.e. help with practical problems. We found that flood-exposed victims who blamed themselves for flood damage were less likely to seek agency assistance than those who did not hold themselves accountable for such damage. It may be that those who blamed themselves for their misfortune felt less entitled to financial assistance than those without this attribution (cf. Comer & Laird, 1975). If future research supports this inference, mental health counseling for disaster victims may need to include among its goals the legitimization of seeking agency relief from the practical problems posed by disaster. Cognitive therapy aimed at redirecting victims' causal attributions for the disaster may be the most effective way of achieving this goal.

Further research is needed to better understand the process by which social support mediates reactions to traumatic events. Our work particularly highlights the need for studies that simultaneously examine perceived control and social support as they affect mental and physical health outcomes. If enhanced sense of control proves to be the basis for the supportive value of social networks, it may also explain victims' preference for seeking assistance from self-help groups and indigenous nonprofessionals rather than from mental health professionals. Because the relationship

198 S. D. Solomon and E. M. Smith

with professionals is asymmetrical and nonreciprocal, it may be perceived as a greater threat to self-esteem and autonomy (control) than is the mutual self-help relationship. Needed are studies that provide sound evidence recording the relative effectiveness (i.e. actual helpfulness) of informal caregivers as compared to professionals (Cowen, 1982), as well as the kinds of help each is best suited to provide.

Acknowledgements

This research was supported by a supplement to the Epidemiological Catchment Area Program (ECA) Cooperative Agreement U01 MH 33883 awarded to Principal Investigators Lee N. Robins and John E. Helzer of Washington University in St. Louis, for research performed with NIMH Principal Collaborators Darrel A. Regier, Ben Z. Locke, and Jack D. Burke, Jr.; the NIMH Project Officer was Carl A. Taube.

The authors gratefully acknowledge the invaluable contributions of Lee Robins and Ruth Fischbach in research design, Linda Cottler and Evelyn Goldring in instrument development, Larry McEvoy in computer programming, and Tom Pryzbeck in statistical analysis.

Requests for reprints should be sent to Susan D. Solomon, Division of Epidemiology and Services Research, National Institute of Mental Health, 5600 Fishers Lane, Room 10C–26, Rockville, MD, 20857. The opinions or assertions contained herein are the private ones of the authors, and are not to be considered as official or reflect the views of the National Institute of Mental Health.

References

Abramson, L. Y. , Seligman, M. E. P. & Teasdale, J. (1978). Learned helplessness in humans: critique and reformation. *Journal of Abnormal Psychology*, **87**, 49–74.
Baum, A., Fleming, R. & Davidson, L. M. (1983*a*). Natural disaster and technological catastrophe. *Environment and Behavior*, **15**(3), 333–54.
Baum, A., Fleming, R. & Singer, J. E. (1983*b*). Coping with victimization by technological disaster. *Journal of Social Issues*, **39**(2), 117–38.
Belle, D. (1982). *Lives in stress: women and depression*. Beverly Hills, CA: Sage Publications.
Brickman, P., Rabinowitz, V.C., Karuza, J., Coates, D., Cohn, E. & Kidder, L. (1982). Models of helping and coping. *American Psychologist*, **37**(4), 368–84.
Cohn, V. (1980, June 7). Waste sites may invade water supply, subcommittee told. *The Washington Post*, A2.
Collins, D. L., Baum, A. & Singer, J. E. (1983). Coping with chronic stress at Three Mile Island: psychological and biochemical evidence. *Health Psychology*, **2**(2), 149–66.
Comer, R. & Laird, J. D. (1975). Choosing to suffer as a consequence of expecting to suffer: why do people do it? *Journal of Personality and Social Psychology*, **32**(1), 92–101.
Cowen, E. L. (1982). Help is where you find it: four informal helping groups. *American Psychologist*, **37**(4), 385–95.

Dweck, C. S. & Wortman, C. B. (1980). Achievement, test anxiety and learned helplessness: adaptive and maladaptive cognition. In H. W. Krohne & L. Laux (eds.) *Achievement stress and anxiety.* Washington, DC: Hemisphere.

Eaton, W. W. & Kessler, L. G. (eds.). (1985). *Epidemiologic field methods in psychiatry: the NIMH epidemiologic catchment area program.* Orlando: Academic Press.

Fischer, C. S. (1982). *To dwell among friends: personal networks in town and city.* Chicago: University of Chicago Press.

Gleser, G. C., Green, B. L. & Winget, C. (1981). *Prolonged psychosocial effects of disaster: a study of Buffalo Creek.* New York: Academic Press.

Gove, W. R. & Hughes, M. (1984). *Overcrowding in the household.* New York: Academic Press.

House, J. S. & Kahn, R. L. (1985). Measures and concepts of social support. In S. Cohen & L. Syme (eds.) *Social support and health.* New York: Academic Press, pp. 83–108.

Kessler, R. C. (1982). A disaggregation of the relationship between socioeconomic status and psychological distress. *American Sociological Review,* **47**, 752–64.

Kessler, R. C. & McLeod, J. D. (1984). Sex differences in vulnerability to undesirable life events. *American Sociological Review,* **49**, 620–31.

Lazarus, R. S. (1966). *Psychological stress and the coping process.* New York: McGraw-Hill.

Lowenthal, M. (1964). Social isolation and mental illness in old age. *American Sociological Review,* **29**, 54–70.

Robins, L. N., Fischbach, R. L., Smith, E. M., Cottler, L. B. & Solomon, S. D. (1986). Impact of disaster on previously assessed mental health. In J. Shore (ed.) *Disaster stress studies: new methods and findings.* Washington, DC: American Psychiatric Press, Inc, pp. 22–48

Robins, L. N., Helzer, J. E., Weissman, M. M., Overaschel, H., Swenberg, E., Burbe, J. & Regier, D. A. (1984). Lifetime prevalence of specific psychiatric disorders in three sites. *Archives of General Psychiatry,* **41**, 949–58.

Robins, L. N. & Smith, E. M. (1983). *Diagnostic interview schedule/disaster supplement.* St. Louis: Washington University School of Medicine, Department of Psychiatry.

Rossi, P. H., Wright, J. D., Weber-Burdin, E. & Perina, J. (1983). Victimization by natural hazards in the United States, 1970–1980; survey estimates. *International Journal of Mass Emergencies and Disasters,* **1**(3), 467–82.

Schulz, R. (1976). Effects of control and predictability on the physical and psychological well-being of the institutionalized aged. *Journal of Personality and Social Psychology,* **33**, 562–73.

Seligman, M. E. P. (1975). *Helplessness: on depression, development and death.* San Francisco: W. H. Freeman.

Shapiro, S., Skinner, E. A., Kessler, L. C. et al. (1984). Utilization of health and mental health services. *Archives of General Psychiatry,* **41**, 971–8.

Shinn, M., Lehmann, S. & Wong, N. W. (1984). Social interaction and social support. *Journal of Social Issues,* **40**(4), 1–9.

Shumaker, S. A. & Brownell, A. (1984). Toward a theory of social support: Closing conceptual gaps. *Journal of Social Issues,* **40**(4), 11–36.

Smith, E. M. (1984). *Chronology of disaster in eastern Missouri* (Contract No. 83-MH-525181). Rockville, MD: National Institute of Mental Health.

Smith, E. M., Robins, L. N., Przybeck, T. R., Goldring, E. & Solomon, S. D. (1986). Psychosocial consequences of a disaster. In J. H. Shore (ed. *Disaster stress studies: new methods and findings.* Washington, DC: American Psychiatric Press, Inc, pp. 49–76.

Solomon, S. D. (1986). Mobilizing social support networks in times of disaster. In C. Figley (ed.) *Trauma and its wake. vol. 2. Traumatic stress theory, research, and intervention.* New York: Brunner/Mazel, pp. 232–63.

Solomon, D. S., Bravo, M., Rubio-Stipe, M. & Canino, G. (1993). Effect of family role on response to disaster. *Journal of Traumatic Stress,* **6**(2), 251–65.

Solomon S. D. & Canino G. J. (1990). Appropriateness of DSM-IIIR criteria for post-traumatic stress disorder. *Comprehensive Psychiatry,* **31**(3), 227–37.

Solomon, S. D., Regier, D. A. & Burke, J. D. (1989). Role of perceived control in coping with natural and technological disaster. *Journal of Clinical and Social Psychology,* **8**(4), 376–92.

Solomon, S. D., Smith, E. M., Robins, L. N. & Fischbach, R. L. (1987). Social involvement as a mediator of disaster-induced stress. *Journal of Applied Social Psychology,* **17**(12), 1092–112.

Taylor, S. E. (1983). Adjustment to threatening events: a theory of cognitive adaption. *American Psychologist,* **38**(11), 1161–73.

Thoits, P. A. (1987). Gender and marital status differences in control and distress: common stress versus unique stress explanations. *Journal of Health and Social Behavior,* **28** (March), 7–22.

Wallston, B. S., Alagna, S. W., DeVellis, B. M. & DeVellis, R. F. (1983). Social support and physical health. *Health Psychology,* **2**, 367–91.

9

Debriefing following traumatic exposure

ARIEH Y. SHALEV

Soldiers are eager to talk, their memory is good, they do so better when together, in groups.
(S. L. A. Marshall, Island Victory, 1944)

Debriefing is a group-oriented intervention in which the major elements of a trauma are reviewed by the participants shortly after the event. Debriefing has been recommended as a stress management technique suitable for groups exposed to traumatic events, and has been practised, as such, by several rescue organizations (Dunning & Silva, 1980; Wagner, 1979; Raphael, 1986; Mitchell, 1981; Bergman & Queen, 1986; Griffin, 1987; Jones, 1985). Although intuitively helpful, the structure of this technique, its goals and its mechanisms of action have not been identified. A systematic description is needed in order for debriefing to become an object of scientific scrutiny and interest. This chapter reviews several debriefing protocols, outlines the principal dimensions of this method, and suggests a framework for future research.

Disasters, wars and traumatic events regularly result in immediate and long-term psychological changes. Among the individuals affected, behavioral and psychiatric responses range from the most pervasive forms of posttraumatic stress disorder (PTSD) to a variety of positive learning experiences.

The immediate reactions to traumatic events include all forms of human suffering and massive attempts to cope with the effects of the exposure. A wide variety of symptoms have been documented including paralyzing anxiety, cognitive disarray, dissociative and conversion reactions, psychological and physiological depletion, and emotional numbing (Bar-On et al., 1986; Weisaeth, 1989; Krystal, 1978; Green et al., 1983). These immediate reactions constitute an urgent appeal for specialized care, indeed for 'every comforting human response' (Raphael, 1986, p. 247) capable of reducing suffering. This is the primary goal of early intervention following trauma.

Typical of this stage is the mobilization of social resources and spontaneous rescue efforts by both professionals and nonprofessionals (Quarantelli, 1986). These efforts draw into the circle of the traumatic exposure other members of society who may themselves become victims. In this way, relatives and friends of the victims may also become secondary victims, reacting to their real and symbolic losses (Jones, 1985; Wright K. and Bartone, P., this volume).

Long-term studies of trauma populations (e.g. Green, 1987; Solomon, Schwarzwald & Mikulincer, 1987; Kulka et al., 1989) show that a substantial number of survivors suffer from the after effects of the trauma for prolonged periods. PTSD is the most widely recognized consequence of trauma but is far from being the only one: a variety of psychiatric disorders including depression, dysthymia, phobias, dissociative disorders, alcohol and drug abuse has been documented, along with profound personality changes, increased physical morbidity, high rates of mortality and uncontrolled reenactments of the trauma by repeated self-exposure or victimization of others. These long-term effects add another goal to early treatment efforts, namely the prevention of posttraumatic morbidity.

Exposure to trauma may occur individually or in randomly assembled groups. For some populations (e.g. police, fire departments and armies) such exposure is predictable, organized, and part of one's professional duty. Despite the protective role of preparation and training (Hytten & Weisaeth, 1989), such 'organized exposure' produces a substantial number of disabling psychological sequelae. A variety of stress disorders have been described among fire fighters (McFarlane, 1988a,b), rescue workers (Dunning & Silva, 1980; Raphael et al., 1983), and combat veterans (Solomon et al., 1987; Helzer, Robins & McEnvoi, 1987; Kaylor, King & King, 1987). Traumatic exposure by professional groups is often repetitive, adding a third goal to early intervention: the prevention of burnout, of anticipatory anxiety, and of inadequate reactions to subsequent exposures.

Very little is known about the short-term, let alone the long-term, outcome of early intervention after group exposure to trauma. Retrospective data, such as Solomon and Benbenishty's (1986) survey of combat veterans of the Lebanon War, which was conducted one year after the war, suggest that early intervention is effective in reducing the incidence of PTSD. Prospective studies are obviously difficult to carry out (e.g. Green, 1986) and are therefore unavailable.

Several studies, however, provide a rationale for early intervention and delineate its optimal timing and its target population. The first line of evidence concerns the pathogenic effects of the secondary stressors that may follow the trauma itself (e.g. Lindy & Grace, 1986). Green (1987) found a strong correlation between the secondary stressors that followed the Buffalo Creek dam collapse (e.g. relocation) and the intensity of stress reactions 14 years after the event. Similarly, Baum, Gatchel & Schaeffer. (1983) considered the ambiguous information which followed the Three Mile Island nuclear leak as a major stressor. Figley and Leventman (1980) described the stressful experience that was generated by the inappropriate 'decompression' which occurred when Vietnam veterans were rapidly transported from the battle field to the continental United States. Interventions which reduce these secondary stressors may improve the long-term outcome after traumas and disasters.

A second line of evidence supporting early intervention is the discrepancy between the population at risk for developing posttraumatic disorders and the scope of the established treatment strategies. The classical model of intervention in exposure of organized groups to trauma has been practiced in most western armies since World War I (Salmon, 1919). These interventions follow the principles of secondary prevention (i.e. treatment of identified patients within medical facilities). Recent research has shown that many trauma survivors develop posttraumatic sequelae without acute disabling symptoms during the trauma exposure. Solomon et al. (1987) found that 16% of 386 combat veterans of the 1982 Lebanon War who had not sought treatment for the psychological effects of the war, suffered from diagnosable PTSD one year later. Similarly, despite the low number of identified stress casualties during the Vietnam War (Bourne, 1969, Ingraham & Manning, 1986) a substantial number of veterans developed PTSD in the succeeding years (e.g. Kulka et al., 1989). Among Israeli veterans of the Lebanon War with delayed PTSD, only 10% have sought specialized help (Solomon et al., 1989). Early interventions which focus on identified patients will address only part of the population at risk.

New modes of intervention conceived as primary prevention and addressing all the exposed population are indicated. In addition, these data add another goal to early intervention: identifying symptomatic patients and providing information about specialized help.

Primary prevention strategies directed at the entire population at risk have been reported by a number of authors (Griffin, 1987; Raphael, 1986; Birenbaum, Copolon & Scharff, 1976; Cohen, 1976; Cohen & Ahearn, 1980). Group *debriefing* has been particularly recommended for organized groups after trauma exposure (Dunning & Silva; 1980; Jones, 1985; Mitchell, 1981; Griffin, 1987; Bergman & Queen, 1986; Raphael, 1986). Immediate and long-term beneficial effects of debriefing have been suggested, but with very little systematic evidence (Bloom 1985).

Past and present forms of debriefing

Task-oriented debriefing

Debriefing is used by numerous institutions in order to gather information and develop 'lessons learned' for the future. The Israel Defense Forces, for example, have systematically debriefed soldiers and commanders after every mission (Gal, 1986) without ever considering this practice a psychological intervention. Other military and nonmilitary institutions, such as the FBI, fire departments, research teams, and business corporations use a variety of meetings with elements of a debriefing format: 'team meetings,' 'problem solving meetings,' etc...

Although apparently of purely instrumental value and not always related to stressful exposure, such forms of debriefing often become part of the institutional culture, acquire a quality of rituals and often mobilize substantial emotions. These meetings fulfil a number of functions that practitioners of psychological debriefing want to achieve. They give meaning to traumatic and stressful events through discussions, comments, citations and rewards. In addition, they integrate the experience into the general framework of the institution and reaffirm the institution's role as a source of meaning and a frame of reference for all action. Professionals who, following a traumatic event, plan a psychological debriefing in an institution which has standard debriefing type meetings (e.g. police, fire departments) need to be aware of such routines, recognize their practical and symbolic value and, when possible, create a link between their own interventions and these routines.

Historical group debriefing

A method of group debriefing following combat exposure was developed during World War II by the chief historian for the US army, Brigadier General Samuel Lyman Atwood Marshall (1900–1977). His method was applied to a large number of combat units during World War II and again in the Korean and Vietnam Wars. Although primarily aimed at gathering historical data, Marshall's method has resulted, according to its inventor, in profound psychological changes among the soldiers debriefed. Because of Marshall's extensive documentation, it is particularly easy to follow his method. Marshall's debriefing technique reflects many of the generic components of the more recent posttrauma and postdisaster forms of debriefing.

Marshall's field notes, located at the US Army Institute of Military History in Carlisle, Pennsylvania, USA, provide vivid description of the method. S. L. A. Marshall served as a reporter in the Korean and Vietnam wars. The extensive documentation of his debriefings include books, (Marshall, 1953, 1956, 1962) transcripts of lectures (Spiller, 1988), field and research notes (Marshall Collection at Carlisle, Marshall Collection at El Paso). His book, *Island Victory* (Marshall, 1944) contains an illustrative account of the development and application of postcombat debriefing. His field notes include several transcripts of debriefing sessions.

Marshall's interest was the study of small unit performance in ground combat. He was especially interested in the 'human factor', those psychological factors that enabled men to act and groups to maintain their integrity (Marshall, 1947). The modern battle field, according to Marshall, presents the soldier with very little positive information and with many ambiguous cues. Infantry soldiers rarely see the enemy, their own buddies are under cover, and the sources of danger and threat (e.g. fire, mines) are hidden. A soldier's capacity to overcome his fears depends, therefore, on his ability to 'feel the presence of others' and maintain a sense of belonging to a group (Marshall, 1947). Marshall was also aware of the individual's inability to identify and make sense of the overall pattern of a combat event in which he participated. Marshall's writings (e.g. Marshall, 1953) contain many descriptions of commanders and soldiers acting and making decisions on the basis of partial information and inaccurate assumptions. Indeed, he grasped one of the major psychological attributes of traumatic events: their chaotic unfolding in the eyes of the individuals involved. Consequently, Marshall believed that the historical truth of combat could only be accessed through reconstruction of group narratives. His method of historical group debriefing was designed to restore a comprehensive description of the combat.

Marshall's debriefing sessions took place on the battle field as soon as possible after the action. All survivors of the battle were present except the medically evacuated. Prior to a debriefing session, Marshall learned the outline of the battle and the specific role played by the unit to be debriefed. Getting acquainted with technical information (e.g. ground, weather, manpower, weapons, food, ammunition, etc.) was considered a sine-qua-non for analyzing the material discussed by the group during the session. The interviewer had to *'study all the available maps'* and *'learn beforehand the larger significance of what the company accomplished – more fully than the company itself'* (Marshall 1944, p. 205).

The sessions opened by informing the group of the procedure and its goals. At that point, superiors were often invited to endorse the session in front of the group and give it their blessing. The instructions defined the group's task as *'describing the combat with all the possible details'* and emphasized the significance, for the Army, of learning from the group's experience. Witnesses were encouraged to speak and to share their experiences with the whole group.

For the duration of the session, military ranks were set aside. Testimonies were, therefore, weighed according to their pertinence to understanding the course of the operation and not to the rank of the witness. *'The word of a superior as to what a man (or a group) did should not be allowed to prevail against the direct testimony of the man himself.'* (Marshall, 1944, p. 204).

A moratorium in time was thus created, during which the hierarchical military structure was temporarily suspended: *'Here you are all equal witness. For the time being we all stand on the same ground. If you hear any man present, whatever his rank, say something which you think is incorrect.... it is your duty to stand up and speak your piece'* (Marshall, 1944 p. 206). Spiller (1988) related this aspect of Marshall's method as a 'democratic interpretation of the battle' and 'genuinely American' and contrasted it with more traditional ways in which military institutions make sense of combat events, where the right to interpret and convey meaning is reserved for officers and commanders.

After a short period of modeling by the military historian, company commanders were often invited to take the lead and conduct the interview: *'If he is fit to lead them in battle, he is fit to lead them in reliving the battle experience.'* (1944, p. 212). The professional leader, however, was always there to remind the commander not to use the session for teaching lessons and to refrain from expressing opinions on a soldier's conduct during the fight.

The reconstruction of the battle, Marshall insisted, had to follow a 'strict chronological path' and uncover the events in sequential order. This structure helped to avoid evasions and to focus the discussion on factual reality rather than on interpretation. Accordingly, all the available information on each stage of the battle was exhaustively collected from all the witnesses. *'No scrap of evidence is too small to disregard at the time of the inquiry. It is often found that the key to all that occurred may be some fact* known to only two or three members of the company which they themselves considered to be of minor import' (Marshall,1944, p. 209).

As a military historian, Marshall was primarily interested in facts rather than opinions. A closer scrutiny reveals, however, that he had a broad concept of what the 'factual reality' was during combat. It included soldiers' thoughts, assumptions and feelings at specific times during the fight and the decisions and actions that followed. It was just as important *'to gather the facts on the moral side of war as on the purely physical side'* (Marshall, 1944, p. 210). The 'group's spirit' was also part of the factual reality. Fatigue, malnutrition and anticipatory intuitions that preceded the engagement were recorded and studied as potential causes of behavior during the action.

Marshall warns future interviewers against discarding any testimony and confronting any witness with disbelief or mistrust: *'The interviewing officer should never cut any witness short or disbelieve in any statement'* (Marshall, 1944, p. 212). Tolerance of ambiguous information was, consequently, the rule and premature closure was systematically avoided. Contradictory statements led to encouraging further clarification and looking for more details. Additional information was never discredited on the basis of earlier statements: *'The record should not be regarded as closed at any time'* (Marshall, 1944, p. 212). Maintaining the integrity of the process (i.e. encouraging openness and communication) was preferable to rectifying misperceptions and achieving a definite version of the events.

The attitude of the interviewer was to be of *'warm interest and respectful attention'*. The interviewer *'should be ever ready with praise'*. *'He cannot obtain the interest of the company and its complete participation unless he conducts himself as a student rather than as a teacher.'*

The death of comrades in combat was of critical importance: *'It will be found, almost without exception, that these men (those who had died) played a conspicuous part in the actions and that the living are especially concerned with being exact in relating what did happen to those who were killed'* (Marshall, 1944, p. 204). The interviewer had to be particularly sensitive to the way in which the death of comrades affected survivors during the battle and during its reconstruction. The memory of the dead added a dimension of seriousness and truthfulness to the process.

Marshall's debriefing sessions are the longest described in the literature and have not been replicated by others. Marshall hoped to avoid any time constraints which would limit the ability to elicit highly complex information of combat events. Ideally, the sessions should have been limited only *'by the time it takes to achieve the desired result'*. Debriefings were continued until the whole picture was obtained. Marshall estimated that seven hours were needed to debrief one fighting day. Allegedly some debriefing sessions took three working days. This attitude toward time, that the unfolding of the process determined of the debriefing, is similar to that of traditional psychodynamic therapy, where the length of the treatment is determined by its course. This attitude may encourage a group process characterized by openness and lack of pressure.

Marshall considered the practice of debriefing as fairly simple. He recommended it for the use of commanders even without formal training. It is clear, however, that he recognized the existence of group resistance and the need to deal with it. He described a group process which opened with an atmosphere of caution and progressed into openness and enthusiastic participation. With some companies a congenial atmosphere could be established *'within ten minutes of the start of an interview'* while in other cases, the interviewing officer had to work patiently with the company for a day or longer before the 'dam breaks'. Marshall believed there was a relationship between difficulties in debriefing and the quality of the unit's leadership: a company with poor leaders was harder to engage in debriefing.

As a military historian, Marshall's principal aim was 'the dissipation of the fog of combat' and obtaining an oral history of the battle. He describes, however, a psychological impact of debriefing on the group, a 'spiritual purge'. This emotional response led to increased self esteem and relief among the soldiers. *'For every unit it was a morale-building experience'* (Marshall, 1944, p. 215), *'Far from objecting to being interviewed about their battle experience, the men usually relish it. It comes as a relief and as partial recognition to them.'* (Marshall, 1944 p. 202)

As far as we know, the emotional reactions of the soldiers to combat, on the one hand, and those encountered during the sessions on the other, were neither elaborated nor reflected upon. However, Marshall did inquire about emotions and affects. 'We asked them not only what they did in the fight but what they actually said and how they felt.' Moreover, in a subtle way, he seems to have turned individuals who had just endured a situation over which they had little control, into active participants shaping the meaning of their recent experience. This process may have had a powerful emotional effect. Similarly, some degree of emotional ventilation may have been facilitated by the sessions.

Marshall's debriefing technique highlights a number of elements that are common to other forms of debriefing (Table 9.1). Among these are: the timing of the intervention, preparation for the session, respect for the

Table 9.1. *Technical principles of S. L. A. Marshall's debriefing method*

Debriefing is carried out on the battle field.

Intervention is immediately after the combat.

All participants take part in the sessions.

Ranks are put aside during the session.

Background information should be learned in advance by the interviewers.

Superiors openly endorse the session in front of the group.

Reconstruction of the event follows strict chronological order.

All the details of the action are collected from each participant.

Conflicting information is tolerated.

Premature closure, early conclusion and teaching lessons are avoided.

The length of the session is limited only by the time needed to obtain the entire narrative of the action.

The participants' emotional reactions and symptoms are not explicitly addressed.

institutional framework, temporary suspension of some of the institution's rules, cognitive reconstruction of the event, tolerance of ambiguous information, integration of grief reactions, use of nonprofessional yet natural leaders, handling resistance to the process and time constraints. Such elements are, explicitly or implicitly, addressed by all debriefing techniques. These elements affect the course of the intervention and its outcome. Four dimensions important to all of the more recent debriefing techniques derive from these elements: (1) appraisal of the stressor; (2) the goals of the intervention; (3) techniques used and (4) the theory of recovery and healing.

Psychological group debriefing

Among the numerous clinicians who have used postevent debriefing for therapy or prevention, the works of B. Raphael (1986) and J. Mitchell (1982, 1983) are the most widely cited. Raphael (1986) formulated guidelines for debriefing teams of helpers involved in disaster rescue after the Granville rail disaster (Raphael et al., 1983) (see Table 9.2). In these sessions the debriefers explored various aspects of the rescuers' experience of the disaster and their responses to it. The description of the original intervention is compelling. 'Sitting around in a group and drinking beer they discussed with the consultant (and in a half joking fashion) a wide range of topics: the frustration of their role and sense of helplessness; the

Table 9.2. *Areas to explore in psychological debriefing of workers and helpers following disasters*

Participants' introduction to, and first knowledge of, the disaster
Personal experience of the disaster:
  Negative experiences and feelings
  Positive experiences and feelings
Relationships to other workers and families
Empathy with other workers and victims
Disengagement from disaster role
Integration of disaster experience

Source: Adapted from B. Raphael, 1986.

fear several had about dying themselves in the narrow space; the terror and revulsion at all these deaths ... the posttraumatic stress reactions of intrusive images, nightmares and fears, the difficulties sharing the experience with their families, and the fact that they could not unload their feelings because immediately after they have finished their work at the rail disaster they were called out to several road accident rescues and were still in an alert, aroused state. As the evening progressed the consultant helped these workers to accept the naturalness of their fears and regain their sense of mastery through discussion, release of feelings and externalization of their experience' (Raphael 1986, p. 255.)

Raphael conceives the goal of debriefing as primarily preventive: 'to help the workers deal with the inevitable stresses so that problems do not arise subsequently'. She recommends formal group sessions. The theory of healing is straightforward: 'The experience is given a cognitive structure and the emotional release of reviewing helps the worker to a sense of achievement and distancing' (p. 286). As with other authors, follow-up data, although anecdotal, is positive; the immediate relief is not measured.

Critical Incident Stress Debriefing (CISD) is similar to B. Raphael's method. It was developed by J. Mitchell (1981, 1982, 1983) and has been applied to several groups of rescue workers (Melton, 1985; Mitchell, 1986). The CISD protocol comprises a series of consecutive phases through which various aspects of the traumatic exposure are explored and worked through by the group (Table 9.3). Ventilation, mobilization of social support, as well as education and identification of symptomatic individuals are used. The focus is on individuals and their reactions and not on the group *per se.* Outcome data which is enthusiastically positive, is again anecdotal and

Table 9.3. *Phases of critical incident stress debriefing (CISD)*

Introductory phase
Facts phase
Thought phase
Reaction phase
Symptoms phase
Teaching phase
Reentry phase

Source: Adapted from Mitchell, 1983.

follow-up data is lacking. However, the explicit structure of Mitchell's protocol has allowed a number of health professionals (e.g. Melton, 1985) to conduct similar debriefing sessions.

Other reports of psychological debriefing are generally similar to Raphael's and Mitchell's (Dunning & Silva, 1980, Wagner, 1979, Bergman & Queen, 1986, Griffin, 1987; Jones 1985), particularly with their focus on individuals and their needs rather than on enhancing group cohesiveness and resilience.

Healing theories related to debriefing

Several theories can contribute to understanding the effects of debriefing. From a psychodynamic point of view, trauma is a breach in the psychic apparatus' capacity to process reactive emotions using the available mental structures (e.g. Benyakar et al., 1989). Consequently both the emotional overload, and the impaired structures must be addressed by the therapist. From this perspective, ventilation and abreaction are the major healing processes to restore the economy of emotions. Ventilation and abreaction facilitate the individual's 'discharge' of his or her overwhelming internal tension, preventing the development of symptoms.

The role of the group process in affecting the damaged psychic structures is more complicated. The basic premise is that during group events several intrapsychic processes and structures are conveyed to the group. The group therefore becomes the source of the individual's stable identity and the site of his or her projected invulnerability and magical protection. When trauma ruptures the individual's links with the group, an intolerable sense of isolation, disarray and helplessness may occur (Dasberg, 1976). Debriefing may correct these effects by reestablishing the mutual exchange between the individual and the group.

Derived from psychoanalytic theory, is Van der Kolk's observation that traumatic memories are stored as iconic recollections rather than as verbal ones (e.g. Greenberg & Van der Kolk, 1987). According to these authors, the persistence of iconic memories precludes further processing of the traumatic experience, a process for which the symbolic function of language is required. Verbalization of recent traumatic experience is, accordingly, an important healing principle. A recent study by Pennebaker and Susman (1988) supports the idea that failure to disclose traumatic experiences can have deleterious effects on health.

Horowitz (1976) has emphasized the similarities between PTSD and grief. The intrusive components of normal grief (Lindemann, 1944) are, according to Horowitz, aborted and repeated endlessly in PTSD. This view emphasizes the therapeutic role of grief processes during debriefing.

H. Krystal's (1978) concept of the 'freezing of affect' and passive surrender to threat are also important psychoanalytic concepts for understanding the debriefing process. Individuals who are incapable of expressing any emotional reactions in early debriefing interventions may be manifesting 'freezing' and may require further help.

Lazarus' coping theory is also pertinent to understanding the effects of debriefing, in particular the concepts of coping strategies and traumatic reappraisal (Lazarus & Folkman, 1984). Appraisal is the process of cognitive assessment of an event. This perspective emphasizes the role of cognitive schemata in modulating stress reactions and potentially in the cognitive reorganization which can take place in debriefing. The role of coping strategies in debriefing is more problematic and may indeed challenge the appropriateness of this technique for all individuals. Some individuals, by virtue of their coping style, may do better when allowed to repress and forget their trauma. Research has shown that denial, repression and avoidance are beneficial for a number of subjects (e.g. Lazarus, 1982). Denial, however, is much less effective when the someone is reexposed; in the case of reexposure, those who seek information appear to fare better than those who avoid it. The possibility of reexposure should, therefore, be considered in planning the degree to which reactions to a traumatic event are worked through during debriefing.

The studies of postevent recollections by E. Loftus (1979) are important to understanding the cognitive processing of trauma and the resulting emotions. The work of Loftus constitutes an important, and often ignored, contribution to the area of traumatic stress. In a series of studies of eyewitness recollections, Loftus showed that memories can be transformed by presenting the subject with new information shortly after an event. Recollections could be either enhanced or compromised, and new objects could be introduced to the recollection. Substituting in the verbal description, for example, the word 'smash' for 'hit' after presenting subjects with a movie of a car accident, can modify the visual image recalled a week later (p. 78). Such modified memories persist for years – constituting the subjects 'real' memory of the event. Thus, Loftus' work shows a possible connection between the content of a traumatic recollection and the events that may follow the trauma. In addition, it provides data in support of early intervention, such as debriefing, in shaping the ways in which the event are remembered.

Social support theory also provides support for group debriefing as a way of enhancing social interactions. Two group phenomena, however, warn against simple assumptions about the beneficial nature of mobilizing group forces following trauma. Both the development of a negative group identity and the all too easy merger of an individual's identity with that of the group can be negative outcomes of the group debriefing.

Scapegoating and outward oriented rage are frequently encountered in groups of victims. These feelings are used to justify various kinds of retaliatory fantasies or activities while, at the same time eternalizing and often glorifying the status of being a victim. This can leave the individual in a regressed status of 'member of a victimized group'. Such an impersonal identity can result in the reaffirmation of social bonding to the group that then, by virtue of projection and hatred, may act out against real or imagined 'enemies' (Lifton, 1973). The history of Nazi antisemitism, and, in particular, the quasispontaneous emergence of the SA gangs out of survivors of World War I's trenches (Fest, 1973) is only one example of this kind.

Another effect of such a merged identity can be to prevent individual recovery. This has been as described in a series of clinical studies of the late Israeli psychoanalyst Hillel Klein (e.g. Klein & Kogan, 1987). Having survived a concentration camp himself, Klein warned against the pervasive effect of adopting a collective identity (i.e. 'holocaust survivor') as opposed to regaining one's own individual identity. The effacement of personal identities, according to Klein, results in the survivors' inability to mourn their own personal losses and come to terms with their grief. Individuation and separation from the collective identity of the group are essential for recovery. Debriefers should be aware of the need to conduct their intervention in a manner that opens access to individual grief – often at the expense of the merging tendencies within the group.

Common elements of debriefing methods

Debriefing protocols differ in their goals, their content, and their techniques. Various goals have been set by different authors including working through emotional overload (Mitchell, 1981, 1983), improvement of group cohesion (Griffin, 1987), teaching coping skills (Bergman & Queen, 1986), initiation and disengagement from the 'disaster role' (Raphael, 1986) and detection of symptomatic individuals (Mitchell, 1983). Accordingly, various aspects of the trauma exposure have been suggested as focal points of the debriefing sessions. Among these are the factual reality of the event (Marshall,1944), the emotional reactions of individuals exposed (e.g. Mitchell,1983), postevent elaboration and attribution (e.g. Bergman & Queen, 1986) and residual symptoms (e.g. Mitchell, 1983). Similarly, various techniques have been applied including cognitive rehearsal (Marshall), ventilation, support and resource mobilization (Mitchell, 1983), education (Raphael, 1986) and active counselling and teaching (Wagner 1979).

In spite of these differences, in practice many parameters of postevent debriefing overlap and all forms of debriefing have a number of elements in common. Debriefing is usually done shortly after a traumatic event. It is usually practised at the site of the action or within the same organizational setting in which the exposure took place. Debriefing is conducted in groups, with individuals who have been exposed to trauma. It always involves a degree of cognitive review of the event and has a factual basis. It includes verbal and emotional exchanges within the group, and results in the sharing of various levels of information and most often in reframing previous views and learning new information.

These commonalities indicate the need that future studies of debriefing examine the following areas: 1) the nature of the trauma; 2) the goals of the intervention; 3) the techniques used in the debriefing; and 4) the inferred mechanism of action of the intervention.

The nature of the trauma includes those elements that precede the intervention and determine the conditions under which it takes place. They must be taken into consideration in planning, designing, and analyzing the outcome of debriefing. They include attributes of the traumatic event (e.g. duration, type of event, etc.), of the group exposed and debriefed, and of the mode of exposure (e.g. passive victims, helpers, perpetrators, etc.).

The goals of the treatment are the behaviors, emotions, cognitive attitudes, and group factors that the intervention intends to change. Whenever possible, practitioners of debriefing should be explicit about the elements of the trauma that they wish to temper. Among the possible targets for the debriefing are:

1. Emotional dyscontrol: disabling affects such as terror, panic, sadness, guilt, sense of failed enactment, numbing and freezing of effect.
2. Cognitive dysfunction related to the state of increased arousal (e.g. narrowing of the cognitive field, inability to concentrate or shift attention, etc.).
3. Shattered cognitive schemata of control, security, invulnerability, etc.
4. Loss of the capacity to enjoy rewarding interpersonal contacts
5. 'Traumatic membrane' effect: perceptual and cognitive dissonance resulting from the subject's inability to disengage from the disaster experience and reestablish a continuity of meaning and experiencing with 'normal' life (Shatan, 1974, Lindy, 1985).
6. Traumatic conditioning: conditioned emotional responses to a variety of cues which may trigger intense negative experiences. Persistence of iconic memories.
7. Impacted grief: the inability to engage in a reparatory process of mourning.
8. Traumatic group effects such as scapegoating, projection, nihilistic and antisocial attitudes.
9. Improper information concerning the event, its outcome and the normal reactions to its occurrence. Several of these phenomena call for specific interventions, the outcome of which can be measured by psychometric instruments that are currently available.

The goals and targets can also be viewed as individual and group effects, both short term and long term. Table 9.4 suggests some of the different individual and group goals of debriefing.

Studies of debriefing must describe the ways in which the intervention is actually carried out and the technical procedures used. The description of the techniques should clearly define those elements of the intervention that are expected to affect outcome and hopefully also the supposed mechanism of action of the intervention. The goals of the debriefing and the techniques used should match the healing theory and the outcome measures chosen.

Conclusions

Despite a growing number of supporters, numerous anecdotal reports, and a strong theoretical rationale, the practice of debriefing needs further empirical study in order to be accepted by professional decision makers involved in stress management. This can only be achieved through empirical research that examines the immediate and long-term effects of this technique. As with other research efforts in the area of trauma, this is far from a simple task. Debriefing is, by definition, practised in situations

Table 9.4. *Goals of psychological debriefing*

For organizations
Improve communication between group members
Enhance group cohesion
Improve readiness for future exposures
Symbolize and attribute meaning to the disaster event
For Individuals
Decrease overwhelming emotions
Decrease cognitive disorganization
Enhance self-efficacy
Facilitate emotional disclosure and return of pleasure
Disengage from the disaster role
Learn new coping skills
Initiate grief process
Legitimize feelings and emotions
Correct inaccurate information

that are hardly conducive to research purposes; one should therefore expect numerous difficulties with regard to measuring the effect of debriefing. Given the current state of knowledge, naturalistic, uncontrolled studies, demonstrating an immediate effect on individuals' symptomatology, distress and wellbeing, may constitute a considerable step forward. The outline suggested in this chapter is an attempt to systematize the study of this technique and to suggest a number of outcome variables for beginning field studies of debriefing.

References

Bar-On, R., Solomon, Z., Noy, S. & Nardi, C. (1986). The clinical picture of combat stress reaction in the 1982 Lebanon War: cross war comparison. In N. Milgram (ed.) *Stress and coping in times of war*. New York: Brunner/Mazel, pp. 97–102.

Baum, A., Gatchel, R. J. & Schaeffer, M. A. (1983). Emotional behavioral and physiological effects of chronic stress at the Three Mile Island. *Journal of Consulting and Clinical Psychology*, **51**, 565–72.

Benyakar, M., Kutz, I., Dasberg, H. & Stern M. J. (1989). The collapse of structure: a structural approach to trauma. *Journal of Traumatic Stress*, **2**, 431–50.

Bergman, L. H. & Queen, T. (April, 1986). Critical incident stress: Part 1. *Fire Command*, 52–6.

Birenbaum, F., Copolon, J. & Scharff, I. (1976). Crisis intervention after a natural disaster. In R. H. Moos (ed.) *Human adaptation: coping with life crises*. Lexington: Heath and Company, pp. 394–404.

Bloom, B. L. (1985) Concluding summary. In *Stressful life event theory and research: implications for primary prevention.* Rockville, MD: NIMH/ ADAMHA p. 98.

Bourne, P. G. (1969). Military psychiatry and the Vietnam war in perspective. In Bourne P. G. (ed.) *The psychology and physiology of stress.* New York: Academic Press, pp. 219–36.

Cohen, R. E. (1976). Post disaster mobilization of a crisis intervention team: the Managua experience. In H. G. Parad, H. L. P. Resnick & L. P. Parad (eds.) *Emergency and disaster management: a mental health source book.* Phildadelphia, PA: Charles Press.

Cohen, R. E. & Ahearn, F. L. (1980). *Handbook of mental health care for disaster victims.* Baltimore: Johns Hopkins University Press.

Dasberg, H. (1976). Belonging and loneliness in relation to mental breakdown in battle. *The Israeli Annals of Psychiatry and Related Disciplines,* **14**, 307–21.

Dunning, C. (1990). Mental health sequelae in disaster workers: prevention and intervention. *International Journal of Mental Health,* **19**, 91–103.

Dunning, C. & Silva M. (1980). Disaster-induced trauma in rescue workers. *Victimology,* **5**, 287–97.

Fest, J. C. (1973). *Hitler.* Ullsteing Verlag: Frankfurt, pp. 171–93.

Figley, C. & Leventman, S. (1980). *Strangers at home, Vietnam veterans since the war.* New York: Praeger Publishers.

Gal, R. (1986). *A portrait of the Israeli soldier.* Westport, CT: Greenwood Publishing Group.

Green, B. L. (1986). Conceptual and methodological issues in assessing the psychological impact of disaster. In B. J. Sowder & M. Lystad, (eds.) *Disasters and mental health: contemporary perspectives and innovations in services to disaster victims.* Washington, DC: American Psychiatric Press, pp. 191–208.

Green, B. L. (1987). Long term consequences of man made catastrophes. In R. J. Ursano & C. S. Fullerton (eds.) *Individual responses to disasters.* Bethesda, MD: Uniformed Services University of the Health Sciences, pp. 39–70.

Green, B. L., Grace, M. C., Lindy, J. D., Titchener, J. L. & Lindy, J. G. (1983). Levels of functional impairment following a civilian disaster: the Beverly Hills Supper Club fire. *Journal of Consulting and Clinical Psychology,* **51**, 573–80.

Greenberg, M. S. & Van der Kolk, B. A. (1987). Retrieval and integration of traumatic memories with the 'painting cure.' In B. A. Van der Kolk (ed.) *Psychological trauma.* Washington, DC: American Psychiatric Press, pp. 191–216.

Griffin, C. A. (1987). Community disasters and post traumatic stress disorder: a debriefing model for response. In T. Williams (ed.), *Post-traumatic stress disorders: a handbook for clinicians.* Cincinnati: American Disabled Veterans Publication, pp. 293–8.

Helzer, J. E., Robins, L. N. & McEnvoi, L. (1987). Post-traumatic stress disorder in the general population. *New England Journal of Medicine,* **317**, 1630–4.

Horowitz, M. (1976). *Stress response syndrome.* New York: Aronson.

Hytten, K. & Weisaeth L. (1989). Helicopter crash in water: effects of simulator escape training. *Acta Psychiatrica Scandinavica,* **355**, 73–8.

Ingraham, L. & Manning, F. (1986). American military psychiatry. In R. A. Gabriel (ed.) *Military psychiatry.* Westport, CT: Greenwood Publishing Group, pp. 25–65.

Jones, D. R. (1985). Secondary disaster victims: the emotional impact of recovering and identifying human remains. *American Journal of Psychiatry*, **142**, 303–7.

Kaylor, J. A., King, D. W. & King, L. A.(1987). Psychological effects of the military service in Vietnam: a meta-analysis. *Psychological Bulletin*, **102**, 257–71.

Klein, H. & Kogan, I. (1987). Life under existential stress 40 years after the Holocaust: therapeutic aspects. *Journal of Psychotherapy*, **1**, 94–8.

Krystal, H. (1978). Trauma and affect. *Psychoanalytical Study of the Child*, **33**, 81–116.

Kulka, R. A., Schlenger, W. E., Fairbank, J. A. et al. (1989). *Trauma and the Vietnam War generation*. New York: Brunner/Mazel.

Lazarus, R. S. (1982). The costs and benefits of denial. In S. Bereznits (ed.) *The denial of stress*. Madison, CT: International Universities Press, pp. 1–30.

Lazarus, R. S. & Folkman, S. (1984). Cognitive appraisal processes. In R. S. Lazarus & S. Folkman (eds.) *Stress appraisal and coping*. New York: Springer Publishing Company, pp. 22–52.

Lifton, R. J. (1973). *Home from the war*. New York: Basic Books.

Lindemann, E. (1944). Symptomatology and management of acute grief. *American Journal of Psychiatry*, **101**, 141–8.

Lindy, J. D. (1985). The trauma membrane and other clinical concepts derived from psychotherapeutic work with survivors of natural disasters. *Psychiatric Annals*, **15**, 153–60.

Lindy, J. D. & Grace, M. (1986). The recovery environment: continuing stressor versus a healing psychological space. In J. Sowder & M. Lystad (eds.) *Disasters and mental health: contemporary perspectives and innovations in services to disaster victims*. Washington, DC: American Psychiatric Press, pp. 147–60.

Lindy, J. D., Grace, M. C. & Green, B. L. (1981). Survivors: outreach to a reluctant population. *American Journal of Orthopsychiatry*, **51**, 468–78.

Loftus, E. F. (1979). *Eyewitness testimony*. Cambridge: Harvard University Press.

McFarlane, A. C. (1988*a*). The longitudinal course of post-traumatic morbidity: the ranges of outcomes and their predictors. *Journal of Nervous and Mental Disease*, **176**, 30–9.

McFarlane, A. C. (1988*b*). The phenomenology of post-traumatic stress disorders following a national disaster. *Journal of Nervous and Mental Disease*, **176**, 22–9.

Marshall, S. L. A. (1944). *Island victory*. New York: Penguin Books.

Marshall, S. L. A. (1947). *Men under fire: the problem of battle command in future war*. New York: William Morrow & Co.

Marshall, S. L. A. (1953). *The river and the gauntlet*. New York: William Morrow & Co.

Marshall, S. L. A. (1956). *Pork Chop Hill*. William Morrow & Co.

Marshall, S. L. A. (1962) *Night drop, the American airborne invasion of Normandy*. New York: Little Brown.

Melton, C. (December, 1985). The days after: coping with the after effects of the Delta l-1011 crash. *Firehouse*, 49–50.

Mitchell, J. T. (ed.) (1981). *Emergency response to crisis: a crisis intervention guidebook of emergency service personnel*. Bowie, MD: R. J. Brady Co.

Mitchell, J. T. (Fall, 1982). Recovery from rescue. *Response Magazine*, 7–10.

Mitchell, J. T. (1983). When disaster strikes ... *Journal of Emergency Medical Services*, **8**, 36–9.

Mitchell, J. T. (1986). Critical incident stress management. *Response!* **5**, 24–5.

Pennebaker, J. W. & Susman, J. R. (1988). Disclosure of trauma and psychosomatic processes. *Social Science and Medicine*, **26**, 327–32.

Quarantelli, E. L. (1986). Community responses to disaster. In B. J. Sowder & M. Lystad (eds.) *Disasters and mental health: contemporary perspectives and innovations in services to disaster victims*. Washington, DC: American Psychiatric Press, pp. 169–79.

Raphael, B. (1986). *When disaster strikes*. New York: Basic Books, New York.

Raphael, B., Singh, B., Bardbury, L. & Lambert, F. (1983). Who helps the helpers: the effect of a disaster on the rescue workers. *Omega*, **14**, 9–20.

Salmon, T. (1919). The war neurosis and their lesson. *New York State Journal of Medicine*, **59**, 933–44.

Shatan, C. F.(1974). Through the membrane of reality: impacted grief and perceptual dissonance among Vietnam Veterans. *Psychiatric Opinions*, **11**, 6–15.

Solomon, S. D. (1986) Enhancing social support for disaster victims. In B. J. Sowder & M. Lystad (eds.) *Disasters and mental health: contemporary perspectives and innovations in services to disaster victims*. Washington, DC: American Psychiatric Press, pp. 115–29.

Solomon, Z. & Benbenishty, R. (1986). The role of proximity, immediacy, and expectancy in frontline treatment of combat stress reaction among Israelis in the Lebanon War. *American Journal of Psychiatry*, **143**, 613–17.

Solomon, Z., Kotler, M., Shalev, A. & Lin, R. (1989). Delayed post-traumatic stress disorder. *Psychiatry*, **52**, 428–36.

Solomon, Z., Schwarzwald, J. & Mikulincer, M. (1987). Frontline treatment of Israeli Soldiers with combat stress reactions. *American Journal of Psychiatry*, **144**, 448–54.

Spiller, R. J. (1988). S. L. A. Marshall and the ratio of fire. *The Royal United Service Institute for Defense Studies Journal*, **133**, 63–71.

Wagner, M. (1979). Airline disaster: a stress debriefing program for police. *Police Stress*, **2**, 16–20.

Weisaeth L. (1989). A study of behavioral responses to an industry disaster. *Acta Psychiatrica Scandinavica*, **355**, 13–24.

10

Relocation stress following natural disasters

ELLEN T. GERRITY and PETER STEINGLASS

The thing is, it makes you realize how fast and easy you can lose everything you've worked a long time to get. You find out that life goes on and that maybe there are more important things than money and possessions. These can be swept away in an instant. Family and friends, your happiness in life, is where it's all at.
(West Virginia mother, 3 months after a flood destroyed her family's home)

Natural disasters account for much of the damage and destruction of homes in the United States. During the years 1965–1985, 531 major natural disasters occurred in the United States resulting in widespread destruction and loss of life (Rubin et al., 1986). This figure represents federally declared disasters including hurricanes and tropical storms, ice and snow events, earthquakes, dam failures, flooding, high winds, coastal storms, tornadoes, and drought. The resulting expenditures of federal money reached $6 billion, with millions more paid by state and local governments.

The total cost of this destruction is estimated to be even higher, about two and a half times the value of building losses. This final figure includes the individual costs borne by disaster victims themselves, estimated to be an additional 75% beyond government estimated figures (Rubin et al., 1986). During this same period (1965–85), the number of dwellings destroyed and damaged is estimated at $1\frac{1}{2}$ million, with floods accounting for about 750 000 of these losses.

Tucker County, West Virginia, one of the communities in our family research study, was only one of the 29 West Virginia counties declared a disaster area in the 1985 flood. The dollar damage to homes, agriculture, businesses, and public property in Tucker County was estimated at $66.3 million. More than 400 families were displaced, and about 90% of the businesses sustained major damage or were totally destroyed (Bittinger, 1985; Teets & Young, 1985, 1987).

220

Home loss affects hundreds of thousands of people each year as a result of these kinds of disaster experiences. Homes can be destroyed instantly – by a tornado or a flood – or more gradually, through the seepage of toxic waste or the impersonal progression of urban development. The ultimate outcome is the same: the home is gone and the family must come to terms with the loss and its consequences. Although much has been written regarding the impact of disasters on individual and community life, little attention has been given to the influence of the home loss itself on family adjustment. Often this loss is accompanied by profound disruption, which affects the internal fabric of family life, social networks, community ties, work routines, financial income, and in the most extreme cases, the physical health or life of family members.

Because homes have enormous psychosocial and practical importance in the lives of families, the loss of a home as a result of a catastrophic event can have a lasting impact on a family. This chapter is devoted to what the loss of a home means to families, and in what ways some families manage to cope with this loss, while others are destroyed by it. Included is a review of relevant psychological and sociological literature on loss of home as a background for this discussion. Interview data is presented about family coping strategies from our study which focused on the mental health consequences of families relocated as a result of a natural disaster. Specifically, interview excerpts are provided from families who had experienced 100% home destruction as a result of a severe flood in a small town in Tucker County, West Virginia. The positive and negative coping styles of families are also addressed in this chapter, in the light of the theoretical considerations as well as the kinds of circumstances which may lead them to seek counseling and other forms of assistance following this serious disruption to their lives. And finally, implications for mental health intervention and future research are discussed.

Our family interviews were part of a study conducted by the Center for Family Research of the George Washington University Department of Psychiatry, 1985–1989. This NIMH funded study focused on how families respond to residential relocation caused by a major natural disaster, and how this response affects the subsequent psychosocial recovery process for family members. During the four years of this study, the project team collected data on site in three communities which experienced a natural disaster that necessitated temporary or permanent relocation of substantial numbers of families in the community. In West Virginia, interview participants were members of 40 families, including a husband, wife, and up to two children between the ages of 8 and 21. Three sets of data were collected over an 18-month period, and included self-report questionnaires, a semistructured family interview, a structured diagnostic interview (the Diagnostic Interview Schedule), and direct behavioral assessments of family interaction (Steinglass & Gerrity, 1990a, b).

As we begin our discussion, a description of one family's experience is presented in greater detail, to help place the experience in a more meaningful context for the reader. In this and other examples, family names have been changed as a safeguard to their identity.

The Webster family

The Webster family had owned their home in a small town in West Virginia for 10 years. Larry Webster was self-employed as a carpenter, while Kathy Webster worked part-time in her inlaws' clothing store and took most of the responsibility for raising their four children. Their situation was similar to many of the families locally: although not wealthy, their expenses were minimal, and their financial status was fairly secure. Their home was paid for, other expenses were few, and little was spent on entertainment, travel, or personal luxuries. Like most families in their town, they had no flood insurance.

The flood waters rose suddenly following several days of rain caused by Hurricane Juan, with the flood level cresting at 21 feet at 3:00am on November 5, 1985. The family left the house, escaping the flood waters by moving to higher ground. They stayed close together during the long night, fearful about their home, their friends and relatives, and their future.

What they saw the next day was shocking. Their home was gone. The depth and force of the flood had washed it completely off its foundation and away. Although the house was later found downstream, most of the remaining contents were watersoaked and unsalvageable. Over the next several weeks, the family made numerous trips to the destroyed home to confront the painful task of sorting through what remained of their possessions.

The Webster family moved three times during the following months, first to stay with Larry's parents, and later to a trailer provided by FEMA (the Federal Emergency Management Agency), and then to their new home. As months passed, family roles and responsibilities shifted. Larry had lost all of his carpenter tools in the flood, and continued to be unemployed. He filled his time repairing and cleaning his parents' store, which had also been severely damaged in the flood. Kathy worked 50–60 hours each week in the store, while struggling with the responsibilities for the care of her family.

Worries about the future were heightened by delays in the response from government agencies responsible for disaster relief.

Family strain between children, parents, and grandparents intensified as two families tried to live together in one home. The children became withdrawn and school grades started to drop. When government disaster loans became available, the long process of building their new home began. Rebuilding was fraught with obstacles such as severe weather, unreliable contractors, unexpected expenses, and lack of help. These obstacles contributed to daily tension and caused the project to be postponed again and again. Moving from living with relatives into a FEMA trailer brought some relief, allowing the family more autonomy, but also forced the family to live in crowded conditions, and to struggle further with bureaucratic regulations.

The problems experienced by the Websters were very similar to those of other disaster victims. The suddenness of the disaster, and the consequent impact on family life forced the family to face unforeseen difficulties and fears that they may not survive as a family. The loss caused immediate changes in the most personal of family routines and interactions, as well as serious adjustment problems as the long-term implications of the loss were encountered. But to fully understand what the loss of home can cause, we will examine what the 'home' itself can mean to a family.

Meaning of home

Since Fried's *Grieving for a lost home* appeared in 1963, the potentially powerful effects of home loss on individuals, families, and neighborhoods became a focus of much social science research. Fried had documented the depth and quality of the loss experience as one which closely resembles profound grief, and for some people, had long-term negative effects on adjustment. For these individuals, 'home' meant much more than the physical or social environment. The home was integral to the sense of self, so much so, that when it was lost, a reorganization of the self became necessary. For many of these individuals, home represented an extension of the self, identity with family, and a symbol of the future. Without the home, all of these things were threatened. In later works (1982*a*, *b*, 1984), Fried continued to explore the loss and relocation experience of these and other families, expanding his investigation of the symbolic and aesthetic properties of the home. Each of these attributes contributing to the meaning of home is potentially the basis for 'place attachment' for individuals and families, which is experienced as the 'positive affective bond that develops between individuals (or groups) and their residential environment' (Shumaker & Taylor, 1983, p. 233).

In the case of home loss, how strong a bond exists depends on the extent to which the needs of the individual or the family are met, the quality of the environment and, more specifically, how invested a family was in staying within a specific community when the loss was experienced. Determination of 'quality' is elusive, however, as it is subjectively determined. How satisfied someone may be with a new environment, even if it appears objectively 'better', may in fact depend upon how much it is like the old environment (Stokols & Shumaker, 1981). Some researchers suggest that one motivation for rebuilding a home on the original, but now hazardous property, is to enhance the familiarity of the new home (Burton, Kates & White, 1978; Kiecolt & Nigg, 1982).

The perception of personal choice as an essential element to what home means is presented in Rapoport's (1985) thoughtful review of the meaning of the home environment. Rapoport makes the case that 'if an environment is not chosen, it is not home' (p. 256). A crisis situation, by definition, often eliminates most of the options in one's ability to choose, while creating situations which have an impact on long-term future adjustment. And in most instances, available choices after sudden home loss continue to be greater for those who had more freedom of choice prior to the loss, for financial or other reasons (Bolin, 1985; Feld, 1973; Trainer & Bolin, 1976).

While an unchosen and truly novel housing environment can become a home, efforts are needed to make this happen, by transforming the key physical and social elements into something personally meaningful (Saile, 1985). The properties of home which can distinguish it from a mere 'house', include *order* (spatial, temporal, and sociocultural), *identity* (spatial and temporal), and *connectedness* (with people, place, past, and future). Sudden change can destroy these qualities, many of which might have been preserved if the change had been slower or more controllable (Dovey, 1985; Werner, Altman & Oxley, 1985). These qualities can apply to sudden destruction of other larger social units, such as neighborhoods, as well (Taylor & Browner, 1985).

In most of the work concentrating on home and attachment, theorists generally agree that individuals can become attached to their sociophysical environment, at varying levels of connection, and this attachment has important implications for both adjustment and loss (Heller, 1982; Shumaker & Conti, 1985; Shumaker & Hankin, 1984; Stokols & Shumaker, 1982; Stokols, Shumaker & Martinez, 1983). Within disaster research, investigators have attempted to look closely at this issue.

Home destruction due to a natural disaster

In disaster research, it has generally been assumed that home destruction which results in involuntary relocation will be associated with substantial short- and long-term evidence of psychosocial maladjustment, or even major psychopathology (Erikson, K. T., 1976a, b; Logue, Melick & Hansen, 1981; Rossi et al., 1983; Trainer & Bolin, 1976). One well-known example is the extensive study of the 1972 Buffalo Creek flood (Gleser, Green & Winget, 1981). The flood was caused by the sudden bursting of an earthen dam which released a tremendous mass of water and debris into Buffalo Creek Valley, in West Virginia. This disaster led to massive property loss, substantial loss of life, and the destruction of the community life. Survivors were relocated in multiple makeshift trailer parks at considerable distances from their original communities. As often happens after disasters, little effort was made to relocate survivors based on prior communal ties or extended family relationships. Relocation sites originally intended as temporary housing became permanent residences for many of the survivors.

The results of this study suggested almost uniform short- and long-term psychopathology in both adults and children. The mental health teams reported short-term reactions in adults, including psychic numbing, sluggishness in thinking and decision-making, anxiety, grief, despair, and severe sleep disturbances. Long-term responses (2 years postdisaster) including physical complaints, survivor guilt, listlessness, apathy, decreased social interaction, and chronic depression. Although this research study had serious scientific limitations (i.e. no comparison group, the interviewees were plaintiffs in a law suit, and interview data was largely clinical and not based on research instruments of established reliability and validity) these findings were compelling enough to warrant follow up investigations. Current studies of Buffalo Creek are attempting to document long-term effects while utilizing comparison groups and reliable measures (Gleser et al., 1981).

Community oriented researchers have incorporated into their studies community level factors, such as cohesion and community responsiveness, believing individual suffering to be absorbed by qualities inherent in the community response (Quarantelli, 1978, 1985). Difficulties arise in separating the effects of home destruction from the multitude of other stressors which occur after disaster events. Recent research studies have attempted to consider social context and personal attributes (e.g. family and social community) as well as characteristics of the disaster (Baum et al., 1981;

Garrison, 1985). In this regard, one of the most interesting studies of the mental health impact of relocation is a study of the long-term effect of Cyclone Tracy, which struck the Australian community of Darwin on Christmas day in 1974 (Milne, 1977). The disaster totally destroyed an estimated 5000 of the 8000 homes in the community. During the 10 days following the disaster, the community population was reduced from 45 000 to 10 500 people, largely as a result of a massive evacuation to communities that could provide medical assistance and shelter. The findings of this study indicated that those respondents who had stayed in Darwin, rather than being evacuated, fared best in their postdisaster recovery; evacuees who never returned to Darwin fared worst. Milne proposed that disaster victims who stay within a familiar community, with an intact social support network, survive much better in the long run than do those who leave their communities.

These researchers have investigated factors which are more specifically related to the home loss experience itself, e.g. severity of the exposure as measured by such factors as length of time spent in temporary housing, and the number of moves required to establish permanent housing (Bolin, 1985). Delays, especially those without sufficient cause or explanation, can contribute to prolonged distress. In disaster situations, disaster victims who lose their home should be assisted in returning to what they perceive as 'home' as soon as possible.

Within the context of research on families, the loss of home takes on a special significance. During the experience of home destruction, the family is exposed in an extraordinary way to their larger physical and social environment. In this instance, researchers have an opportunity to examine how families function during a crisis situation and to document the range and variability of family response (Bolin, 1982; Clason, 1983; Raphael, 1986; Solomon, 1986, 1989; Solomon et al., 1987).

Families and loss of home: a conceptual framework

How the experience of the family is understood is largely dependent on the theoretical and conceptual foundation of the research. Our research was most strongly influenced by four perspectives: family systems theory (Steinglass, 1987); social construction theory as applied to families (Reiss, 1981); attribution theory (Abramson, Garber & Seligman, 1980); and cognitive approaches to stress and coping models (Lazarus & Folkman, 1984) (See Table 10.1.) How these approaches relate to the disaster experience and home loss, is briefly reviewed.

Table 10.1. *Theoretical approaches to family research on home loss*

Theoretical approach	Key elements	Key citation
Family systems theory	Organization Morphogenesis	Steinglass, 1987
Social construction theory	Family paradigm	Reiss, 1981
Attribution theory	Personal vs. universal helplessness	Abramson et al., 1980
Stress and Coping Theory	Appraisal Emotion focused coping Problem focused coping	Lazarus & Folkman, 1984

Family system theory

Family systems theory is built on the assumption that families, as open systems, maintain their internal constancy through a continuous exchange and flow of information with their larger environment (Steinglass, 1987). Such operating principles as constancy, adaptiveness and change, order and organization, subsystems, boundaries, and permeability, all contribute to an understanding of how a family may function during a crisis. The organization within the family itself, as well as the interaction of the family and the environment, are of particular importance, at times more important than the influence of specific characteristics. According to this theory, a family may begin to malfunction after a crisis because the family system itself is unable to cope with the sudden change, rather than because of the specific impact of the new experience. Within the family system, individual members are constrained and shaped in their behavior by the nature of their relationships with others in the system.

Furthermore, core constructs within family systems theory help to provide an understanding of the family crisis of home destruction. In a functional family system, the membership is made up of 'those individuals whose constancy of contact and relationships produce predictable patterns of functional behavior' (Steinglass, 1987, p. 36), which can be relied upon for system 'organization' and maintenance. After a severe crisis, family members could rely on one another to behave in predictable patterns during the adjustment and resolution of the crisis period because of this 'organization'. A second concept central to family systems theory, 'morphogenesis', has to do with change and growth. Morphogenesis is the process by which a system responds to an event that is disrupting family stability, and which may lead to changes in the organization. First-order change may generate realignments of family elements; second-order change (often occurring after a serious crisis or problem) may involve complete restructuring of the system. The better the quality of information within the family system, and the more clearly it is communicated from one member to another, the greater the capacity of the family to grow and function effectively following a crisis.

Social construction theory

Another approach to understanding families in crisis has been developed by Reiss and his colleagues (Reiss, 1981). At the core of the Reiss model is the construct of the 'family paradigm'. Reiss proposes that, just as individuals develop social constructions about the world in which they live, families *as groups* also develop such constructions. These shared underlying assumptions about reality, in combination, make up a family's 'paradigm'. In general, families can be distinguished in three ways: (1) in their conception of safety or danger about the world; (2) in their belief about whether the world treats the family as a group or as isolated individuals; and (3) in the extent to which the families experience the environment as novel or familiar.

Social construction theory proposes that a family's coping response to stress is determined by the family's cognitive and emotional appraisal of the event, by the efficacy of the family's own response, and by the relationship of the event to the family's concept of its development (Reiss & Oliveri, 1980). Based on this theory, in one instance a family might initially respond to sudden home destruction by viewing the loss as a family issue, taking responsibility for responding to the event, and focusing on current, not past, family issues arising from the experience. Alternatively, another family may focus on its 'victimization', leaving individual members isolated in their experience, and make little effort to respond to this new information.

Attribution theory

Within attribution theory, the concepts of personal and universal helplessness are relevant to the process by which disaster victims seek to understand why a tragic event has occurred to them. The concept of 'universal helplessness' is characterized by the belief that an outcome is independent of all of one's own responses as well as the responses of other people (Abramson, Garber & Seligman, 1980). On the other hand, if an individual believes that desired outcomes are not contingent on their own responses, but that others have the capacity for such responses, a sense of 'personal helplessness' results, along with a feeling of responsibility, low self-esteem, and the potential for long-term maladjustment. Some victims believe strongly, despite evidence to the contrary, that it was their 'personal helplessness' that led to the disaster and that others would not have failed as they did. The important relationship is between the uncontrollability of the event and the perception of responsibility and failure by the individual.

Stress and coping

The coping process, as defined by Lazarus and Folkman (1984), also includes concepts which are useful to understand the responses of families following severe crises. In particular, the process of 'appraisal', whereby an individual judges an event to be a harm/loss situation, a threat, or a challenge, has an important impact on future actions. While these categories are not mutually exclusive – for example, home destruction can be viewed simultaneously as a severe harm and a challenge – the process of appraisal has proven to be a predictor of whether coping was oriented toward emotion regulation (emotion focused coping) or toward doing something to relieve the problem (problem focused coping) (Rochford & Blocker, 1991).

In situations which have a high degree of uncertainty, Lazarus predicts that direct action will decrease, and information seeking will increase. If these actions are not available as options, individuals may then resort to intrapsychic strategies (Silver & Wortman, 1980). In some cases, appraising an event as a challenge may result in problem focused coping, i.e. directing one's activities to solving problems, or cognitive reappraisal of the event through reinterpretation or developing new standards (Wortman & Silver, 1987). In other cases, appraising the event as harmful or as a threat may result in emotion focused coping, such as avoidance, distancing, or displacement of emotion.

Family coping

Our interviews with families following the loss of their home revealed many examples of both positive and negative coping strategies. After experiencing the disaster, families frequently attempted to make sense of what happened, and to behave in such a way as to make their understanding meaningful in their daily life. Whether or not the family's attempts to recover from such serious crises lead to functional or dysfunctional adjustment is an important concern for those offering both short- and long-term assistance to victims of home destruction. What follows are examples of the range of reactions appearing among flood victims whose homes were completely destroyed (See Table 10.2).

Functional family coping

For many families, the shock of home destruction generated a period of adjustment leading toward eventual recovery, as they attempted to make sense of the event in terms of their past and future life together. For some family members, the struggle focused on understanding what had happened in their lives; others directed their energy toward very specific coping activities.

Our interviews with families revealed three positive coping strategies. These were: (1) the reordering of priorities, especially the redefining of material possessions as having less meaning than in the past; (2) personal and fairly constant immersion into recovery activities, directed toward safeguarding what could be saved, and letting go of what could not; and (3) the development of a new understanding of the meaning or purpose of life; for many, a new relationship with God, or a realignment with one's family or social world. These coping strategies are illustrated in the following interview excerpts. (Note that the reference to time with each quotation indicates the time which has elapsed since the flood occurred.)

Reordering of priorities

The reordering of priorities as a coping strategy was frequently mentioned by family members. During the conjoint interview, family members focused on the ways in which the disaster had affected the home life and relationships within the family and the community, expressing their feelings about what was most difficult about the disaster and whether there had been any kind of positive outcome. Family members would often describe how the disaster had changed their outlook on what was now important to them, and what was no longer important.

Married couple, with two small children (at 2 months postdisaster)

Material things don't mean as much to me. I look at my kids and I think I don't need anything else. I was living with my mother and she would get upset if something got

Table 10.2. *Functional and dysfunctional family coping strategies*

Functional strategies	Dysfunctional strategies
1. Reordering of priorities	1. Displacement of emotion
2. Personal immersion into recover activity	2. Avoidance of social contact
3. Reinterpretation of meaning	3. Family conflict

broken and I would think, 'so what? I've lost my whole house. Why are you upset about a doll being lost, or a dish being broken?' (Wife)

I think we've learned to appreciate everything we have more. I just don't see it as something that can easily be replaced. Anything we get we are more appreciative of having. (Husband)

Same couple (at 16 months)

It seems like we don't work at the house. I don't know . . . before, the house had to be perfect as far as remodeling and working in the yard. We don't do near as much of that. Like it's not as important any more, it seems to me . . . Because it can all go in a minute. (Husband)

I think I'm less materialistic than before. Before I thought I'd never move again. Now, I think I could. I might have to. (Wife)

Married couple, with two small children (at 2 months)

It makes you stop and think. I have a lot today, but tomorrow I may not have anything. The family was OK . . . no injuries or anything. We were all together. It changes your outlook on life a lot. It makes you appreciate things more. Things you didn't appreciate before. If you can enjoy today, do it, because you never know what tomorrow may bring. Right? (Husband)

We don't put our priorities on our possessions now. We know that's not the most important thing because we can have them one day and one day they're gone. But our family, we were just happy that nobody was injured and that everybody was still able to be together. (Wife)

Woman, with three children (at 16 months)

I've changed, material-wise . . . You stop and realize and you think that we could have lost part of the kids. We could have lost ourselves. At least we're still together as a family. I think you learn to appreciate one another more.

Older married couple, with a teenage son (at 3 months)

Losing the things I lost, I don't put the value on material things now that I did before, and I don't intend to in the future. There were things I thought I had to have that I didn't need. In the future I think I'll be more careful in buying and not just have a lot of things cluttering up the house. All those things were just in a matter of hours gone. It took you 20 years to put in that house. I've talked to different people that really, losing their material things had really affected them bad. To me, none of us lost our lives or got injured, and that's really more important. (Wife)

Young couple, with one son with a chronic illness (just after the flood)

The jobs seem more important now than they were. Before, our home was paid for, and we had no heating expenses, all we had were utilities and food, so it was pretty cheap living. Now it would be more important if one of us lost a job. Whereas before it wouldn't have been such a big deal if it had happened before. (Wife)

Personal immersion into recovery activity

Personal immersion into recovery and other kinds of activity was another way family members adjusted to the sudden change in their lives. Rather than focusing on what was irretrievably lost, some families avoided introspection and became more involved in the activities of cleaning, repairing, rebuilding, planning, and organizing, in order to eventually achieve a stability which had been taken from them.

Young couple, with two small children (at 14 months)

It's like ... you do everything for existence. You don't do anything for enjoyment because it takes so much of your time to do the basics. I don't think we'd be so worried about the home if it wasn't for the kids. We're worried about them having something to call home more than we are I think.

Older couple, with a teenage son (at 2 months) [showing desire to immerse in work]

You can't do nothing in that trailer. You can't have pictures on the walls, you can't put underpinning on the trailer, you can't do this, you can't do that ... We've got a year. But it's agonizing to wait until next December to do anything, to know anything ... You can't paint or do anything.

Reinterpretation of meaning

Development of a new understanding of the meaning of life in a deeper or more abstract way was one of the cognitive strategies undertaken by some families following the destruction of the home. For some of the families this meant a renewal of their spiritual faith, turning to God to provide an explanation for what had happened to them. For others, the trust was placed in the relationships with their immediate family or their larger social world to provide a purpose for their future life. Some saw this renewal as a return to traditional values; others felt it was a beginning of a new understanding of what life meant, even if it resulted in a rejection of what they had believed before the disaster.

Elderly couple, in poor health, with a teenage daughter (Mary), (at 2 months)

The hardest thing for me was knowing I was going to have to give up the house because my brothers and sisters had been raised there, my mother and dad they were gone, and I had Mary on tapes from the time she was a baby and all the pictures. But I just said, 'God, you've got something better for me, and I can't dwell on it.' so in a day or so I just let that go by. I knew if I dwelled on it, it would be that much harder and it wouldn't do me a bit of good because there wasn't any way I could do anything about it. It was gone and that was it. So I just told God to take care of it and He did for me ... so I just believed in that and He let me know I was going to have another home and that's the only thing that's just been in my mind. I'd say 'well, you just wait and see,' because I knew that He just wouldn't let that happen and lose everything not to give me something better. I just felt that He maybe had to get that out of my life for me to see other things a little bit ... I just said 'God, my home's gone, you know it, and you will eventually replace what I need in my life.' That has always, from the day of the flood, been my motto. (Wife)

We have just tried to keep Mary's life normal. We were always used to getting things for her and letting her do things so she had a normal life, and right now we just can't give her everything like we planned on. But I'd rather do without something myself to be able to see that she can do something. (Wife)

My cousin ... he came in and helped me with my work. Then we sat down and talked a long time after we got done. It just really made me feel good. They want to help, you know. (Husband)

What really helped me; I go to church. Faith in the Lord and I read His word and if I hadn't had that, I don't know, and seeing the people come and help. I do a lot of reading of the Bible. That's all I care about is reading the Bible. That gives me strength. (Husband)

Older couple, with a teenage son (at 3 months)

I think it would prepare us for the future, things that may happen in the future. There for a few months after the flood, it was just like we had been in a war or something . . . A lot of us wouldn't be able to handle the situation, so it gave us a little bit of insight as to what we might be facing the future. We might have to cope with a situation like this again.

Young woman, one son with a serious illness (at 16 months)

I guess with the flood, it lets you know that life goes on. Even when a disaster does hit, it's not the end of the world. It gives you faith that God does give you a way to carry on. We had this one little picture . . . and the flood waters didn't get to it. It was pictures on the mailbox and it said something to the effect that if His eyes are on the sparrow, wouldn't he also take care of you? We've always been taken care of, even after the flood. We got through everything.

I think I'm going more into an Appalachian outlook. The Appalachian family typically clans together and shuts the rest of the world out. I don't know how to explain that, but you know what I mean. You're born here, you're raised here, and you die here, and you forget there's another world out there. You start out with another identity. I think I'd just as soon be a little hermit and stay here. It seems safer.

Middle-aged couple, with teenage children (at 15 months)

I guess maybe in the back of your mind, you're thinking, 'really, do you really want to stay here the rest of your life? Do you want to go on living here? Do you want to try again?' Sometimes I really didn't. (Wife)

It was the perfect time for us to have gotten out, but somebody had to be here to help get the store going again, do all the work up there and get it opened back up. My grandparents were getting old. (Husband)

Dysfunctional family coping

Not all family coping strategies were effective in producing positive family functioning. Negative patterns appeared with some families, evident at both the earlier (4 month) and later (16 month) periods of recovery. These included: (1) displacement of emotion about the disaster toward other people or things perceived as responsible, not only for the disaster, but also for the inability of the family to return to their preflood state; (2) avoidance of family, especially extended family, resulting in a sense of isolation; and (3) family conflict, expressed in anger and unresolved daily arguments. Eventually, the inability to effectively communicate becomes the source of continued family problems.

Displacement of emotion

Displacement of emotion resulting from the loss is often noted as a temporary reaction after sudden shocks. However, some families continued to divert all grief and painful emotions onto those they deemed responsible for the disaster itself or for their continuing problems.

Teenager (at 16 months)

Before the flood I hardly got into trouble. I used to have a job working at the drug store. As soon as the flood hit that messed me up. Then we moved out of town and I got to hanging around with the wrong people. I broke into a store and I just got sent off. That's what happened after the flood ... and I see it as caused by the flood. If it hadn't happened, I wouldn't have been in this institution and I wouldn't have broken into the store.

Young woman, with small children (at 15 months)

It's a positive change for me in that I'm getting to be home with the baby, but as far as I wonder what my future is going to be, it's negative that way. I gave up my job, and it seems like I gave up everything.

Young woman, one son with serious illness (at 16 months)

It was a loss of faith in the government, that the employees in the system would be so incompetent and everything would get so messed up and all the red tape that you'd be out of your home and didn't have anything. We moved a total of four times to our present home, and that's a lot of disruption.

The government representative was the worst. She just made us feel like we were scum, that we didn't even know how to take care of a place. That was the main problem. She was the main reason we got thrown out of the trailer, it was at her recommendation. . . . One day things got hot and heavy ... and my husband is short-tempered. Not long after we got the eviction notice ... it was the next month after they had an argument.

Middle-aged woman, with three children (at 3 months)

Here about a week ago, I got up in the middle of the night thinking about a bowl of flowers my sister-in-law had on a table in the restaurant when the flood hit. It was about 3:00 or 4:00 in the morning. I couldn't go back to sleep, I worried about those flowers, 'where are those flowers?' And why, I don't know, to me it's just a silly little thing. It really had no effect on me. It was flowers in her restaurant, not in my house, but I couldn't go back to sleep because of worrying about this bowl of flowers.

Young couple, with two small daughters (at 16 months)

The rich got richer and the poor got poorer. It's the way it's going to be, and that's the way it's going to stay. (Husband)

But I know one woman, I won't mention her name, but she has so taken advantage of this, and I know as well as I'm sitting here that she was putting on a big show. That's what it was. (Wife)

Avoidance of social contact

Some families withdraw from their extended family, isolating themselves as a family or as individual members from their connections with the social world. Although often perceived as necessary to protect the family from difficulties with friends or relatives, the withdrawal can lead to the family becoming isolated in their experience and severing all chance for future healing.

Young woman, with small children (at 3 months)

My family is the most difficult thing about my experience with the flood. They have the attitude that this is your lot in life, you have to accept it.

Young woman, with a son with a serious illness (at 16 months)

It's true that you can't go home again, and it was real uncomfortable living with my parents. As a matter of fact, I hardly go visit her anymore. I visit outside, but to eat supper, play dominoes, spend time, whatever, I've only done it twice since the holidays [3 months], and we're only a mile apart. It just made me back off from her and not be as close. I think I had more than my fill of her. Even though I appreciated having a place to live it was under her rules and her dictates and her moods.

Young woman, with two small daughters (just after the flood)

The hardest thing ... I said something about going through the flood, and she says 'Well, I lived through it with you.' I said, 'No, you haven't. You don't know the first thing about it.' Then she said, 'Well, you need to take them to church more often. You need to take them to church. You need to take them to church.' Which I know. We need to go to church more often.

Young couple, with two small daughters (at 16 months)

Our relationship with our relatives has gotten worse. It sure hasn't gotten any better. It's gotten worse. (Husband)

Family conflict

In some families, the conflicts appear among their own family members. But instead of leading to communication and eventual resolution, the anger is expressed in daily quarrels, effectively eliminating the possibility of the rebuilding of the home on an emotional level.

Middle-aged woman, with three children (at 16 months)

He's not working. I hate it. I literally hate it. Because we're in this new house now. I've worked almost the whole 20 years we've been married. When I first started out working I didn't have to. Now I have to, I literally hate it. . . . I hate the responsibility of all the bills. Then coming home, of course, he's been helping with the laundry and trying to get the kids to help with picking up around the house, but it's not always done. But there's other ways that I want to do things, you know. There's things I want to do, that I want to be home to do. When I come home from work, I'm just too tired . . . It's the same old thing day in and day out. I hate it.

Young couple, with two small children (at 16 months)

You're not doing much at all for my parents anymore. You're never there to do it. (Wife)

No, I'm always over there. (Husband)

This is going to be Divorce Court. (Wife)

When it snows, who goes over there and shovels the snow? I'm doing things now that your father would have done in the past, simply because I was down the road two miles. Rather than have me run up. But now, he sees me in the yard, and he yells over and says come over here. (Husband)

I'm not being mean, but that you would think that when we think it's just the opposite. (Wife)

Yeah. I'll have to start making a list. Maybe I should report in before I do something. (Husband)

Older couple, with a teenage son (just after flood)

We're having a time coping with our son. He's having a time. He's the only one not coping. We can cope, but he's having an awful time adjusting.

Mental health intervention

Crisis model/field intervention

Mental health services to individuals and families who have lost homes because of disasters are, like other disaster services, generally based on a crisis model, with emergency services organized quickly for short-term intervention. The National Institute of Mental Health has funded a variety of programs for disaster victims which have frequently involved collaboration with the Center for Mental Health Studies of Emergencies, the Public Health Service, and the Federal Emergency Management Agency (FEMA) (Lystad, 1985b).

Services are organized around several practical principles. (1) Provide mental health services in different settings for different phases of the emergency; (2) Give special attention to high-risk victims, e.g. children, physically handicapped, elderly; (3) Offer services for disaster workers who may develop trauma reactions as a result of exposure to disaster stressors; and (4) Develop programs adapted to cultural and regional realities. Services provided early in the emergency attempt to meet the practical as well as emotional needs of families who have lost their homes, and are often initially administered within emergency shelters.

As a rule, mental health services are organized around the primary principles of other kinds of crisis intervention provided in the field (Myers, 1989). Unlike noncrisis services, emergency mental health workers ideally work closely within the overall system of disaster relief. For example, a mental health worker may assist a family with its request for emergency housing, and, while doing so, will deal with the immediate psychological impact of this stressor on the family. This assistance may take place at the site of the destroyed home, at the home of relatives, in a FEMA trailer, or at an emergency shelter. As noted by Tierney & Baisden (1979), 'The need for food, clothing, and shelter can be just as much of an emergency to a family as the need for impartial mediation in an angry family dispute' (p. 42). This approach reflects the need to respond to the varying levels of response and the stage of adjustment of the family.

The specific phase of the intervention will determine the nature and scope of the mental health services to individuals who lose their homes. Early on, the shock of the loss combines with the serious immediate needs of replacement shelter. Later, families struggle with the responses of individual members to the loss, as they attempt to maintain or recreate family cohesion and build a new home. Individual members may differ in their response to the disaster and in coping style. If communication breaks down at this (or any) point, family recovery is threatened. Finally, mental health workers must be alert for delayed or long-term reactions and continue to provide services for families (Bornstein & Clayton, 1972; Horowitz, 1983, 1985; Wilson, Smith & Johnson, 1985). Crisis intervention teams can be involved in the training of local mental health professionals who will continue services after crisis teams have left the community.

Since disruption of housing after a disaster often leads to the dissolution of social support, an important goal of crisis intervention is to mitigate the effects of this disruption (Aneshensel & Stone, 1982; Bolin, 1986; Crabbs & Heffron, 1981; Lystad, 1985a; Solomon, 1986, 1989). Social support disruption is caused by either death, or relocation as a result of evacuation, temporary housing, frequent relocations, lack of transportation, or a breakdown in communication systems. In large-scale disasters, fragmented networks may be bolstered by the emergence of a 'therapeutic community' made up of disaster relief agencies, local disaster committees, church groups, and the less formal support of outside volunteers (Bolin, 1989; Drabek et al., 1975). In smaller disasters, victims may find it necessary to turn to medical or mental health professionals for psychological support (Tierney & Baisden, 1979; Waeckerle, 1991).

Mental health workers need to be more aware of the possibility that the destruction of the home may cause a short- or long-term grief reaction. The disruption of the neighborhood and extended family relationships may interfere with the mitigating effect of current social support. Supplementing social support networks is one example of mental health intervention, but equally important is giving families the opportunity to freely express their feelings in a nonjudgmental climate and assisting them with finding meaning in their experience (Janoff-Bulman, 1985; Silver & Wortman, 1980).

Children

Often, intervention with families is made in the form of outreach to children. Because the perception of stigma associated with contacting mental health professionals exists in some communities, children can be an important link between mental health workers and families facing serious difficulties in crisis situations (Stewart, 1985). This link is manifested in a number of ways. First, the reactions of children to the disaster are often watched closely by the family and the community. Children are seen as especially vulnerable, with their direct and indirect expressions of distress often difficult to interpret. Secondly, schools are very often the center for community intervention on the part of local leaders, mental health workers, teachers, and parents. Discussion among adult members of the community will center at first on the needs of the children, but then move fairly easily to the needs of the families and the community. Finally, while parents may hesitate to ask for psychological assistance for themselves, they will ask for such services for their children. Once initiated, family intervention can proceed. Many disaster intervention programs have developed materials to help families cope with the reactions of their children (e.g. American Red Cross, 1981; Doudt, 1981; Farberow & Gordon, 1981; Lystad, 1985*c*). These materials are generally available to families at disaster related community meetings soon after a disaster.

While contact with children may initiate mental health support to families, it is the family itself which is the first resource for the child. Whether the intervention is originally made with an adult or a child, eventually the family should be seen as the basic unit for intervention. The impact of the home destruction is felt by every member of the family, and within the family system, the reaction and coping style of each member will affect every other member. In communities where extended families play important roles, other relatives may be included as well, especially in those instances where relatives are providing temporary housing for the victim family (Harris, 1991). Research on the effects of temporary housing has most frequently examined the role of relatives (Davis, 1977; Loizos, 1977; Trainer & Bolin, 1976). Bolin (1982, 1985) showed that after a period of about one month, the relationship between the victim family and relatives begins to deteriorate, with interpersonal conflicts increasing as a result of crowding and financial problems. Temporary housing provides more privacy to the victim family but has features which can also contribute to stress, including relocation at some distance from the original home, transportation problems, and difficulties in obtaining needed services. FEMA trailers, often used as a temporary shelter by families, also generate problems among families. These problems are a result of inadequate construction, lack of timely responsiveness from agency representatives, difficulties in getting or keeping the trailer for the time period it is most urgently needed, location away from the original neighborhood, and the haphazard design of trailer communities. Difficulties are prolonged when families do not receive information regarding permanent housing, long-term loans, or contractor availability. Children can be profoundly affected by such long-term consequences of home disruption, and mental health professionals need to take these environmental realities into account when planning intervention strategies.

Intervention and research implications

Since all of the families described in this chapter experienced 100% home destruction, most were unable to use the process of sorting through belongings and memories to more slowly process their grief. It is unclear

Table 10.3. *Mental health intervention strategies*

Crisis model/field intervention
1. Respond to immediate practical needs
2. Mitigate impact on social support network
3. Monitor delayed and long-term reactions

Children
1. Link to families
2. Support family resources
3. Extend services to other relatives

Intervention and research implications
1. Targeting specific groups
2. Research/provider collaboration
3. Values and attributions
4. Methodology

whether families who have the opportunity to move back into their original homes are able to use this experience to help their adjustment. Those who have no home to return to have only their relationships and their thoughts to begin the process of recovery. It is here that these individuals and families begin to meet the challenge of their future lives and where intervention can begin.

Whether the ability to process one's loss is therapeutic or not is only one of several research questions which should be considered in future disaster projects (See Table 10.3).

Other research directions include:

Targeting specific groups

While we have focused on families in our study, most disaster studies have involved individual adults, or, in some cases, children. Additional groups which may be in need of special intervention efforts include: a) identified cultural groups whose perception of the disaster may be markedly different as a result of past experiences with disasters or differing attitudes about home; b) business owners or employees who have lost their livelihood, but not necessarily their homes, in a disaster; c) relatives of victims who help (or hinder) the recovery of victim families; d) emergent community leaders who come forward to lead recovery, but often discontinue their leadership role when the crisis period is over; and e) emergency workers.

Research/provider collaboration

The collaboration between emergency mental health teams, the local mental health agency, and disaster researchers deserves further exploration to determine the most effective way to provide needed services quickly. In many instances, disaster researchers can play an important mental health role while conducting research, particularly for those victims who may resist seeking traditional services despite being under severe stress. Participation in a research study carries much less stigma. It nevertheless provides an opportunity for participants to share their concerns and difficulties in an atmosphere that can be an important first step in the appraisal of stress and the formulation of coping strategies. Our research study provided the opportunity for families to discuss together for the first time the experiences they had individually and jointly shared during the disaster and afterwards. For many, the discussion provided understanding, comfort, and a chance to attach some meaning to their experiences.

Values and attributions

The role of personal values, attributions, and perceptions as they influence the adjustment of families who lose their homes is an important research area. Longitudinal studies extended to later in life might further explore the ways the disaster served as a turning point in the family's life. Cognitive strategies play an important role in postdisaster adjustment. Careful documentation of these strategies with current disaster victims can inform future intervention efforts.

Methodology

In disaster research, one continually seeks the right questions, methods, and approaches to capture precisely what is a profound experience that changes people's lives in dramatic ways (Solomon, 1989). Combining a human approach with scientific principles requires constant vigilance that the proper balance is achieved. Creative interdisciplinary approaches are needed in both mental health intervention and in research so that the families' needs are met, and the information can inform future efforts in both areas.

Conclusions

The experience of home destruction in a family's life calls forth many of the more extreme human emotions: grief, anger, dread, despair, as well as courage, selflessness, gratitude, and hope. In the context of natural disasters, the experience of home loss is only one of a multitude of events contributing to a family's emotions and future adjustment. But it is within the context of such events that the loss of one's home can carry with it profound symbolic meaning and consequent deep emotional pain which may affect the future of the individual family. It is important that efforts continue to be directed at research that will address the complexity of the disaster experience, maintain appropriate levels of rigor and scientific principles, and respect the unique experiences of families who undergo such losses.

Acknowledgements

This research was supported by Grant No. R01 MH40376 from the National Institute of Mental Health.

References

Abramson, L. Y., Garber, J. & Seligman, M. E. (1980). Learned helplessness in humans: an attributional analysis. In J. Garber & M. E. P. Seligman (eds.) *Human helplessness: theory and applications*. NY: Plenum Press.

American Red Cross. (1981). *Family disaster plan and personal survival guide*. Washington, DC: American Red Cross.

Aneshensel, C. S. & Stone, J. D. (1982). Stress and depression: a test of the buffering model of social support. *Archives of General Psychiatry*, **39**, 1392–6.

Baum, A., Gatchel, R. J., Aiello, J. R. & Thompson, D. (1981). Cognitive mediation of environmental stress. In J. H. Harvey (ed.) *Cognition, social behavior, and the environment*. Hillsdale, NJ: Lawrence Erlbaum, pp. 513–33.

Bittinger, W. (ed.) (1985). *Killing waters: the great West Virginia flood of 1985*. Terra Alta: CR Publications.

Bolin, R. C. (1982). *Long-term family recovery from disaster*. (Program on Environment and Behavior, Monograph No.36). University of Colorado: Institute of Behavioral Sciences.

Bolin, R. C. (1985). Disasters and long-term recovery policy: a focus on housing and families. *Policy Studies Review*, **4**(4), 709–15.

Bolin, R. C. (1986). Disasters and social support. In B. J. Sowder (ed.) *Disasters and mental health: Selected contemporary perspectives* (DHHS Publication No. 85–1421). Washington, DC: National Institute of Mental Health, pp. 150–7.

Bolin, R. C. (1989). Natural disasters. In R. Gist & B. Lubin (eds.) *Psychosocial aspects of disaster*, NY: Wiley, pp. 61–85.

Bornstein, P. E. & Clayton, P. J. (1972). The anniversary reaction. *Diseases of the Nervous System*, **33**, 470–2.

Burton, I., Kates, R. W. & White, G. F. (1978). *The environment as a hazard.* NY: Oxford Press.

Clason, C. (1983). The family as a life-saver in disaster. *International Journal of Mass Emergencies and Disasters*, **1**(1), 43–62.

Crabbs, M. A. & Heffron, E. (1981). Loss associated with a natural disaster. *Personnel and Guidance Journal*, February, 378–82.

Davis, I. (1977). Emergency shelter. *Disasters*, **1**(1), 23–40.

Dovey, K. (1985). Home and helplessness. In I. Altman & C.M. Werner (eds.) *Home environments*. NY: Plenum Press, pp. 33–64.

Doudt, K. (1981). *Helping your child cope with disaster*. New Windsor, MD: Church of the Brethren.

Drabek, E. E., Key, W. H., Erickson, P. E. & Crow, J. L. (1975). The impact of the disaster on kin relationships. *Journal of Marriage and the Family*, **37**(3), 481–95.

Erikson, K. T. (1976a). *Everything in its path*. NY: Simon & Schuster.

Erikson, K. T. (1976b). Loss of communality at Buffalo Creek. *American Journal of Psychiatry*, **133**(3), 302–5.

Farberow, N. L. & Gordon, N. S. (1981). *Manual for child health workers in major natural disasters* (DHHS Publication No. 81–1070). Washington, DC: NIMH.

Feld, A. (1973). Reflections on the Agnes flood. *Social Work*, **18**(5), 46–51.

Fried, M. (1963). Grieving for a lost home. In L. J. Duhl (ed.) *The urban condition: people and policy in the metropolis*. NY: Basic Books.

Fried, M. (1982a). Endemic stress: the psychology of resignation and the politics of scarcity. *American Journal of Orthopsychiatry*, **52**(1), 419.

Fried, M. (1982b). Residential attachment: sources of residential and community satisfaction. *Journal of Social Issues*, **38**(3), 107–19.

Fried, M. (1984). The structure and significance of community satisfaction. *Population and Environment*, **7**(2), 61–86.

Garrison, J. L. (1985). Mental health implications of disaster relocation in the United States: a review of the literature. *International Journal of Mass Emergencies and Disasters*, **3**(2), 49–65.

Gleser, G. C., Green, B. L. & Winget, C. (1981). *Prolonged psychosocial effects of disaster: a study of Buffalo Creek*. NY: Academic Press.

Harris, C. J. (1991). A family crisis-intervention model for the treatment of post-traumatic stress reaction. *Journal of Traumatic Stress*, **4**(2), 195–207.

Heller, T. (1982). The effects of involuntary residential relocation: a review. *American Journal of Community Psychology*, **10**(4), 471–92.

Horowitz, M. J. (1983). Post-traumatic stress disorder. *Behavioral Sciences and the Law*, **1**(3), 19–20.

Horowitz, M. J. (1985). Disasters and psychological responses to stress. *Psychiatric Annals*, **15**(3), 161–7.

Janoff-Bulman, R. (1985). The aftermath of victimization: rebuilding shattered assumptions. In C. R. Figley (ed.) *Trauma and its wake: the study and treatment of post-traumatic stress disorder*. NY: Brunner-Mazel, pp. 15–35.

Kiecolt, K. J. & Nigg, J. M. (1982). Mobility and perceptions of a hazardous environment. *Environment and Behavior*, **14**(2), 131–54.

Lazarus, R. S. & Folkman, S. (1984). *Stress, appraisal, and coping*. NY: Springer.
Logue, J. N., Melick, M. E. & Hansen, H. (1981). Research issues and direction in the epidemiology of health effects of disasters. *Epidemiology Review*, **3**, 140–62.
Loizos, P. (1977). A struggle for meaning. *Disasters*, **1**(3), 231–9.
Lystad, M. (1985*a*). *Facilitating mitigations through mental health services after a disaster*. Paper presented at the American Bar Association International Symposium on Housing and Urban Development after Natural Disasters, Miami, Florida.
Lystad, M. (1985*b*). Mental health programs in disasters: 1974–84. In M. Lystad (ed.) *Innovations in mental health services to disaster victims* (DHHS Publication No. 86–1390). Washington, DC: NIMH, pp. 1–7.
Lystad, M. (1985*c*). Special programs for children. In M. Lystad (ed.) *Innovations in mental health services to disaster victims* (DHHS Publication No. 86–1390). Washington, DC: NIMH, pp. 150–60.
Milne, G. (1977). Cyclone Tracy: I. Some consequences of the evacuation of adult victims. *Australian Psychologist*, **12**, 39–54.
Myers, D. G. (1989). Mental health and disaster: preventive approaches to intervention. In R. Gist & B. Lubin (eds.) *Psychosocial aspects of disaster*, NY: Wiley, pp. 190–228.
Quarantelli, E. L. (ed.). (1978). *Disasters: theory and research*. Beverly Hills, CA: Sage.
Quarantelli, E. L. (1985). An assessment of conflicting views on mental health: the consequences of traumatic events. In C. R. Figley (ed.) *Trauma and its wake: the study and treatment of post-traumatic stress disorder*. NY: Brunner-Mazel, pp. 173–215.
Raphael, B. (1986). *When disaster strikes: how individuals and communities cope with catastrophe*. NY: Basic Books.
Rapoport, A. (1985). Thinking about home environments: a conceptual framework. In I. Altman & C. M. Werner (eds.) *Home environments*. NY: Plenum Press.
Reiss, D. (1981). *The family's construction of reality*. Cambridge, MA: Harvard University Press.
Reiss, D. & Oliveri, M. (1980). Family paradigm and family coping: a proposal for linking the family's intrinsic capacities to its responses to stress. *Family Relations*, **29**, 81–91.
Rochford, E. G. & Blocker, T.J. (1991). Coping with 'natural' hazards as stressors. *Environment and Behavior*, **23**(2), 171–94.
Rossi, P. H., Wright, J. D., Weber-Burdin, E. & Pereira, J. (1983). *Victims of the environment: loss from natural hazards in the United States, 1970–1980*. NY: Plenum Press.
Rubin, C. R., Yezer, A. M., Hussain, Q. & Webb, A. (1986). *Summary of major natural disaster incidents in the United States, 1965–1985*. (Special publication No. 17). Boulder, CO: University of Colorado, Natural Hazards Research and Application Information Center.
Saile, D. G. (1985). The ritual establishment of home. In I. Altman & C.M. Werner (eds.) *Home environments*. NY: Plenum Press, pp. 183–212.
Shumaker, S. A. & Conti, G. J. (1985). Understanding mobility in America: conflicts between stability and change. In I. Altman & C. M. Werner (eds.) *Home environments*. NY: Plenum Press.
Shumaker, S. A. & Hankin, J. (1984). The bonds between people and their

residential environments: theory and research. *Population and Environment*, 7(2), 59–60.

Shumaker, S. A. & Taylor, R. B. (1983). Toward a clarification of people–place relationships. In N. R. Reimer & E. S. Geller (eds.) *Environmental psychology: Directions and perspectives*. NY: Praeger Publishers.

Silver, R. L. & Wortman, C. B. (1980). Coping with undesirable life events. In J. Garber & M. E. P. Seligman (eds.) *Human helplessness: theory and applications*. NY: Academic Press, pp. 279–341.

Solomon, S.D. (1986). Mobilizing social support networks in times of disaster. In C. Figley (ed.) *Trauma and its wake*. NY: Brunner-Mazel, vol. 2, pp. 232–63.

Solomon, S. D. (1989). Research issues in assessing disaster effects. In R. Gist & B. Lubin (eds.) *Psychosocial aspects of disaster*, NY: Wiley, pp. 308–40.

Solomon, S. D., Smith, E. M., Robins, L. N. & Fischbach, R. L. (1987). Social involvement as a mediator of disaster-induced stress. *Journal of Applied Social Psychology*, **17**(12), 1092–112.

Steinglass, P. (1987). A systems view of family interaction and psychopathology. In T. Jacobs (ed.) *Family interaction and psychopathology*. NY: Plenum Press, pp. 25–65.

Steinglass, P. & Gerrity, E. (1990*a*). Forced displacement to a new environment. In J. D. Noshpitz & R. D. Coddington (eds.) *Stressors and the adjustment disorders*. NY: Wiley, pp. 399–417.

Steinglass, P. & Gerrity, E. (1990*b*). Natural disasters and post-traumatic stress disorder: short-term versus long-term recovery in two disaster-affected communities. *Journal of Applied Social Psychology*, **20–21**, 1746–65.

Stewart, S. (1985). Families. In M. Hersen & S. M. Turner (eds.) *Diagnostic interviewing*. NY: Plenum Press, pp. 289–307.

Stokols, D. & Shumaker, S. A. (1981). People in places: a transactional view of settings. In J. H. Harvey (ed.) *Cognition, social behavior, and the environment*. Hillsdale, NJ: Erlbaum.

Stokols, D. & Shumaker, S. A. (1982). The psychological context of residential mobility and well-being. *Journal of Social Issues*, **38**(3), 149–71.

Stokols, D., Shumaker, S. A. & Martinez, J. (1983). Residential mobility and personal wellbeing. *Journal of Environmental Psychology*, **3**, 5–19.

Taylor, R. B. & Browner, S. (1985). Home and near-home territories. In I. Altman & C. M. Werner (eds.) *Home environments*. NY: Plenum Press, pp. 183–212.

Teets, B. & Young, S. (1985). *Killing waters: The great West Virginia flood of 1985*. Terra Alta, WV: CR Publications.

Teets, B. & Young, S. (1987). *Killing waters II: West Virginia's struggle to recover*. Terra Alta, WV: CR Publications.

Tierney, K. J. & Baisden, B. (1979). *Crisis intervention programs for disaster victims in smaller communities*. Rockville, MD: National Institute of Health.

Trainer, P. & Bolin, R. (1976). Persistent effects of disasters on daily activities: a crosscultural comparison. *Mass Emergencies*, **1**(4), 279–90.

Waeckerle, J. F. (1991). Disaster planning and response. *New England Journal of Medicine*, **324**(12), 815–21.

Werner, C. M., Altman, I. & Oxley, D. (1985). Temporal aspects of homes: a transactional perspective. In I. Altman & C. M. Werner (eds.) *Home environments*. NY: Plenum Press, pp 1–32.

Wilson, J. P., Smith, W. K. & Johnson, S. K. (1985). A comparative analysis of PTSD among various survivor groups. In C. R. Figley (ed.) *Trauma and its wake: the study and treatment of post-traumatic stress disorder.* NY: Brunner-Mazel, pp. 142–72.

Wortman, C. B. & Silver, R. C. (1987). Coping with irrevocable loss. In G. R. VandenBos & Bryant (eds.) *Cataclysms, crises, and catastrophes: psychology in action.* Washington, DC: American Psychological Association, pp. 187–235.

11

Group reactions to trauma: an avalanche accident

PAL HERLOFSEN

Avalanches have been a threat to humankind for as long as man has lived and travelled in mountainous areas. Only gradually over the centuries, and through devastating experiences were safe paths found through mountainous areas. Today, as many more areas are available to people less qualified and trained to master and judge the mountains, the danger of avalanches is much greater. This is particularly true in countries where cross-country skiing and alpine sports are popular. The majority (60%) of avalanche victims in Europe are skiers who usually are caught in avalanches when skiing outside marked boundaries. Other victims are caught in avalanches while merely travelling through a danger area by car or working in an avalanche area. As a consequence, huge sums of money have been invested in safety measures along the most travelled and vulnerable routes.

Avalanches are not only caused by sliding snow. Extremely dangerous rock and mud avalanches sometimes follow earthquakes, flooding, or heavy rain. These avalanches can cause disasters in areas where people are not expecting or prepared for such devastation. Volcanic eruptions with lava flow can bury whole communities. Avalanches may lead to other disasters such as floods caused by rivers damming-up, e.g. in Columbia, 1983 when 30 000 people died (Baskett & Weller, 1988; Lima et al., 1987).

In this chapter, I will concentrate on the physical, psychological and sociological hazards of snow avalanches, as it would be too ambitious to describe responses to all types of avalanches in a single chapter. This chapter will examine responses to avalanches, and the broader issue of the impact of *unexpected* natural disasters on groups and communities.

Avalanche disasters

Since ancient times, the Alps in Europe have had a reputation for dangerous avalanches. In 218 BC, the Carthaginian general Hannibal lost

248

half of his 36 000 men in the Alps. Perhaps the greatest known avalanche disaster occurred in 1970 in Peru (Oliver-Smith, 1979). Nearly 18 000 people were killed. The avalanche was triggered by an earthquake which released a combination of ice and earth which buried the town and surrounding areas of Yungay. The organizational stability of the entire community and region was disrupted.

Perhaps the most bizarre avalanche disaster of recent times was man-made and occurred during World War I. Austrian and Italian soldiers, fighting for the control of the Dolomite Mountains, observed that shellfire triggered avalanches in the area. Both sides soon began directing their guns into the high mountaintops where great snow masses hung. Avalanches crashed down into the mountain beds and in two days of fighting, using avalanches as weapons, an estimated 18 000 men died (Curr, 1982).

Avalanches of this magnitude have not been seen in North America even though quite a few people have lost their lives over the years. The worst avalanche accident in the United States, which resulted in the loss of 96 lives, occurred in 1910 when two trains were buried near Stevens Pass in Washington. Several days later, 62 people died in Canada when railroad workers clearing a railroad track from a previous snow avalanche were caught by a new avalanche (Churchill, 1923–31).

Recently, the Utah Avalanche Forecasting Center (UAFC) recorded all avalanche activity in the US between 1982 and 1987. Schaerer (1987) reported the occurrence of 145 avalanches involving 188 individuals. Of these people, 91 (48%) were trapped in the avalanche. Twenty-one people required medical attention and 12 were killed (13%). Of the 12 who died, 11 were completely buried. On the international level, the International Rescue Commission (IKAR) systematically registers information on snow avalanches. In Switzerland, data from the Institute for Avalanches from 1960 to 1974 indicated that only one out of 10 persons buried in an avalanche managed to survive.

Over the last 10 years, 69 people have died in avalanches in Norway (out of a population of 4.2 million). Of those who died, 21.7% were women and 78.2 % men. In one year alone, 1986, 21 persons died in avalanches. The number of deaths varies tremendously from year to year, depending on weather conditions and human exposure (Grossman et al., 1989; Ramsli, 1974).

Causes of avalanches

The ultimate cause of an avalanche is most often a combination of factors. The three most prominent are the quality and consistency of the snow, the

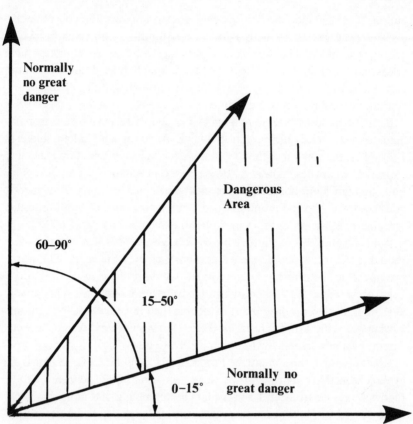

Fig. 11.1. Angle of terrain and risk of having an avalanche.

wind and the temperature, and the physical outline of the terrain. The single
most important factor for the release of an avalanche is probably the angle
of the terrain. Avalanches have been seen in areas with from 10 to 60 degree
inclines. Most avalanches occur in areas with 15 to 50 degrees of incline; for
most practical purposes 30 to 55 degrees is the range of most concern. These
figures are affected by a variety of factors such as wind, temperature,
snowfall, tree growth, etc. Angles of 30 to 35 degrees often result in larger
avalanches, whereas angles near 50 degrees often cause smaller, but more
frequent, ones unless the terrain has many natural obstacles such as
unevenness or dense trees (Fig. 11.1).

The weather, primarily the temperature and wind, are a major concern in
the prediction of avalanche risk. Most avalanches are released during, or
immediately after, heavy snowfalls (50 cm in 24 hours or a snowing
intensity of 2.5 mm/hour). The amount of snow necessary to release an

avalanche depends on whether heavy winds are present. If the relative velocity of the winds is 8–10 meters per second, snow will drift easily and, as a consequence, will build up behind natural obstacles in the terrain. The danger of an avalanche, therefore, will be greater. Even in winters with little snow, an avalanche danger can exist if the weather has been windy and snow has been transported and packed into exposed areas.

The last consideration concerning avalanche risk is the quality of the snow, i.e. the type of snow crystals and whether there are different layers in exposed areas. This again is dependent on the variation in temperature and on the amount of snow accumulation. Dry new snow often has huge particles of little weight which can easily create an avalanche hazard after a heavy snowfall. Wet new snow has heavy particles stuck together, creating the possibility of an avalanche. Hail is dangerous because it produces slippery sheets between snow layers. Frost can also reduce the friction between the various layers. Crust on the surface of the snow can create an icy, slippery surface increasing the possibility of an avalanche.

The causes of an avalanche are thus found in a wide variety of constantly changing and interacting factors. As a consequence, it is difficult, if not impossible, for casual travelers to predict the potential danger of an area unless actual on the spot examination has taken place. Even in an avalanche prone area with a reliable local warning system, it is extremely difficult to absorb the information and process the threat. This has been well demonstrated by D. Butler in his paper on the Southern Glacier National Park in Montana (Butler, 1987).

Mechanisms of death

The grim statistics for the survival of victims caught in avalanches are due to a number of factors.

Traumatic injuries

Avalanches, regardless of type, have a relatively high velocity; some dry powdery avalanches have their velocities clocked at over 200 mph. Survivors caught in an avalanche report moving from the surface to deeper levels many times during the 'travel' downwards. This explains many of the blunt trauma injuries found in both the survivors and the dead. Fractures, dislocations and internal bleedings are the most common injuries. The blast itself can cause emphysema to the lungs, and bursting of the eardrums. Data from the UAFC Statistiisk Arbok (1991) indicate that nine out of ten fatally injured, as well as survivors, evidence blunt major trauma. This percentage varies with the type and velocity of the avalanche.

Asphyxia

A common finding on autopsy is asphyxia resulting from body compression with acute respiratory and circulatory failure, and food remnants in the mouth and larynx probably due to external abdominal compression from the surrounding snow. Wet snow avalanches are the most dangerous because of their weight and force. If a person is completely buried, the chances of survival depend upon the duration, the depth of burial and the type of avalanche: dry floe avalanche or a slab avalanche composed of dry snow or wet heavy particles.

Both types of avalanche are dangerous. The first, dry-floe, causes a blastlike effect. The snow particles act like a heavy gas penetrating the nose and mouth. The victim suffocates if he does not manage to cover his face. Immobilization, with even a minor restriction on the ability to breathe caused by compression, is enough to cause death. Heavier, wet particles of snow will, to some extent, penetrate every opening. But the cause of death will be asphyxia from compression of the body, making it impossible to move the thorax. Wet particles also create a 'face mask' which makes it difficult to breathe. General hypothermia gradually sets in but this condition, in isolation, is not a killer. Temperature will fall slowly and, as a consequence, the body's need for oxygen decreases. Clothing, the availability of oxygen, and the physical condition of the person trapped are all important factors in survival. It is extremely important to realize that an avalanche victim, or, for that matter, anyone suffering from hypothermia, may look dead but may not be dead. Core body temperature can stabilize around 32 degrees Fahrenheit for some time and the victim will survive, provided correct resuscitation is started. Severe hypothermia is seen if the temperature falls below 32 degrees core temperature (Stalsberg et al., 1989).

The clinical signs and symptoms of hypothermia include: cold cyanotic skin and mucous membranes; markedly decreased heart and respiratory rates; and alterations in mental status ranging from apathy and poor concentration to coma. Apnea occurs at 24 degrees and asystole at 15 degrees.

The unconscious avalanche victim with hypothermia should not be handled roughly and should be kept in a horizontal position, otherwise s/he can become hypovolemic. Further loss of heat should be prevented through removal of extremely wet clothes, and shelter from the wind. If possible, oxygen should be given and cardiac activity monitored because of the danger of arrythmia. Warm fluids should be administered. It is important to keep in mind that warming up the victim externally creates the risk of opening up arteriovenus shunts. The ultimate goal is to get the victim rapidly to the hospital. Incredible stories of people surviving for days under the snow are most often explained either by the density of the snow or by their body having been sheltered by wreckage that created an air pocket in the snow. If the temperature remains low, and the person can avoid creating an icelike surface on the inside of the pocket, it is possible to survive for quite some time.

Psychosocial considerations

Large accidents or disasters give rise to a variety of psychosocial reactions in individuals and groups (Malt, 1986). The many faces of disaster will be particularly manifested in the groups most directly exposed and involved, i.e. the survivors, next of kin, leaders, and rescuers. Other groups, such as medical personnel and pathologists doing a huge number of postmortems, may also be affected. In Norway, models were developed for psychosocial support services following community, company, and communication disasters (Weisaeth, 1991).

Not surprisingly, the major part of research done hitherto focuses on individual reactions within the groups mentioned. There is a substantial literature on human reactions to large accidents or disasters. With the introduction of the posttraumatic stress disorder as a psychiatric diagnostic category in DSM-III (1980), there is a marked improvement in the diagnosis of symptoms and reactions of to trauma. It is, therefore, disappointing that a 'treatment of choice' for PTSD seems long in coming. We still tend to treat specific isolated symptoms in the disorder both by behavioral/psychological and pharmacological means. The complexity of the disorder is reflected in areas such as the phenomenology and specificity which are not yet well understood.

One major area that has not sufficiently been explored concerns the effect of group cohesion during the postdisaster period. It is recognized that the individual often is able to use the group for support and help during, and in the weeks subsequent to, a crisis or disaster and will benefit tremendously from a psychological working through (Heller & Swindle, 1983). Whether empirical and scientific proof is available to show that group cohesion *before* a dramatic life threatening event will provide better protection against stress, thus enabling individuals within the group to cope better, is more doubtful. Traditionally, attention has been focused on the individual's capacity for coping and working through. However, the importance of being a member of an already established group before a traumatic situation strikes is well established and practically implemented in organizations like the Army, fire brigades, etc. Systematic research where defined groups have been involved is harder to find. This is primarily due to the fact that it is not practical to keep closed groups exposed to large accidents or disasters together, both in the immediate postdisaster period and for some weeks afterwards to work through their experience in a meaningful way. It is also both complicated and organizationally very difficult to do a scientific study on survivors immediately after a large accident, keeping them together without outside interference, and making use of the group process. However, an avalanche in Northern Norway in 1986 provided the opportunity to study a group of survivors immediately after a large accident. This chapter will report findings from the work with the direct victims.

The avalanche

A military NATO winter exercise called Anchor Express was held in 1986; 23 000 men took part. The location was near Narvik, Troms County in Northern Norway, and the valley in which the accident happened was named Vassdalen. It is a long, narrow, roadless valley with rather steep sides. One can pass through by means of an old track, walking in summer or skiing in winter. The avalanche, as could be seen later, only touched the edges of this track. Unfortunately, due to the heavy equipment to be transported, a new path was forged in the snow that was closer to the mountain side. This was done by army engineers. Strategically, the exercise involved moving a mechanized battalion through this valley as a flank maneuver, a task considered very difficult under winter conditions. Geographically, the area in which the exercise was carried out was known to have a potential risk for avalanches, but this danger was absent until the period shortly before the exercise started. Weather conditions deteriorated during the last 2 weeks before the exercise; huge amounts of snow fell and temperatures varied from -2 °C to -34 °C. Wind intensity also shifted. Then, three days before the exercise was scheduled to start, temperatures rose again with more snow and a change in wind direction. This resulted in an increased avalanche risk, only partly discovered by experts already present in the exercise area. The avalanche accident that occurred in the initial phase of the exercise struck a platoon of 31 young Norwegian servicemen from an engineering corps, and caused 16 deaths. Fifteen other members of the platoon had been kept in reserve outside the avalanche area.

The avalanche which the platoon experienced while progressing through a mountain valley was a 'slab avalanche'. The velocity was approximately 35 m/s and the volume 20 000 m^3 with an average depth of 2.5 m, maximum 8 meters (Report to the Norwegian Parliament (Om Skredulykken i Vassdalen) no. 68, 1986–87). The density of the snow was slightly above 400 kg/m3, being thicker towards the edges. Of the 31 soldiers, 17 were completely buried, 13 were partly buried, and one was not buried at all. Six of the 13 managed to start a search for their comrades immediately, gradually digging out those who could be seen. During the one hour period in which the survivors were in isolation before help could reach them, they were able to organize a random search over the avalanche area. Two men set off after only 5–10 minutes in order to bring help, and had to cover approximately 4 kilometers on foot before the alarm could be given.

After one hour, rescue personnel with dogs arrived, and it was quickly established that 17 soldiers were still missing. The last survivor was found and brought out 3 hours after the avalanche impact. Three soldiers were badly injured and could not participate in the rescue activities. One experienced emotional trauma; he, however, was protected by his comrades and given an easy task to perform, i.e. to stand in one place to mark the central point during the search. The remaining 16 bodies were eventually found without evidence of life after they had been under the snow for from 80 minutes to 74 hours.

The disaster victims

In Norway, military service is compulsory and 80% of Norwegian males perform military service as conscripts throughout the country, the majority in Northern Norway where this accident occurred.

The soldiers in the platoon were between 19 and 26 years old, with an average age of 21 years. The conscripts selected for an engineering company are well qualified from civilian life, i.e. the majority have passed their junior college exam or have acquired some professional training.

At the time of the exercise, they had completed 8 months of their 12-month tour. The majority lived in southern Norway and most of them had not been home for approximately 1½ months. They were scheduled to go on leave right after the exercise and most had made calls to their families before leaving the barracks expressing doubts about the weather conditions.

The platoon can be divided into the following groups:

1. the dead, 16 soldiers (including 2 NCOs).
2. the survivors, 15 soldiers (1 NCO).
3. the remaining members of the platoon, the 15 soldiers who were left outside the avalanche exposed area as reserves.

Members of the last group were left to themselves the whole of the next day as they were too few to be mobilized for an effective search party. Little or no information was directed their way, and they learned about the accident by listening to military radio frequencies and later to the national radio service (NRK).

In this way, they were very much exposed to their own fantasies and, gradually during that afternoon, became frustrated and anxious. Their officers held a meeting with all of them at 0030 that same night and announced the names of the dead and missing. Despair, sorrow and hopelessness were dominant and very few, if any, slept that night. Time was spent talking and sharing feelings and waiting to hear if others had been found.

On the disaster site, the survivors had been evacuated by helicopter and track vehicles. Nine were admitted to the Light Field Hospital (LFSH), and six to local hospitals. Of the latter, two stayed in civilian hospitals for up to 2 weeks, while the remainder were sent home as they had injuries preventing them from finishing their military service.

Method

In addition to the clinical material, self-report questionnaires were used to assess stress reactions at different points in time. The following instruments were applied as they are often used in Norway and particularly in disaster situations: The General Health Questionnaire (20 question version), the State Anxiety Inventory (12 item version), the Impact of Event Scale and, the Posttraumatic Stress Scale (PTSS-10) (Holen, 1990).

The PTSS-10 scale is especially effective when screening disaster populations for psychiatric risk cases among survivors (Malt & Weisaeth, 1989). The scale has ten items, and there are only two choices in the version used – yes or no. The items were qualified one by one by factor analysis. PTSS-10 usually correlates very well with the GHQ (Weisaeth, 1989).

These four questionnaires were given to the survivors and the remainder of the platoon after 3 days, 40 days, and 60 days. The data collected later became important as confirmation of our clinical observations and reports received from officers and soldiers.

Acute reactions

When the men were brought out, they were all affected by hypothermia. In addition, some had dislocations or broken limbs. All of them had been thrown around when engulfed in the avalanche and, thus had extensive bruises. Emotionally, they were drained in the sense that they had mask-like faces, spoke in hushed voices, and were reticent to communicate with their surrounding circle. They obviously suffered from regression; this was considered functional for their ego and was encouraged during the first 24 hours.

Survivors, on the first day of the aftermath, expressed a shock reaction with blank faces, paralyzed movements, hushed voices, and a lack of ability to express feelings. Gradually, during the first night, sobbing broke out and comfort from medics was sought. The only female medic present at the LFSH became the most sought-after helper, and her presence seemed to calm the soldiers down with her feminine sympathy. During the night, they stayed close together in one ward and moved the beds so close that they literally touched one another. Fear and anxiety were gradually verbalized, but they remained mostly quiet. Following this, the group was 'restructured' in the sense that they were treated as adult men and the care work was gradually withdrawn. Then they became more reflective. Feelings of passivity and isolation were rather pronounced during the first day but gradually disappeared during the second day. The intense closeness and feelings of sharing strong bonds were replaced by other group phenomena.

Within 36 hours, the survivors were relocated to their barracks, and rejoined the 15 soldiers who had not been exposed to the avalanche. From this point on, the two groups (26 men in total, later 28) were kept together to facilitate and maintain the working through process occurring within the group or platoon. During the first 3–6 days the survivors and the nonexposed comrades struggled to find a common ground on which to function rationally. This became evident when they spent long hours into the night discussing who should go to which burial and who should represent them in the media and other meetings. Through this process, a new sense of purpose was gradually established, very much under the influence of the memories of their dead comrades.

For the group not exposed to the avalanche, the first 36 hours were very different. They had been getting little or no attention, had not been part of the rescuers who were searching for the missing soldiers, and only got information from the radio news bulletins. This lack of personal attention from superiors aggravated their natural feelings of aggression, anxiety, and sorrow for their lost comrades. Sleeping was impossible and mental arousal was high. As mentioned above, they were all relocated to their barracks within 36 hours and the platoon was reestablished. However, different phenomena surfaced gradually over the next week. After 2–3 days, aggression surfaced strongly and was directed outwards, primarily towards journalists, as the group felt the reports about what had happened were not accurate. The aggression became so intense, they actually looked for journalists to beat up. Aggression was also directed towards those responsible in the military command. In these situations it was important to enforce suitable social behavior.

As mentioned, the group *not* hit by the avalanche was aggressive; they seemed to have more intense feelings than the group who survived. It was as if the nonexposed group *competed* in exposing emotions and aggression, and struggled to identify with the survivors. People from the outside had difficulty identifying the avalanche survivors from the nonexposed group. Even direct questioning produced evasive answers from the nonexposed group. This phenomenon lasted for 1 to 2 weeks, but then gradually disappeared. This emotional 'letting off steam' by the nonexposed group with their aggressive, demanding behavior could later be affirmed through analysis of the questionnaires the platoon had completed on the third day.

The avalanche survivors and the nonexposed group were encouraged to perform their regular duties with shorter days and less intensity, and to sleep in their previous rooms that now had empty beds. They also packed the dead comrades' gear in the locker rooms and sent it back to the families. When the next of kin came to Bardufoss for a memorial service, the platoon met them and exchanged words of comfort. This proved very meaningful to both the survivors and next of kin, and continues to be an experience that is treasured. The platoon members were encouraged to participate in burial ceremonies at each dead soldier's hometown some days later.

Intervention

As the accident happened in a military setting, it was natural to use the well established military intervention principles of 'proximity, immediacy and expectancy' as the model for crisis intervention (Belenky, 1987). This was easy to achieve, whereas in a civilian setting, responsibility for drawing up plans for survivors in the aftermath of a large accident entails a very careful analysis of what tools or services – local, governmental, health or social – are available.

In the latter case, it is crucial to first concentrate on what is the best choice available. This should occur before one becomes too reality oriented and finds one's initiative crushed under the lack of social services, money, health professionals or other practical problems. One should strike a balance between the individual's need to be confronted with reality and his/her need and longing for support and care. The value of anticipatory guidance is well documented and implicated in Norwegian disaster intervention models (Hytten, 1990; Malt & Weisaeth, 1989).

In our military setting the men were thus provided with early anticipatory guidance about stress reactions that enabled them to recognize feelings both in themselves and in others. Individually, they saw a psychologist or a psychiatrist once or twice. They were allowed more consultations if they wanted, but very few used this opportunity. In addition, two group sessions were held within the first week both to monitor their working through and to give general information. Here instructions were also provided on how a psychological working through was done. Group sessions were repeated three times for the same purpose during their remaining 2 months of duty and were used to assess the current mental health of the platoon. With the additional help of a 'watching bridge' concept, i.e. close and extensive contact in the sense of caring for and looking after one another, much of the aftercare was left to the group members in the platoon itself.

In order not to disturb the hierarchy of the platoon, the military psychiatrists/psychologists deliberately kept a low profile. The emphasis put on their advisory role reassured the officers. Cooperation became smooth and uncontroversial; the NCOs and officers maintained their roles as leaders, and the basic structure of the platoon was not disturbed.

Results

As previously described, symptoms according to what we see in posttraumatic stress disorder (PTSD) were present in many soldiers in both groups in the immediate aftermath. It was clinically surprising that the intensity and severity of reactions seemed to affect the nonexposed group more heavily than those actually taken by the avalanche. This clinical finding was confirmed when the results of the questionnaires were analyzed. If we look at Table 11.1, the posttraumatic stress score shows this difference clearly even though it was often not possible to demonstrate a clear and statistically significant difference because of low power, i.e. low number of soldiers. The same tendency was evident in the Impact of Event Scale. This scale is divided into two parts, measuring both intrusion and avoidance. The results are seen in Table 11.2 and Table 11.3.

Results from both the questionnaires (GHQ and STAI) demonstrate the

Table 11.1. *Posttraumatic stress score*

	N	Mean	SD	Min	Max
Group					
Avalanche	15	2.80	2.54	0.00	8.00
Reserve	15	4.20	2.37	0.00	9.00

Table 11.2. *Intrusion*

	Impact of event scale				
	N	Mean	SD	Min	Max
Group					
Avalanche	15	10.60	8.51	0.00	26.00
Reserve	14	12.86	6.99	1.00	29.00

Table 11.3. *Avoidance*

	Impact of event scale				
	N	Mean	SD	Min	Max
Group					
Avalanche	15	7.87	6.33	1.00	21.00
Reserve	15	12.80	6.82	1.00	26.00

same tendency, i.e. that the reserve group experienced more severe and intense psychological reactions to the avalanche accident. Gradually, however, over a period of two months, the two groups swopped places in regards to the symptoms. At the follow-up one year later, the nonexposed group showed very few signs of posttraumatic symptomatology. The statistical computations were performed using SAS version 6.04 under AOS/VS on a MV 400.

Discussion

What is the explanation for these rather surprising findings? The enforced passivity of the nonexposed soldiers during the first days had obviously been traumatic as they had no chance to work through their emotional state. They had no reality to be confronted with because of a lack of

Table 11.4. *Trauma experience*

Soldiers	Avalanche exposed	Not exposed
Danger:	Present	Not present
Injury:	Present Some serious	Not present
Conflict:	Present Save oneself – look for others	(Not) present Stay together – go search for friends
Loss	Present	Present

information and thus were subjected to fantasies and uncertainty about the dimensions of the accident. Similar findings have been made in two other studies (Weisaeth, 1990; Weisaeth & Lie, 1990). One concerned merchant gas and oil tankers going into the Arabian Gulf during the Iran/Iraq War. The sailors were passive with no offensive weapon and had to 'sit it out', i.e. had to control and repress their own aggression. The other, concerning UN peacekeeping forces, also revealed similar results.

To understand this seemingly paradoxical result, one needs to examine the two different traumatic experiences suffered by the avalanche exposed and not exposed soldiers. If one analyzes the traumas, one can list the following traumatic experiences that they were wholly or partially exposed to (Table 11.4).

Whether support should be offered on an individual basis with counseling and therapy, or by focusing more on the setting and the surroundings as in group therapy, is in our view highly dependent on the preexisting group structure. The experience from an oil rig accident is that support from colleagues is valued more highly than other support during the first half year – 1 year after the disaster (Holen, 1990). In this avalanche accident, the platoon itself and the fact that they had been together 8 months underlined the intensity of the social dynamics. Social network in the platoon consisted of the same elements as in civilian life, but fellow servicemen were present and available at all times. The following diagram can be drawn:

Civilian life	*Army life*
Family	Family
Friends	Friends in the platoon
Colleagues	Squad members
Neighbors	Roommates

Bearing this in mind, it seems clear that the opportunity to positively influence the social dynamics of the group will be rather good in a military situation.

The social network consists of two important factors:

1. How extensive it is, i.e. how many are actually available.
2. The quality. The quality can be measured by emotional availability, closeness, perseverance, and refractoriness.

Within a platoon where cohesion is strong, personal friends, colleagues, and fellow squad members were present. Family, however, will be missed. The quality elements in '2' are also available. This should ensure that the group itself is characterized by cohesion and dedication, thus becoming an excellent emotional working place. However, the leaders' task will be to constantly guard the group's borders as the balance between fight/flight is delicate and potentially destructive. The group must be a safe place to express emotions and care for one another. But the leader must also lead, i.e. make demands from the group and enforce army regulations. The group's social behavior should also be closely observed.

Generally speaking, treatment groups can be divided into three categories (Foulkes & Anthony, 1957):

1. Activity groups
2. Therapeutic groups
3. Psychotherapeutic groups

The first category contains groups whose active role in the disaster may have had a therapeutic effect on the participants. This might not have been the original intention. In the second category, therapeutic groups are given tasks to perform with a specific therapeutic purpose. The psychotherapeutic group is based on the following principles of treatment (Bloch & Crouch, 1985):

1. The group relies on verbal communication.
2. Every individual member is ensured room for change.
3. The group itself is the main body for psychological work.

In the present case, we found that the optimal working through was provided by a combination of elements from all three categories. With the structure already present, it was important to ensure that the working through of the event guaranteed each individual enough scope for active individual participation. It was also important that he considered his participation to be the necessary therapeutic factor ensuring change. The possibility for individual support, mutual acceptance, and reassurance concerning self-identity strengthened the individual's emotional defenses. At the same time, the group itself gradually helped different individuals exercise or practise social control, so that 'letting off steam', as in the journalist witch hunt, could be avoided (Klein, 1985). The leadership, i.e. the officers, had to exercise great self-restraint to 'keep their hands off' as group processes became intense and violent action could be triggered off.

The group process shifted from a state of dependency towards fight/ flight and ended up with pairing. Theoretically, this can be understood in the context of group analytic thinking, particularly through the Basic Assumption Theory. It is interesting to note that the group will, according to the theory, oscillate from stage to stage depending on a variety of factors. W. R. Bion (1961) was the first to formulate this Basic Assumption Theory, which was developed during the Second World War in a psychiatric military hospital. The theory is useful in understanding the group dynamic processes in groups affected by a common problem, and to some extent left to work with it. The regression and dependency observed in the survivors during the first few days indicated that the leaders needed to provide protection and nourishment, both in a material and spiritual sense. Emotional availability became a new challenge for the officers which could be integrated into their thinking at an early stage. It could be elaborated on as the survivors entered the action-prone stage, i.e. fight/flight, when aggression surfaced easily as demonstrated by their angry feelings towards the journalists. Flight was also prominent in that many wanted to avoid the burial ceremonies.

For the nonexposed group, the initial insecurity and shock quickly evolved into fight/flight, and later pairing, as they tried to become closer to the survivors. New friendships and loyalties were formed, privileges fought for, e.g. in connection with who would represent them in different matters, and strong feelings of envy surfaced. This threatened cohesion, potentially ending in fights. The oscillation between these three stages, seen in both groups but often at different times, became less pronounced over a period of one month. By this time, the platoon had integrated both groups and had been rebuilt as a working group, i.e. a regular engineering platoon. Difficulties could still surface but were handled by the platoon or company with more ease.

Conclusions

The most interesting finding is the marked difference between the two groups immediately after the avalanche particularly in view of the totally different kinds of trauma they were exposed to. Also interesting is the lack of PTSD in both groups at the 17 month follow-up. Individual symptoms were seen but no one could be diagnosed as suffering from PTSD according to DSM-III-R criteria. Feelings of vulnerability were present but, at the time, of no clinical significance. Time will show whether this will become more important over the years. For the nonexposed group, the passivity and group processes can account for the reactions seen during the first weeks. Later, during the working through, the intensity of emotions faded away and was replaced by a mourning process, leading to a complete recovery. The emotions in the exposed group gradually grew and flattened out during the first 2–5 weeks, then diminished.

The lack of PTSD is more difficult to explain. A combination of factors proved important. First, the pre-existing group structure and the insight into one's own and others' emotions allowed group processes to develop. Another important factor was the struggle with the bereavement process, gradual coping with aggression, and a command structure that was aware and willing to let emotions be played out in the group context. Finally, intervention by military mental health professionals, both in an advisory capacity and in a practical working through, was also crucial.

The most important lessons learned are that, in any crisis, unexpected behavior patterns can be activated and become quite severe in the presence of guilt, rage, and helplessness (loss of comrades) (Lindemann, 1944). The task to contain the major part of the surfacing emotions can be done in a group, provided enough room is given to its members to work with their inner feelings and also the outer world. Leaders should be advised to enforce limits, allowing ample reality testing.

Guiding the process of satisfactory working through psychological trauma in a group setting should not be considered a hopelessly daunting challenge. In the present case, the main tool used to cope with emotions was the group itself. Support, gradual insight into one's own and others' emotions, and the struggle with denial, aggression, and sorrow were features strongly present in the platoon. Thus, 'treatment' had to be incorporated in the planning and carrying out of the daily routines which the platoon had to perform.

Knowledge of group processes can indeed be a powerful tool and should be integrated in support programs, particularly when closed groups are affected by physical and psychological trauma.

References

Baskett, P. & Weller, R. (eds.). (1988). *Medicine for disasters*. London: Butterworth & Co. Ltd.

Belenky G. (ed.) (1987). *Contemporary studies in combat psychiatry*. New York: Greenwood Press.

Bion, W. R. (1961). *Experiences in groups*. London: Tavistock Publications.

Bloch, S. & Crouch, E. (1985). *Therapeutic factors in group psychotherapy*. London: Oxford University Press.

Butler, D. (1987). Snow-avalanche hazards: the nature of local knowledge and individual responses. *Disasters*, **11**(3), 214–20.

Churchill, W. (1923–31). *The world crisis*. London: Butterworth & Co., Ltd, vol. 2.

Curr, D. (1982). Avalanches, the white terror. *National Geographic*, **162**(3), 290–305.

Foulkes, S. H. & Anthony, E. J. (1957). *Group psychotherapy*. London: Maresfield Reprints.

Grossman M., Saffle, J., Thomas, F. & Temper, B. (1989). Avalanche trauma. *The Journal of Trauma*, **29**(12), 1705–9.

Heller, K. & Swindle, R. W. (1983). Social networks, perceived, social support, and coping with stress. In R. D. Felner, L. A. Jason & Moritsugu, J. et al. (eds.) *Preventive psychology: theory, research and practice in community intervention*. New York: Pergamon Press.

Holen, A. (1990). *A long-time outcome study of survivors from a disaster*. Dissertation, University of Oslo. Department of Psychiatry. Faculty of Medicine. Falck Hurtigtrykk a/s. Oslo.

Hytten, K. (1990). Studies on stress and coping: psychosocial and physical dangers. Establishment and manifestations of negative and positive response outcome expectancies. Medical Faculty, University of Oslo.

Klein, H. (1985). Some principles of short-term group therapy. *International Journal of Group Psychotherapy*, **35**(3)

Lima, B. R., Pai, S., Santacruz, H., Lozano, J. & Luna, J. (1987). Screening for the psychological consequence of a major disaster in a developing country: Armero, Colombia. *Acta Psychiatric Scandinavia*, **76**, 561–7.

Lindemann, E. (1944). Symptomatology and management of acute grief. *American Journal of Psychiatry*, **101**, 141–8.

Malt, U. (1986). Biopsychological aspects of accidental injuries. Dissertation, University of Oslo, Faculty of Medicine, Oslo.

Malt, U. & Weisaeth, L. (ed.). (1989). Traumatic stress: Empirical studies from Norway. *Acta Psychiatrica Scandinavica*, **80**(Suppl.), 63–72.

Oliver-Smith, A. (1979). The Yungay Avalanche of 1970: anthropological perspectives on disaster and social change. *Disasters*, **3**(1), 95–101.

Om Skredulykken i Vassdalen (5. mars 1986). St. Meld. nr. 68 1986–87. (About the Avalanche accident in Vassdalen 1986). In Report to the Norwegian Parliament no. 68, 1986–87. Forsvarsdepartementet (Department of Defense) Oslo.

Ramsli, G. (1974). Avalanche problems in Norway. In G. F. White (ed.) *Natural hazards – local, national, global*. London: Oxford University Press, pp. 175–80.

Schaerer, P. (ed.). (1987). Avalanche accidents in Canada. *Avalanche News*, **23**,

Stalsberg, H., Albretsen, C., Gilbert, M. et al. (1989). Mechanism of death in avalanche victims. *Virchows Archiv A Pathological Anatomy*, **414**, 415–22.

Statistisk Arbok (1991) Oslo. (*Statistical Yearbook of Norway, 1991*, The Central Bureau of Statistics of Norway), pp. 72–5. Fabritius a/s.

Weisaeth, L. (1989). Torture of a Norwegian ship's crew. *Acta Psychiatrica Scandinavica*, **80**(355), 56–62.

Weisaeth, L. (1990). Stress on UN military peace keeping. *WISMIC Newsletter*, **2**(2), 15–18.
Weisaeth, L. (1991). The psychiatrist's role in preventing psychopathological effects of disaster trauma. In A. Seva (ed.) *The European handbook of psychiatry and mental health*. Barcelona: Editorial Anthropos, pp. 2342–58.
Weisaeth, L. & Lie, T. (1990). Post-traumatic stress reactions in sailors exposed to terror attacks. In *Proceedings from the Second International Conference, Wartime Medical Services*. Stockholm, pp. 158–69.

12

Community responses to disaster: the Gander plane crash

KATHLEEN M. WRIGHT and PAUL T. BARTONE

Several theoretical approaches or models are available to those interested in studying community responses to disaster and trauma. Unfortunately, recent experience with disasters proves that these models are overly restrictive. This chapter draws on observations following a major military air disaster to develop a new, expanded model of the impact on communities from such events. This model avoids the key restrictions of earlier models.

One critical restriction of community disaster models is the principal level of analysis that is adopted. Some models focus on individuals within the community, and aggregate individual reactions to form a picture of community response. Others view the community as a social unit that must be considered as a separate entity. These different views are usually assumed to be mutually exclusive, leading to a debate over which is more correct (Melick, 1985; Quarantelli, 1985; Powell & Penick, 1983; Tierney, 1986).

Tierney (1986) summarizes the controversy about theoretical orientation. Each orientation focuses either on a group or an individual level of analysis to the exclusion of the other. Those researchers who assume a community perspective conclude that psychological effects following disaster are minimal and short term, and that poor outcomes arise from inadequate disaster planning and resources on the part of community organizations (Quarantelli, 1985). The alternative orientation is a 'psychological trauma' perspective. It concludes that the catastrophic nature of the event and the subsequent trauma of dealing with the experience and its aftermath result in significant, adverse, and typically long-term psychological effects (Erikson, 1976; Lifton & Olson, 1976).

Another important restriction of community disaster models relates to disaster victim classification models. Existing models typically restrict their perspectives to the disaster site and to the immediate postimpact phase. Potential 'victims' at risk for traumatization are identified on the basis of maximum exposure (Berren, Beigel, & Ghertner, 1980; Dudasik, 1980; Frazer & Taylor, 1982). Current orientations and classification models thus fail to adequately describe the complexity, duration and potential spread of the effects of disasters on communities. This is especially true as communities become more 'global'.

The Gander military air disaster

On December 12, 1985 a chartered airliner stopped at Gander, Newfoundland to refuel. Shortly after takeoff, the aircraft stalled and crashed into the forest at the end of the runway, exploding on impact, and killing all on board. The snowy crash site cut a long swath of burned and broken trees and debris. Bodies, equipment, and personal possessions were strewn over a wide area. The flight carried 8 aircrew and 248 US Army soldiers, members of the elite 101st Airborne Division from Ft Campbell, Kentucky. They were returning home after six months of United Nations peacekeeping duty in the Sinai desert. The families of these soldiers awaited their homecoming, and a number of them gathered in the Brigade gymnasium at Ft Campbell to prepare for the celebration.

Word of the tragedy reached Ft Campbell headquarters shortly after the crash. During the next frantic hours, confirmation of the flight manifest began and families were notified to assemble in the Brigade gymnasium for an announcement. At Gander, Department of Defense personnel worked with Canadian officials to recover the bodies, equipment, and victims' personal possessions. Over the next few days the bodies and personal effects were transported with formal military escort to Dover Air Force Base, Delaware, the largest mortuary in the Department of Defense. The extensive mortuary and body identification process continued for two months and directly involved more than a thousand professional and volunteer participants.

The Army dead included one-third of the battalion representing US Armed Forces in the Sinai. Approximately one-third of these soldiers were married and lived at Ft Campbell, a tightly knit military community straddling the border between Kentucky and Tennessee. The crash shattered the community and deprived 36 children of their fathers. It was the US Army's deadliest single-incident tragedy in peacetime and the worst aviation disaster ever to occur on Canadian soil (Wright, 1987).

Individuals, groups, and organizations affected by the Gander crash extended far beyond the borders of the Ft Campbell community. Those most profoundly affected had significant relationships with the victims, such as next of kin, leaders, and other unit members (Bartone & Wright, 1990). In addition, Gander crash site workers, Dover mortuary personnel, and many organizations and individuals were profoundly affected by their experiences (Bartone et al., 1989; Garrigan, 1987; Harris, 1986; Radke, 1987; Ursano et al., 1988).

Observations and interview data following the Gander crash revealed an unexpected level of complexity in the communities affected by the disaster. The Gander report (Wright, 1987) summarizes the observations of a small research team that documented the experiences of affected individuals and groups immediately following the crash. The research concluded that an adequate model of human response to disaster should include at least four factors: variation in responses over time; individual, group and formal organizations as levels of analysis; effects on multiple community sites resulting from the extensive and intricate nature of postdisaster participant involvement; and a broadened concept of individuals and groups at risk following exposure to trauma (Ingraham, 1987*b*).

The report concludes that military disasters frequently involve more than one community as a result of the nature of military operations and organizational structures. In the case of the Gander crash, three different community sites were directly affected: the crash site at Gander, Newfoundland; the mortuary site at Dover Air Force base; and the victims' home base site at Ft Campbell, Kentucky. Although these were the predominant sites, families and friends of the victims were located in many different civilian communities throughout the nation. In addition, the crash affected military communities around the world. The military is constantly alert to the risk of death due to combat operations or training accidents. This crash was particularly difficult owing to the heightened awareness of danger and loss, the nature and extent of attachments within the military community, and the fact that the crash occurred during the Christmas season.

Many of those affected by the Gander crash were neglected by the health care providers and helpers. During crisis times, attention focuses on the bereaved; primarily the immediate family. Many individuals who are profoundly affected, and who could profit from professional consultation, are overlooked. Many of the senior leaders who were critical in uniting and focusing the community after the crash fell into the category of the neglected. Other neglected or overlooked groups included the different service providers, for example, the body handlers at the mortuary, security police at the crash site, military officers assigned to assist each bereaved family, and chaplains.

The model of the disaster community that developed following the

Gander crash was an effort to incorporate these complexities. The model focused on the participants' degree of involvement in postdisaster events to capture the dynamic nature of an emerging disaster 'community of meaning' that was not restricted by time or place. This community of meaning evolved over time following the crash, but was invisible as a specific place in time prior to the event. The criteria for classifying potential victims shifted from on-site direct exposure to the disaster and its immediate effects, to a more inclusive perspective focusing on participant involvement. 'Involvement' was identified by individual and group activities, roles and relationships that developed following the crash, and the shared meaning of the traumatic event (Wright et al., 1990). As the research team documented observations during the six-month period, the outlines of an expanded disaster community emerged. The shift in perspective identified individuals, groups and organizations who had peripheral contact with the disaster sites and the immediate victims, but who were profoundly touched by the event.

It was apparent that the affected groups were clustered in three geographical sites: (1) Gander, Newfoundland (the crash site); (2) Dover Air Force Base (the site of the mortuary where body identification occurred); and (3) Ft Campbell, Kentucky (home base of those killed). At the crash site, search and recovery of bodies and body parts was a ghastly process that involved heating the frozen ground to free burned, charred, and mutilated remains from the icy landscape. The body parts were carefully numbered, tagged, and placed in plastic bags for transport to the Dover mortuary. Most of this work was accomplished by teams of Army 'graves registration' personnel, who labored at the task for about two weeks. They were assisted by elements of the Royal Canadian Mounted Police, and by local rescue and fire personnel. Families of the dead were strongly discouraged from coming to the crash site. Canadian Aeronautics Safety officials were present to collect data pertaining to the cause of the crash. Senior leaders and officials from the US Army and Air Force directed the body and equipment recovery operation. Garrigan (1987) found that over half of the Army body recovery workers showed symptoms of posttraumatic stress disorder (PTSD) three to four weeks following their experiences.

At Dover, literally hundreds of volunteers and professionals labored for over six weeks to process and identify the 256 human remains. Despite the refrigeration in the mortuary, putrid odors grew worse daily. Many workers reported feeling unable to rid themselves of the smell, even after leaving the mortuary. One volunteer claimed, 'I've taken four showers today, and I still don't feel clean'. This sense extended beyond the workers themselves, in many cases. The wife of another morgue worker required him to change his clothes before coming into the house after working in the mortuary all day. Besides these Army, Air Force, and civilian morgue workers, many less centrally involved people were affected at Dover. Leaders and officials had a difficult time coordinating the efforts of different services and agencies. Normal Air Force operations at Dover were suspended for a time due to the excessive demands represented by this massive body identification operation. Community workers, teachers, and clergy volunteered to assist in any way possible. The event dominated the military and civilian community at Dover throughout the Christmas holiday, and into January and February.

In the days following the crash, most of the families of the dead gathered at Ft Campbell and waited there for news of the body identification process. Here, the impact of the loss was most apparent. Grief stricken family members, leaders, friends, and fellow soldiers mourned the death of their comrades. Even those who were strangers to the dead were affected. As one of those working in the personnel office described:

I went on about my duties pretty much as usual. The work has to go on, and someone has to do it. All the memorial services, all the crying families didn't bother me. I live across the street from one of the soldiers who died in the crash. From right out my window, I can see his house, and his car is still parked in front where he left it when he deployed to the Sinai. It hasn't moved! It takes a long time to get rid of big things like cars, I guess. I see it every morning, just where he left it. I know he won't be coming to get it. That car, it's like a silent reminder. That's the only thing that bothers me.

It was also clear that individuals in Washington, DC who were involved in coordinating responses were profoundly affected. For example, one of the individuals responsible for managing casualty assistance efforts to families told this story:

I'm very religious, Catholic. After Gander, I just stopped going to Mass. I couldn't believe in God anymore. The God I believed in would never let anything so horrible happen. These young men were among the best in the world, it just didn't make sense. I still can't understand it. How could God just let them all die like that?

As the disaster community developed in scope and complexity, it was helpful to organize the research observations using a diagram that consisted of a series of concentric circles, radiating out from a center point representing the dead. Fig. 12.1 represents this model graphically.

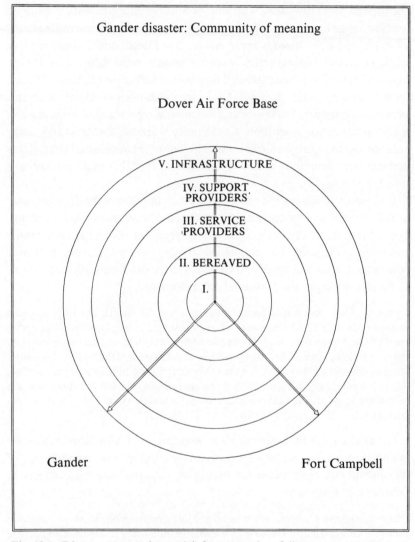

Fig. 12.1. Disaster community model: five categories of disaster community members.

The Gander disaster community

Wright et al. (1990) identified five categories of disaster community members using the expanded model. Each category was represented by a circle and placed in the diagram according to their involvement with the dead and the bereaved, and their relationships with members of the adjacent circles. The first two circles included the bereaved, those who had significant attachments to or involvement with the dead victims. Next of kin, friends, commanders, and surviving troops from units sent to the Sinai desert met these criteria. They were found to be at highest risk for psychiatric distress.

The third circle included the service providers who had direct contact with one of the disaster sites and with the bereaved or the dead. Their exposure to, and involvement with, the adjacent circles of the bereaved and the center point representing the dead, identified them as being at risk. This is consistent with the current literature that considers disaster responders as 'hidden victims' (Hersheiser & Quarantelli, 1976; Jones, 1985; Raphael, 1984; Taylor, 1983; Taylor & Frazer, 1981). Service providers frequently are traumatized by their disaster experiences, especially those experiences relating to body recovery and identification, and work with grieving families. Research observations following the Gander crash supported the high risk status of service providers, and their obvious distress during and after their work with the Gander victims and the victims' next of kin.

The Royal Canadian Mounted Police and graves registration personnel from several US Army posts, who worked at the Gander crash site on body recovery operations, reported various PTSD symptoms (Garrigan, 1987; Harris, 1986). Professional and volunteer workers involved in body identification at the Dover mortuary reported sleep disturbances, anxiety, and distressing dreams (Ursano, 1987; Ursano et al., 1988). Workers at the Family Assistance Center at Ft Campbell who helped bereaved families also reported trouble sleeping, and some sought psychiatric help. Many officers who assisted the next of kin showed increases in symptoms directly related to duration and intensity of exposure to bereaved family members (Bartone, 1987; Bartone et al., 1989). Through the reports of these officers, we gained insight not only into their own reactions, but also into the reactions of the family members they assisted. One assistance officer reports:

I drove the mother to the airport so she could attend the memorial service at Ft Campbell. The stepfather wanted to go, but they didn't have the money. We couldn't arrange for the Army to pay, since he wasn't next of kin. The man cried in the car coming back from the airport. I'll never get over that.

The fourth circle of the model included support providers. These individuals and organizations worked in the background of the disaster, providing instrumental or affective support to the service providers. These participants had indirect contact with the dead or the bereaved. Their primary involvement was with those who formed the first echelon of support to the primary victims. Their activities, roles and relationships involved them vicariously in the actual experience of the Gander crash.

However, they became significant members of the expanded disaster community. Several examples of support providers were those community members who lived at, or near, one of the disaster sites and volunteered their services and assistance, such as at Dover. Also at this level of involvement were those who managed and directed the service providers, such as the chief of the Army Community Services office at Ft Campbell, and the head of Red Cross services on Post. Both of these men reported feeling profoundly disturbed, but consciously delaying expression of their own feelings in order to better care for their staff, and provide support to their clients. Also in the category of support providers are those who made up formal and informal support systems for the service providers. This included family, friends, coworkers, supervisors, and counselors, as well as those who listened to or spent extra time with the more directly exposed disaster workers. For example, the Chaplains at Ft Campbell worked with almost no sleep for the first five days following the crash, ministering to the grieving. Throughout this period, they held support sessions with each other to manage their own grief and distress.

Finally, the fifth circle included members of the infrastructure. They were officials at the highest levels of the military and government who performed critical roles in coordinating the overall response to the Gander crash. They influenced communication, operations, and the organization of disaster resources. They had significant responsibilities for decision making during the crisis, continual exposure to information requiring coordination from the different sites affected by the crash, and high visibility. Individuals and groups in this circle maintained the outer boundary of the disaster community, controlling access, and communication, between this community and the rest of the nation.

The Gander crash not only affected those within the immediate confines of Ft. Campbell, the stricken community that directly suffered losses, but also reverberated throughout a much broader social system. The new 'disaster community' evolved in response to a major catastrophe, and had no meaning as a fixed place in time. Individuals, groups, and organizations emerged over time and became included within this community. Examples from two different circles within the model capture the complexity of participants' responses and illustrate the evolving disaster community. The first example describes the commanders and leaders of the soldiers killed at Gander who are represented in the circle of the bereaved. The second example is the Family Assistance Center. Many different groups of service providers from the third circle of the model worked with the bereaved next of kin at the Center. Both examples are illustrated in Fig. 12.2. They highlight the complex development of roles, relationships and activities,

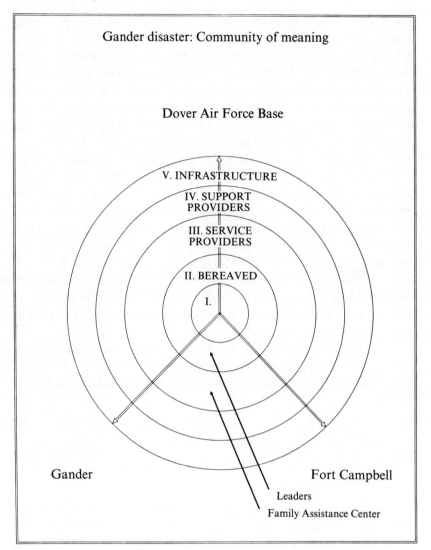

Fig. 12.2. Two examples of participants and their involvement in the disaster community.

and the shared meaning of the event that identify the participants and their involvement.

The bereaved: critical leaders and events in community mourning

Ingraham (1987*a*) describes the grief of several leaders at Ft Campbell and their critical role in integrating and focusing the stunned community following the Gander crash. He emphasizes the importance of key community leaders assuming the role of 'grief leadership' in the mourning process. He hypothesizes that group recovery following traumatic losses depends, in part, on the group's ability to mourn the loss of valued members through public rituals, and to comfort and insure the welfare of immediate survivors and next of kin (Ingraham, 1989). Correspondingly, these leaders operated within a context of significant events that facilitated mourning and encouraged solidarity in the Ft Campbell community. For example, there was a planned family reception in the Brigade gymnasium where families awaited the soldiers' homecoming on the morning of the crash. The Brigade Commander assumed a key role in grief leadership as he told the assembled families what had happened. He made critical, emotionally laden announcements about the crash, assuring families that information would be passed on to the community as soon as it became available. He focused on the importance of not being alone in grief and empathized with those who had lost friends and family. His capacity to express his own grief helped both families and soldiers to do the same. Those assembled in the gymnasium that morning were able to respond to him, and subsequently to one another.

The Presidential Memorial Service four days later was another significant event unifying the community in the mourning process. The Division Commander led families and soldiers in both their grief and their resolve to go on.

In this terrible tragedy, there are three things we must do. First, we must mourn the loss of our fallen soldiers, sons, daughters, husbands, and feel the pain of that loss. Second, we must care for their families, who need our support now more than ever. And finally, we must rebuild our unit and our strength so that we can go on with our lives, our jobs, our mission.

He emphasized the importance of the President 'sharing our sorrow', and joined the President in greeting the bereaved families and expressing condolences. The President underscored that he represented the American people and that he had come to mourn with the community because the nation was grieving as well. He and the First Lady touched and talked to each of the family members and many of the Task Force soldiers gathered at the Memorial Service. The Division Memorial Service occurred in the week following the tragedy and was significant in the participation of the entire Ft Campbell community, including adjacent towns' people. At this service the Division Commander remembered each 'Fallen Eagle' by reading his or her name, rank, and home state, followed by a single cannon shot. Several months later, a Silent Tribute Service occurred after the last victim was buried. The Division Commander directed a one minute sounding of the Post sirens, followed by a two minute silent tribute honoring the 248 soldiers lost in the crash.

The preceding events illustrate how the initial shock from the Gander crash was transformed into a mourning process involving the entire Ft Campbell community. The key commanders' activities and critical role in grief leadership helped affected individuals focus on identification with the group. As observed in other postimpact disaster communities, repeated acknowledgement of the common experience of grief and loss involving the community as a whole, established relationships and strengthened bonds among group members (Form et al., 1958; Mileti, Drabeck & Haas, 1975; Raphael, 1986; Tierney & Baisden, 1979). A series of significant public rituals continued to emphasize the community experience of loss and reinforced affective bonds among those who remained. During this process, the formal roles, relationships, and organizational boundaries within the community shifted to more informal linkages established on the basis of involvement in the postdisaster community. These linkages provided the foundation for developing instrumental and affective layers of support and maintaining the social fabric of the community.

The service providers: The Family Assistance Center

The shift in formal roles and relationships, the blurring of explicit organizational boundaries, and the relaxing of rules and regulations, all occurred within a community united by their sharing of loss. These changes permitted several creative and flexible interventions following the Gander crash. For example, the Family Assistance Center was a unique, ad hoc phenomenon materializing at Ft Campbell in response to a crisis situation that could not be handled independently by existing service facilities. As soon as news of the crash reached the Post, personnel and resources organized and assembled at the Eagle Conference Center. This facility provided a central location and convenient access for bereaved families. Various support facilities and offices on Post sent representatives to the Family Assistance Center to coordinate available resources. The Chaplains' Office, the Mortuary Affairs Office, the Veterans Administration, the Red Cross, Army Mutual Aid, Army Community Services, the Judge Advocate General's Office, and the Mental Health Services all provided handpicked teams of service providers to staff the Center.

There was little time for planning meetings, and few questions about what to do as staff assumed initiative in response to the crisis. The immediate priority was to install telephone hot lines to verify the flight manifest, locate and inform the victims' next of kin, and provide accurate status reports to those calling the Center. The pace increased over the course of the morning, and relevant service agencies were established amidst a crescendo of telephone calls and the arrival of bereaved families. Activity shifted to the Family Assistance Center from the Brigade gymnasium where families received official word of the crash as they assembled for the originally planned homecoming celebration.

Scores of military and civilian personnel, many of them volunteers, staffed the Center around the clock. They gave information, advice, and comfort to grieving and distraught family members. Upstairs, a private room was available with a mental health specialist who provided onsite private counseling and support for families in grief, as well as for exhausted staff as the situation became progressively more hectic over the first few days. Even though the magnitude of the event stunned the community, an immediate response was required. During the postimpact phase, there is little time for disaster responders to deal with their own grief and anguish as they comfort bereaved survivors (Barton, 1969; Duckworth, 1986; Dunning, 1988; Durham, McCammon & Allison, 1985; Hartshough & Myers, 1985; Siporin, 1976). At Ft Campbell, however, an extremely functional and creative organization emerged to respond to bereaved families. Mental health outreach was available for families and overwhelmed staff. The Family Assistance Center was a practical intervention providing efficient service to the victims' next of kin, and offering a stress management technique for the service providers.

Relaxing organizational boundaries and changing traditional roles and activities resulted in an effective community intervention that emerged in response to community members in crisis. Other Ft Campbell community agencies demonstrated similar shifts during this time. For example, in the immediate aftermath of the crash, a Casualty Coordinating Team was activated on Post. The purpose of the team was coordination of Post and community service providers responding to the crisis. The team represented key community and organization leaders. Their integration facilitated an organized response in the aftermath of the tragedy. The official (Gander) After Action Report (1986) documents these interventions and recommends them for future mass casualty events. They demonstrate the initiative and creative changes that can emerge when a community undergoes crisis. At Ft Campbell, layers of community support developed as surviving members worked together and shared the experience of grieving for those lost at Gander. This context, fostered by key leaders, encouraged intense personal involvement of community members and the development of creative solutions.

Conclusions

Community transformation occurs in response to a particular set of circumstances that brings people together in a common pursuit over a period of time (Panzetta, 1971). For the Ft Campbell community, the transformation occurred in response to the significant losses sustained by its members following the Gander crash. These tragic circumstances provided the context of meaning that changed the activities, roles, and relationships within the community. The dramatic precipitating event and the shifts observed in the community hours after the crash occurred, might imply a temporary, fragile transformation. However, the extent of traumatic loss sustained by the community is insufficient to explain the type of reaction observed. It was characterized by the emergence of mutuality and shared experiences in support of community members. As observed over other disasters (Erikson, 1976; Lifton & Olson, 1976; Shore, Tatum & Vollmer, 1986), the situation could have deteriorated into one of chaos and dysfunction, creating the destruction, temporary or otherwise, of a formerly unified community.

Key commanders, as they mourned the loss of their soldiers, appeared to influence the positive transformation described for Ft Campbell. As described above, these leaders focused the community on shared values and common goals, uniting them in the significance of their mutual experience of loss and bereavement. Their focus was articulated by meaningful public rituals that fostered a sense of integration and solidarity. The unified community then could proceed with activities and plans that would sustain Ft Campbell through the crisis, and maintain it once the crisis had ended. This transformation provided the backdrop for supporting the bereaved and reconstructing the psychological life of the community in the aftermath of significant traumatic loss.

Table 12.1 provides a summary of key leader actions in the aftermath of disaster and the apparent effects of those actions on the community. In the early period of shock and disbelief, community leaders reassure families and survivors by conveying accurate information, dispelling rumors, and providing a calm and controlled role model for others to follow. Following this phase, leaders reinforce a sense of order and stability by establishing a framework within which rebuilding efforts can proceed efficiently. They also organize and assist with memorial services that show respect for the

Table 12.1. *Summary of key leader actions and impact on community recovery from disaster*

Leader Actions	Community effects
Public announcements and appearances	Provides useful, accurate information; Reestablishes a sense of order/control
Press briefings	Reassures families, others
Other statements	Dispels rumors
Calm demeanor	Sets model for others to follow
Establishes controls, policies	Provides framework for organizing volunteer efforts efficiently
Organizes memorial services	Demonstrates respect for dead
Attends funerals, grieves	'Gives permission' to grieve
Offers assistance to families	Shows concern, establishes climate of healing, community support
Guides, doesn't 'micromanage'	Communicates trust in others' abilities; fosters cooperation, initiative
Describes loss in positive terms: heroic sacrifice, a gift to community, an opportunity to learn, recognizes contributions of survivors and helpers	Starts to redirect community energy into rebuilding effects
Outlines goals for future	Reorients to future objectives; targets prospective missions

dead, affirm the loss to the community, and acknowledge the need to grieve. By providing special assistance to families of the dead, leaders demonstrate concern and establish a community climate of helping and healing. A sense of cooperation, trust, and initiative is fostered by leaders who guide and support, but allow subordinates to function independently. Finally, leaders encourage community members to focus on positive lessons learned from the disaster by emphasizing the sacrifice and contribution of victims and survivors. In this way the loss can begin to energize efforts to rebuild for a brighter future.

Using the expanded model of the disaster community to organize the wide range of participants who become involved following a disaster may help resolve some of the controversy noted in the disaster literature (Tierney, 1986). Broadening the perspective helps identify individuals, groups, and organizations by what they did, and categorize their experiences based on their postdisaster involvement. This goes beyond the constraints of time and place inherent in current disaster victim classifications (Dudasik, 1980; Frazer & Taylor, 1982). It also addresses the levels of analysis controversy. Those placed in the different circles of the model are included based on the nature of their roles, activities, and relationships in the disaster community. These criteria encompass individuals, groups, and organizations participating at different levels, and provide an in-depth description of a disaster event across the participants' experience. The objectives are to begin to differentiate dimensions of stress and phases of recovery.

Observations over time and across different sites following the Gander crash captured the richness of experience as a 'community' evolved in response to crisis. Reconfiguring the participants of the disaster community based on an interconnecting system of activities, roles, and relationships reveals a complex network of individuals and groups. The model can alert a community to the possibility that the consequences of disasters can be dispersed throughout a much wider social system than was previously assumed. Using the more complex orientation has the advantage of identifying individuals and groups at risk for psychiatric distress following disaster. This orientation also can help focus resources for preventive community interventions (Crabbs & Heffron, 1981; Mitchell, 1983; Mitchell, 1986; Williams, Solomon & Bartone, 1988). Using individual, group, and organizational levels of analysis, across time and place, provides a method for identifying principle stress points, as well as the layers of support that maintain a community in times of crisis. This focus permits identification of individuals and groups who may operate in the background of crisis events, but who contribute significantly to the work of others. Such information is essential for any evaluation of a community's resources and potential to respond to, and recover from, crisis.

Acknowledgements

The views of the authors do not necessarily reflect the positions of the Department of the Army or the Department of Defense (para 4–3, AR 360–5).

References

After Action Report: 101st ABN DIV (AASLT). (1986). *Task Force 3-502 (MFO) Airliner Disaster (12 Dec 85*. Ft. Campbell, KY: Department of the Army Headquarters 101st ABN DIV (AASLT).

Barton, A.H. (1969). *Communities in disaster; a sociological analysis of collective stress situations*. New York: Doubleday and Company.

Bartone, P. (1987). Casualty affairs and survivor assistance officers. In *The human response to the Gander military air disaster: a summary report*.

Division of Neuropsychiatry Report No. 88-12. Washington, DC: Walter Reed Army Institute of Research, pp. 23–5.

Bartone, P. & Wright, K. (1990). Grief and group recovery following a military air disaster. *Journal of Traumatic Stress*, **3**(4), 523–9.

Bartone, P., Ursano, R., Wright, K. & Ingraham, L. (1989). The impact of a military air disaster on the health of assistance workers: a prospective study. *Journal of Nervous and Mental Disease*. **177**(6), 317–28.

Berren, M. R., Beigel, A. & Ghertner, S. (1980). A typology for the classification of disasters. *Community Mental Health Journal*, **16**(2), 103–11.

Crabbs, M. A. & Heffron, E. (1981). Loss associated with a natural disaster. *The Personnel and Guidance Journal*, **59**(6), 378–81.

Duckworth, D. H. (1986). Psychological problems arising from disaster work. *Stress Medicine*, **2**, 315–23.

Dudasik, S. W. (1980.). Victimization in natural disaster. *Disasters*, **4**, 329–38.

Dunning, C. (1988). Intervention strategies for emergency workers. In M. Lystad (ed.) *Mental health response to mass emergencies: theory and practice*. New York: Brunner/Mazel, pp. 284–307.

Durham, T. W., McCammon, S. L. & Allison, E.J. (1985). The psychological impact of disaster on rescue personnel. *Annals of Emergency Medicine*, **14**(7), 73–7.

Erikson, K. T. (1976). *Everything in its path: destruction of community in the Buffalo Creek flood*. New York: Simon & Schuster.

Form, W. H., Nosow, S., Stone, G. P. & Westie, C. M. (1958). How victims help themselves. In W. H. Form & S. Nosow (eds.), *Community in disaster*. New York: Harper & Brothers, pp. 54–82.

Frazer, D. C. J. & Taylor, A. J. W. (1982, December). The stress of post-disaster body handling and victim identification work. *Journal of Human Stress*, **8**(4), 5–12.

Garrigan, J. L. (1987). Post-traumatic stress disorder in military disaster workers. In *The human response to the Gander military air disaster: a summary report*. Division of Neuropsychiatry Report No. 88-12. Washington, DC: Walter Reed Army Institute of Research, pp. 7–8.

Harris, S. L. (1986, September). *The impact of the Gander military air crash on the RCMP (Royal Canadian Mounted Police)*. (Available from Health Services Officer, RCMP. 'K' Division, PO Box 1774, Edmonton, Alberta, T5J 2P1, Canada).

Hartshough, D. H. & Myers, D. G. (1985). *Disaster work and mental health: prevention and control of stress among workers*. (DHHS Publication No. (ADM) 87-1422). Rockville, MD: National Institutes of Mental Health.

Hersheiser, M. R. & Quarantelli, E. L. (1976). The handling of the dead in a disaster. *Omega – The Journal of Death and Dying*, **7**(3), 195–209.

Ingraham, L. H. (1987*a*). Grief leadership. In *The human response to the Gander military air disaster: a summary report*. Division of Neuropsychiatry Report No. 88-12. Washington, DC: Walter Reed Army Institute of Research, pp. 10–13.

Ingraham, L. H. (1987*b*). Conclusions. In *The human response to the Gander military air disaster: a summary report*. Division of Neuropsychiatry Report No. 88-12. Washington, DC: The Walter Reed Army Institute of Research, pp. 37–9.

Ingraham, L. H. (1989, April). Leading through loss: grief leadership in the Army. Paper presented at the Army Leadership Conference, Center for Army Leadership, Kansas, City, MO.

Jones, D. R. (1985). Secondary disaster victims: the emotional effects of recovering and identifying human remains. *American Journal of Psychiatry*, **142**(3), 303–7.

Lifton, R. J. & Olson, E. L. (1976). The human meaning of total disaster: the Buffalo Creek experience. *Psychiatry*, **39**, 1–18.

Melick, M. E. (1985). The health of post-disaster populations: a review of the literature and a case study. In J. Laube & S. A. Murphy (eds.), *Perspectives on disaster recovery*. Norwalk, CT: Appleton-Century-Crofts, pp. 179–209.

Mileti, D. S., Drabeck, T. E. & Haas, J. E. (1975). *Human systems in extreme environments: a sociological perspective*. Boulder, CO: Institute of Behavioral Science, University of Colorado.

Mitchell, J. T. (1983). When disaster strikes: the critical incident stress debriefing process. *Journal of Emergency Medical Services*, **8**, 36–9.

Mitchell, J. T. (1986). Critical incident stress management. *Response*, **5**(5), 24–5.

Panzetta, A.F. (1971). The concept of community. *Archives General Psychiatry*, **25**, 291–7.

Powell, B. J. & Penick, E. C. (1983). Psychological distress following a natural disaster: a one-year follow-up of 98 flood victims. *Journal of Community Psychology*, **11**, 269–76.

Quarantelli, B. B. (1985). An assessment of conflicting views on mental health: the consequences of traumatic events. In C. Figley (ed.), *Trauma and its wake*. New York: Brunner/Mazel, pp. 173–215.

Radke, A. (1987). The mental health response. In *The human response to the Gander military air disaster: a summary report*. Division of Neuropsychiatry Report No. 88-12. Washington, DC: Walter Reed Army Institute of Research, pp. 32–6.

Raphael, B. (1984). Rescue workers: stress and their management. *Emergency Response*, **1**(10), 27–30.

Raphael, B. (1986). *When disaster strikes: how individuals and communities cope with catastrophe*. New York: Basic Books.

Shore, J. H., Tatum, E. L. & Vollmer, W. M. (1986). Psychiatric reactions to disaster: the Mount St. Helen's experience. *American Journal of Psychiatry*, **143**(5), 590–5.

Siporin, M. (1976). Altruism, disaster, and crisis intervention. In H.J. Parad, H. L. P. Resnick & L. P. Parad (eds.), *Emergency and disaster management: a mental health sourcebook*. Bowie, MD: Charles Press, p. 217.

Taylor, A. J. W. (1983). Hidden victims and the human side of disasters. *Undro News*, 6–10.

Taylor, A. J. W. & Frazer, A.G. (1981). *Psychological sequelae of Operation Overdue following the DC-10 aircrash in Antartica*. (Victoria University of Wellington Publications in Psychology No. 27). Wellington, New Zealand: Victoria University.

Tierney, K. J. (1986). *Disaster and mental health: a critical look at knowledge and practice*. Paper presented at the Italy–United States Conference on Disasters, Disaster Research Center, Newark, DE.

Tierney, K. J. & Baisden, B. (1979). *Crisis intervention programs for disaster victims: a sourcebook and manual for smaller communities*. (DHHS Publication No. (ADM) 83-675). Rockville, MD: National Institutes of Mental Health.

Ursano, R. (1987). Dover Air Force Base mortuary operations. In *The human response to the Gander military air disaster: a summary report*. Division of Neuropsychiatry Report No. 88-12. Washington, DC: Walter Reed Army Institute of Research, pp. 5–7.

Ursano, R., Ingraham, L., Wright, K. & Bartone, P. (1988, May). Psychiatric

responses to bodies. Paper presented at the 141st Annual Meeting of the
American Psychiatric Association, Montreal, CAN.
Williams, C., Solomon, S. D. & Bartone, P. (1988). Primary prevention in
aircraft disasters: integrating research and theory. *American Psychologist*,
43, 730–9.
Wright, K. (ed.). (1987). *The human response to the Gander military air disaster: a
summary report*. Division of Neuropsychiatry Report No. 88-12.
Washington, DC: Walter Reed Army Institute of Research.
Wright, K. M., Ursano, R. J., Bartone, P. T. & Ingraham, L. H. (1990). The
shared experience of catastrophe: An expanded classification of the disaster
community. *American Journal of Orthopsychiatry*, **60**(1), 35–42.

Part IV
Responses to trauma across the life cycle

13

Children of war and children at war: child victims of terrorism in Mozambique

JON A. SHAW and JESSE J. HARRIS

On the southeastern rim of Africa, northeast of South Africa, east of Zimbabwe and bordered by the Indian Ocean lies the 'shattered land' of Mozambique. Mozambique has suffered the consequences of war, famine and drought. Of the approximate 14.6 million natives, it is estimated that 6.5 million require international food aid, with 3.2 million dependent on free emergency food. Robert Gersony, in his 1988 report to the Department of State, noted that approximately 2 million refugees have fled their homes. The Mozambique Red Cross estimates that the majority of these refugees are children. Fifty percent of the population is reported to be under 15 years of age. (Uqueio, personal communication)

There is increasing awareness and sensitivity to the plight of 'children in a warring world'. In the last few decades there has been a significant change in the nature and intensity of war. Armed conflicts around the world have been increasingly characterized by low intensity and episodic conflict, the employment of guerrilla armies, and the victimization of the civilian population. Dyregrov et al. (1987) have suggested that 80–90% of all casualties in the current spectrum of armed conflicts are civilians.

In his monograph, *Children of War*, Rosenblatt (1983) states that, 'there are places in the world like Northern Ireland, Israel, Lebanon, Cambodia, and Vietnam that have been at war for the past twenty years or more . . . the children living in these places have known nothing but war in their experiences. The elements of war, explosions, destructions, dismemberments, eruptions, noises, fire, death, separation, torture, grief, which ought to be extraordinary and temporary for any life are for these children normal and constant.' Certainly, this is true of children living in Mozambique.

The war in Mozambique has raged since 1976, when the Mozambique National Resistance (RENAMO) was formed, initially at the behest of the Rhodesian Intelligence Agency and subsequently supported by the South

Africa's Department of Military Intelligence. RENAMO has made little effort to win the hearts of the people or even to hold territory and is predominantly motivated to destabilize the government of Mozambique. By 1985, Isaacman, a professor of African history, estimated that 1800 schools and 25% of the health clinics were destroyed and that approximately 325 000 children had died as a result of the war (Isaacman, 1987). RENAMO has successfully waged a guerrilla war by attacking railroads, roads, and electricity lines. They initiated hit and run attacks on villages seizing arms, ammunition, uniforms, medicine, and, more recently, children. Children have been captured, used as porters, coerced into military training, and forced to participate in guerrilla attacks on other villages. Currently, RENAMO controls virtually 80% of the country with the exception of major cities and province capitals.

On 31 December 1987, the American Ambassador declared that a 'disaster' existed in Mozambique and that the country was eligible for aid from the Office of Disaster Assistance. The ambassador requested, on behalf of the government of Mozambique, that the United States Office of Foreign Disaster Assistance send a child psychiatrist and a social worker to Mozambique with the intent of providing evaluation and consultation to approximately 50 village children. The children were 6–16 years of age, had been kidnapped by the guerrilla forces (RENAMO), forced into military training, and coerced into participating in military activities against their own villages and government forces. A number of these children were recaptured by government forces. Some of the children spent as long as four years with the guerrillas. The government was concerned about their capacity for rehabilitation and expressed fears that a whole generation of children would be lost to the guerilla forces.

Trauma in children has been defined as 'any condition which seems definitely unfavorable, noxious, or drastically injurious 'to their development' (Greenacre, 1952). The exposure to war with its multiple adversities is a significant interference with the child's development. Yet the cognitive immaturity, plasticity, and adaptive capacities of the child have often veiled the effects of war in a certain obscurity. There is a conflicting and controversial literature debating the existence, frequency, and configuration of psychiatric morbidity in children exposed to war.

It is surprising how often children and adolescents are reported to adapt to the conditions of war with little evidence of manifest distress. Anna Freud and Burlingham (1943) noted that children over two years of age, who had witnessed air raids over England in WW II, were able to distinguish between falling bombs and anticraft weaponry, and that, after three years of war the idea of fighting, killing and bombing had ceased to be extraordinary and were accepted as a part of everyday life. Gillespie (1942) described as a remarkable feature of the English home front, the low incidence of child psychiatric casualties compared to the number anticipated. Yet Dunsdon (1941) found that children remaining under fire in Bristol, England demonstrated eight times more incidence of psychological distress when compared to those evacuated.

There are contradictory reports from Israel regarding the effects of shelling on youth. A study of the dreams and sleep habits of Israeli youth on a border town subject to terrorist activities indicated that they slept longer, and had fewer dreams, manifesting fewer horror, sexual and aggressive themes than did their counterparts in a nonborder town. Using measurements of anxiety, Rofe and Lewin (1982), and Ziv and Israeli (1974) discovered that children from frequently shelled Kibbutzim were no different from nonshelled Kibbutzim. There is some evidence that communal solidarity, group cohesion, and common purpose shared by civilian and military participants of war, may provide protection against anxiety (Zuckerman-Bareli, 1982). Milgram and Milgram (1976) compared pre- and wartime measurements of anxiety during the Yom Kippur War and demonstrated that the general level of anxiety in fifth and six graders doubled. There was, however, no predictable relationship between wartime stress and anxiety, but rather a correlation with being a boy and/or being an upper middle class child, and anxiety level.

Some of the confusion regarding the responsivity of children to the exposure of the chaotic violence and life threat of war is explained by developmental effects. The preschool child living within the security of a constantly available and supporting family often mirrors the family response to the stressor. Where there is parental injury, exaggerated parental emotional response, premorbid parental psychopathology, reversal of the dependency role, and excessive intolerance of the child's proclivity to regressive behavior, there may be an emotional derivative effect on the child.

The young child lacks the cognitive capacities available to the adult. His theories of causality are egocentric. Children are rarely able to talk about their frightening experiences. Unable to transform their internal conflicts and feelings into words, they are expressed in repetitive reenactments, intrusive visual images, trauma specific fears, aggressive and regressive activities, and other behavioral states (Terr, 1991).

Several observers studied children as the victims of war (Carlin, 1979, 1980; Arroya & Eth, 1985; Lin, Masuda & Tazuma, 1984; Sack, Angell &

Kinzie, 1986; Kinzie et al., 1989; Dyregrov et al., 1987). There is considerable evidence that the posttraumatic effects are serious and enduring. Sack
et al. (1986), noted that 50% of the Cambodian war refugee children had a
diagnosis of posttraumatic stress disorder (PTSD). There was considerable
comorbidity. Other prominent diagnoses were major depressive disorder,
generalized anxiety disorder, and intermittent depressive disorder. In a
three year follow-up study, 48% continued to exhibit PTSD and 41%
depression. The course was variable with eight subjects having PTSD at
both interviews, while eight subjects had a variable course (Sack et al.,
1986). Arroya and Eth (1985) studied 30 refugees, less than 17 years of age,
who had taken flight from Central America and who were referred to a
mental health clinic. Many had been separated from their families. Often
the parents had preceded the child to this country, leaving the child behind
with relatives. The child was left with the perception of having been
abandoned to the repeated violence of war. The investigators noted that
approximately 33% of these youngsters exhibited posttraumatic stress
disorders. Other diagnostic categories included adjustment disorders,
separation anxiety disorder, somatoform disorders, major depressive disorder and dysthymia.

Dyregrov et al. (1987) studied the effects of war in Uganda on a cohort of
adolescents and noted their resiliency in the face of extreme stress. There
was a proclivity for these adolescents to identify with the 'helper pro-
fessions', and to prepare in an anticipatory way for future positions in a
society hopefully without war or violence. They exhibited little evidence of
'identification with the aggressor'. The children often expressed a wish to be
doctors, lawyers, etc. The authors noted that adults who killed, robbed, and
maltreated the villagers were regarded as strangers, 'belonging to an army
hated for its cruelty and lack of discipline'. They appeared to be rejected as
role models. The authors add a word of caution, however, describing
themes of uncertainty, depression, and anxiety beneath the manifest coping
and adaptive strivings of these youth.

Consultation

Upon entry into the country, the authors were met by representatives of the
American Embassy. An Italian Child Psychologist with the Italian Aid
Program had interviewed many of the children. She noted that they were
placed in 'Centro de Lhanguene', a temporary shelter, a Catholic school,
where they were being housed and provided some opportunities for
schooling, play, and reeducation. While she noted that many of the children

had been beaten and tortured by RENAMO, suffered from malnutrition, experienced losses of family members, and in some instances participated in attacking and killing villagers, she felt that the children were not experiencing psychiatric problems.

We soon met with the Mozambique Vice-Minister of Health and the Deputy National Director of Health. There was a controversy in the government as to whether the children should be treated as prisoners of war or as victims of war. There was disagreement as to the treatment approach. How long should the children be kept at a 'special center' for treatment? Should they be returned to their families, placed for adoption, or assigned to group homes till they reached maturity? They expressed fears that these children would grow up to be delinquents and criminals without loyalty or fidelity to the country. They communicated their concerns that children who had participated in killing would come to enjoy their aggressivity and would prey on their fellow citizens. The Vice-Minister requested a treatment plan be provided the ministry.

Evaluation

The children were housed at 'Centro de Lhanguene', a catholic school in downtown Maputo, the capital of Mozambique. The Director of the center introduced the group of refugee boys, who were marched before us, dancing to the sound of music. They were led by one of the older boys into portraying, in dramatic form, their experiences in captivity, the innocent killing of a village woman, and their eventual triumph over the guerrilla soldiers. They sang songs glorifying the revolution and the need to win victory over the 'bandidos'. There was a marked contrast between those children who were with the center 4–8 weeks and those who had just been captured by government forces and brought to the center. Approximately ten new arrivals were sitting off by themselves separate from the group. Their heads were shaved to remove lice. Protuberant abdomens, a sign of malnutrition, were evident among 20% of the arrivals. They exhibited tattered clothing, bare feet, frozen emotionality, passivity, and a lack of relatedness with each other. They seemed resigned to whatever would be imposed upon them.

It was decided to evaluate 11 of the children individually and to meet with a larger group of 20 for the purpose of acquiring drawings related to several themes, i.e. the worst moment of captivity, the moment you were freed, and what you would like to be in the future.

Individual evaluations

The children were evaluated through an interpreter who spoke both Portuguese and the native tribal dialect common to the southern provinces. Questions were taken from the parent's version of the Diagnostic Interview for Children and Adolescents (DICA-P) (Reich & Welner personal communication), and the revised Frederick and Pynoos PTSD Reaction Index Scale (Pynoos personal communication). The limitations of language and the need to translate from English to Portuguese, and frequently to a tribal dialect, made the use of instrumentation unreliable. While it was possible to make clinical judgments as to the existence of manifest psychiatric morbidity, the limits of enculturation of the instruments made it difficult to derive empirical data.

Table 13.1 depicts the presence of posttraumatic symptomatology along the three dimensions of mood, intrusive thoughts/imagery, and ego restrictions using a four point scale. There is a suggestion of a relationship between the length of captivity and the severity of posttraumatic symptomatology.

Clinical vignettes

A few clinical vignettes are presented to illustrate the spectrum of experiences associated with these children's victimization by war.

Israel (Fig. 13.1) is a handsome 12 year old boy who was originally from Gaza province. He was captured by RENAMO in May, 1987, and held a prisoner for three months. The village where he lived was surprised and overrun by the 'bandidos' who proceeded to loot and to take him and six others (including his mother, sister, and niece) prisoner. They were immediately forced to serve as porters, carrying food, sugar, rice, ammo, and radios to the 'bandido' village. They marched for approximately 14 hours and went without food or water for 24 hours. They were told that, if they cried out or wept they would have their ears and/or fingers cut off with a machete. They continued to walk for two days before they reached the 'bandido' village.

They were guarded at all times. Israel was not allowed to see or talk with his mother or other family members. They were told that they would be kept captive until Independence day. Israel was assigned as an aide to a 'bandido' lieutenant and he was responsible for carrying and providing water. He felt that the bandits were always angry with him.

Soon after reaching the village, he was forced to participate in military training every morning from sunrise to noon. They were required to train,

Table 13.1. *Mozambique children*

	Age	Time captivity months	Time free months	Mood	Intrusive images	Ego restriction
Alfonso	12	1	6	+	+	+ +
Pauli	16	1	2	+ +	+ + +	+ +
Carlos	16	2	6	+	+	+ +
Angelo	14	2	5	+	+ +	+
Josai	14	2	6	+ + + +	+ + +	+ + +
Israel	12	3	5	+	+ +	+
Fernando	15	6	14	+ +	+ + +	+ +
Carlos J.	10	6	3	+ + + +	+ + +	+ + + +
Firinice	6	6	1.5	+ + + +		+ + + +
Vasco A.	15	24	2	+ + +	+	+ + +
Ernesto	10	48	1.5	+ + + +	+ + +	+ + + +

and if they failed to do so, they would be beaten. If they performed well, they would be given water.

Israel reported a repetitive dream which he has experienced since his captivity. In the dream he is running away from the bandido camp to his home in the village. When he arrives, his brother asks him, 'How did you know how to get home?' He responds, 'How can anybody not know the way home'.

Approximately two months after his capture he learned that his mother had escaped. In the third month he escaped with a group of five boys. They pretended to be playing a game and gradually worked their way out to the periphery of the camp where they suddenly ran away. He was held prisoner and interrogated by the government forces for three months before he was sent to the center. His mother is back in her village, but he refuses to return home, preferring to stay in the safety of Maputo, away from the 'bandidos'.

Firinice, a six year-old boy, was accosted by the bandidos at a river near his home. He was forced to lead them to his home where he was made to set fire to his family's hut. As his parents fled, they were killed and decapitated. His parents had been leaders in the militia. A man wrapped a Frelimo flag around the mother's head and noted that, 'This is what Frelimo buys you.' All his older siblings were killed. This account of Firinice's story occurred only months after his recapture by Frelimo. For many weeks he was virtually mute, unresponsive, emotionally frozen, and passively malleable, complying with whatever was expected of him.

Josai (Fig. 13.2) is an anxious and nervous 14 year-old boy who made a

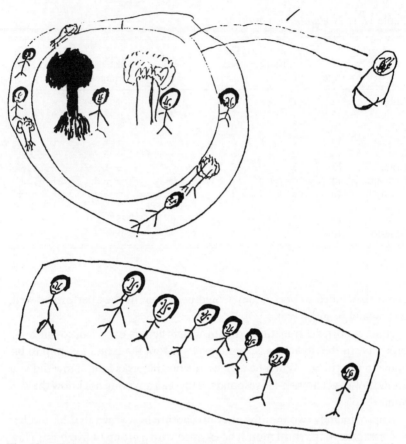

Fig. 13.1. This drawing by Israel portrays the enemy camp in the circle and the captives being guarded and held prisoner away from the camp.

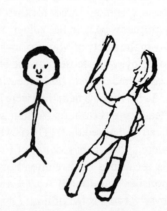

Fig. 13.2. Josai's drawing demonstrating the time when the 'bandido' cut off the fingers of his left hand and left ear. Notice the dimunitive size of the helpless child before the threatening machete. Initially drawing in red (on the colored original), he quickly switched to a less emotionally loaded color.

conspicuous effort to hide his left hand as well as to present a profile that would keep his left ear out of visual awareness. The four digits of his left hand were chopped off with a machete and a good portion of his left ear had also been removed. In a reticent manner he described how 'bandidos' had entered his village, killed his father and demanded to know which villagers were in the militia. When he responded that he did not know, they proceeded to cut off his fingers and subsequently his left ear. He has a recurring dream in which Bandits catch him while he is running away. They ask him, 'Why do you run away? We want you to kill government forces. If you don't, we're going to kill you.' He often thinks of revenge and imagines how he would cut off the hand of the man who attacked him.

Ernesto is a slightly built 10 year-old boy with signs of malnutrition who spent four years with the bandidos. The 'bandidos' attacked his village, overran it, and set up their headquarters. His parents soon joined the 'bandidos'. Ernesto initially served as a porter, but he was subsequently forced into military training. He learned to fire an AK-47 and participated in attacks on other villages. He denied killing anybody, noting that the recoil of the rifle would knock him down. After four years, his guerrilla band was defeated by government forces and he was taken captive. They treated him as a bandit and wanted to kill him. As a prisoner of war he was incarcerated for approximately six weeks in an army jail. He was beaten many times before he was released to the 'Centro de Lhanguene'.

Ernesto graphically described his experiences as a 'bandido', and how at one point, he refused to participate in training and was threatened with death. Just before being killed, another bandit killed the one threatening him and the victim's brains flew out all over Ernesto. He described a repetitive dream of being watched by the bandits, who kill him and he sees his own funeral.

Fernando is a 15 year-old boy with a deformity of the neck suggesting a rupture of neck muscles, resulting in his head being tilted over to the side. He related the injury to being forced to carry a 50 kg load on his head as a porter, while being held captive.

He admitted to participating in a number of attacks and killing six people. He exhibited little remorse or regret. He was preoccupied with being big and strong, expressing a wish to be a soldier and to drive a big truck. Both his parents had been killed, and at the time of his capture he was living with his grandparents. The village was surprised by child warriors with guns. As many of the villagers fled, they ran into an ambush and were killed by the adult 'bandidos'.

After being captured, he was taught to fire an AK-47 and served as a

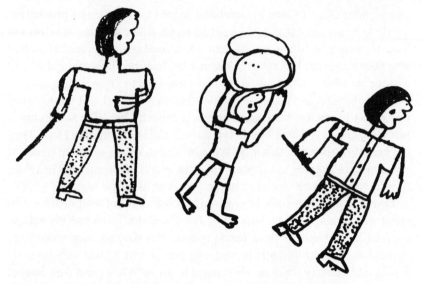

Fig. 13.3. This drawing by Vasco Albamo showing him being forced to be a porter carrying food to the base camp being guarded by two 'bandidos'.

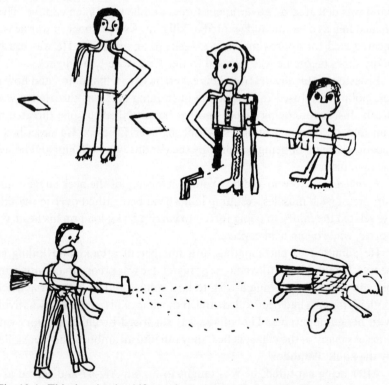

Fig. 13.4. This drawing by Alfonso demonstrates two scenes. The upper scene shows a man having his leg cut off after he tried to escape. The lower scene shows the 'bandidos' killing innocent people they meet in the forest.

guard for the prisoners. To prove his loyalty to the bandidos, he was forced to kill a prisoner or be killed himself. He participated in attacks on several villages, killing three villagers, and reports that in his last firefight he killed three bandits. It was difficult to judge the veracity of this statement as he wanted to ingratiate himself with the government army. On one occasion, he indicated that he did it on purpose. On another occasion, he suggested it was an accident in which he killed them in a cross fire and subsequently fled fearing retribution. Upon his capture he was treated as a POW. He was held in an army jail for ten months. The government forces were afraid that he would return to the 'bandidos'. He was interrogated and tortured by Frelimo. There were scars on the inner aspects of his calves where a stick had been bored into his muscle. He was more afraid of Frelimo than he was of the bandits. Upon his release from jail he was sent to 'Centro de Lhanguene' where initially he carried a stick with him at all times to ensure his safety.

Vaso Albamo (Fig. 13.3) is a tall 15 year-old athletic boy, who wants only to play soccer. He was taking care of a herd of 13 cows when he was surprised by 'bandidos' who took him prisoner and appropriated his herd. He lived with the bandits for two years. He served as a porter and was trained as a guard. He denied ever killing others, although he participated in numerous attacks on villages. He spoke of the safety he experiences in the 'Centro de Lhanguene' and how he never wants to go back to the country. He has a repetitive dream of being beaten and waking up afraid. He described the group life in the center as 'we live like brothers, we have the same problems, we love each other, we dance, sing and play football.'

Alfonso (Fig. 13.4) is a 12 year-old boy, who was held captive with the 'bandidos' for one month. He was kidnapped by the guerrillas while working in the field along with his father, mother and brother. They fired shots into the ground warning them not to try to escape. He was forced to be a porter, carrying water and to participate in military training. His mother's hand was cut off. One day while he was supposed to carry water to the base, he escaped. He returned to the village where he was turned over by the villagers to the government forces. He expressed feelings of sadness concerning the whereabouts of his parents. He feared going home as he would be taken once again by the 'bandidos'.

Discussion

What are the psychological consequences of war and armed conflict on those children who were abducted by guerilla bandits, and forced into

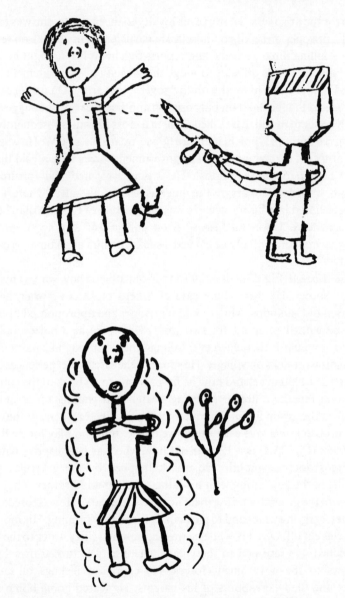

Fig. 13.5. This scene by the younger Carlos depicts the killing and burial of his aunt by the 'bandidos'.

military activities to become the 'pupils of war?'. In some instances, these children not only participated in military action, but also killed others.

The child who was forced to participate in military activities and atrocities is similar to other victims of overwhelming disastrous life events. He may manifest posttraumatic stress symptomatology with its peculiar configuration of ego restrictions, disturbances in arousal, and a propensity to experience intrusive imagery and repetitive thoughts associated with the stressful experience (Terr, 1979, 1983, 1985, 1991; Pynoos & Nader, 1988).

The child's psychological response to an overwhelming stressor is determined by biological and psychosocial risk factors, the level of emotional and cognitive development, the degree of exposure to the stressor with its particular intensity and duration, the degree of injury or life threat, the losses of family members, and the disruption of the continuity of community/school/family (Pynoos & Nader, 1988). The essence of the traumatic situation is the particular meaning that the stressful experience has for the individual and the difficulty in processing that experience into his or her preconceived cognitive view of the world (Horowitz, 1974; Shaw, 1987; Ulman & Brothers, 1988).

The children in Mozambique were exposed to multiple stressors, i.e. life threats, witnessing brutal killings, physical beatings, dislocation from village life, enforced migration, separation from loved ones, exposure to marginal sustenance with food and water, coercive military training, and participation in military attacks on villages with the killings and assaulting of innocents.

The children were forced to be aggressive and violent in war when all they wanted to do was to take flight from violence. The normal child struggles to achieve control over his aggressive and destructive impulses. He controls his impulses by both conscious and unconscious self-regulation. The child who is forced to be aggressive at a time when he is learning to control aggression is traumatized in a particularly cruel manner. How much more traumatized is the child who is forced to aggressively attack members of his own family and village. The youngster who is exposed to sudden violence at a time when he is struggling to control his own aggression is in danger of having his own control over his aggressive impulses undermined and becoming more aggressive himself. We know that children who have been abused often grow up to abuse their own children (Dodge, Bates & Pettet, 1991). They identify with the 'aggressor'. Children exposed to war and conflict situations are reported to have a propensity to outbursts of hostility and aggression. Dyregrov et al. (1987) noted that as war and violence become an integral part of the child's life there is a risk that these children will become the 'pupils of war'. Fernando, the 15 year old boy, cited above, expressed a desire to be a soldier, yearning for a sense of powerfulness that would protect him from the captors and violent forces around him.

It is apparent that the exposure to the sudden realities of mutilation and death, the realistic limitations of the protective power of loving parents, and the sudden and unexpected impact of violence and brutality may undermine the child's illusion of safety. The child's reaction to the traumatic situation is greatly influenced by his underlying fantasy life, and his interpretation of events. When overt traumatic experiences resonate with an underlying fantasy, the experience may lead to a fixation on the trauma, in contrast to those traumatic experiences which are interpreted as incidental (Greenacre, 1952). This fixation may, in turn, lead to a compelling need to repeat the traumatic experience in a continuing effort to achieve mastery over the traumatic situation.

The peculiar brutality of the 'bandidos' in Mozambique is evident in their kidnapping of children from local villages, coercing them into military training, and forcing them to fight against their own villagers and families. Failure to comply resulted in the cutting off of an ear, the fingers of one's hand or even death.

An evaluation of 11 of these children, who were recaptured by government forces, indicated a high frequency of posttraumatic stress symptomatology, dysphoria, and anxiety. There was a proclivity for these children to see themselves as victims of war. There was a tendency, nevertheless, to identify with future career patterns where they would be helpers to other 'victims'. They thought of themselves as future priests, doctors, and bureaucrats. A few imagined working in the mines in South Africa where they would be able to make enough money to support themselves and their families. With one exception, the children indicated they did not want to be soldiers, but rather yearned for peace and freedom from war. Although separated from their families who lived in the country controlled by the 'bandidos', the majority asked to remain in Maputo, the capital of Mozambique, where they would be free from the risk of recapture.

It is also apparent that there is considerable variation in the child's response to the trauma contingent upon the intensity, type and duration of the traumatic experience, the degree of participation in forced military activities, victimization by mutilation, the witnessing of the killing of parents, family members, and other villagers, the child's developmental phase, and his particular subscribed measuring to these experiences.

Table 13.2. *Prevention-intervention plan*

Phase I	Assessment and evaluation Physical and nutritional status Emotional and mental status Coping and adaptive style Severity, duration and type of traumatic exposure Inventory of losses Current stressors Child's definition of the situation
Phase II	Participation in a residential therapeutic program Security and protection Normal school experience Social and group activities Recreational opportunities Range of therapeutic experiences Ongoing assessment
Phase III	Reintegration in the community

A prevention-intervention program

A written 'Psychosocial Treatment Plan for Children Traumatized by War at the Centro de Lhanguene' was presented to the government of Mozambique. The primary features of the program are noted in Table 13.2. The objective was to provide a transitional psychosocial program to facilitate the child's reorganization of his life, enabling him to once again meet the normal developmental expectations of childhood and be an effective participant in communal and family life.

Phase I focuses on assessment and evaluation procedures. Upon referral of a child to the 'Center', the first task is to assess the child's physical and nutritional needs. Next is the assessment of emotional and mental status, i.e. posttraumatic symptomatology, and dysphoria, etc, followed by assessments of: level of maturity, cognitive capacities, the social and family situation; the severity, duration and type of traumatic experiences; current stressors; and coping and adaptive style. An inventory of the child's losses should be conducted, i.e. loss of community, home, mother/father, siblings, neighbors, and body mutilations, etc. Finally, the child's definition and understanding of the traumatic situation should be determined.

Phase II focuses on the child's active participation in a therapeutic residential treatment setting in which one can feel safe and protected. The 'Center' will provide an organized program that encourages participation in a *full* schedule of events that includes practical living arrangements, normal schooling, organized play, sports, group and social activities. The child should have an opportunity to express his feelings and to reexperience the traumatic situation through the safety of play, dance, song, drawings and conversation.

Preferably, a mental health professional who is familiar with posttraumatic symptomatology can work with the child individually or in a group experience in an effort to facilitate abreaction, reconstruction of the traumatic situation, and 'working through'.

The 'Centro de Lhanguene', was particularly skilful in its use of group play and dance to facilitate the child's sense of mastery over the feeling of helplessness that is the essence of the traumatic situation. In a form of psychodrama, the child participants would enact their experiences in captivity through song and dance, turning passive into active; achieving mastery over the experience of helplessness before their captors.

The *younger* children are given an opportunity to draw or play out their experiences and then to talk about them. So that he won't be alone with his feelings, the child is encouraged to verbalize general feelings, questions, and concerns. It is sometimes helpful to provide emotional labels for common reactions such as, 'you are feeling guilty', 'you think you should have done more to resist', 'you are afraid of your anger', 'you want to have revenge', etc. Clarification for confusion is provided. The *older* child is encouraged to express his fears, anxiety, anger, and sad feelings. He needs to talk about the event, to discuss his guilt, shame, grief, and sense of helplessness in being forced to do something he did not want to do.

If he has killed, he must talk about the feelings he experienced when he killed. Did he feel sadness, shame, guilt, or even a sense of power. The child needs to have the opportunity to mourn and grieve, to experience shame and guilt over his betrayal of his own standards of morality, and to be reassured, when possible, that he could not realistically have done anything else without being killed or mutilated himself. Fantasies of revenge and impulses toward aggressive, reckless behavior need to be discussed. There should be encouragement to share bad dreams and worries.

All children need to have emotional support from the group. They can do this by sharing experiences and talking about traumatic events with each other in a group setting. Realistic information is provided about what happened to him, the family and village, how it happened, and what he might expect in the future. Throughout, there is an ongoing *assessment* of the child's *emotional response* to the rehabilitation program, and his *capacity to maintain* progressive development.

Phase III focuses on the reintegration of the child into the community. As the child begins to reorganize his life, to 'work through' his traumatic situation and to enhance his progressive adaptive capacities, plans are made for a more permanent setting. Emphasis must now be placed on finding an extended solution. Psychosocial evaluation will determine the choice of a social setting for the child. Primary emphasis should be placed on returning the child to his family. If this is not possible, consideration of adoption or foster home placement should be given. A program should be developed to follow these children into the future. It will rarely be necessary to refer a child to a group home or institution.

The proposed prevention and intervention program was accepted by the government of Mozambique and is currently being implemented under the leadership of Neil Boothby, PhD (Duffy, 1989).

Conclusions

Mozambique suffered the effects of an enduring civil war. The government of Mozambique requested psychiatric consultation to develop a prevention intervention program (PIP) for children who were kidnapped by 'bandits' and forced into military activities against their own villages and government. Following evaluation and consultation a three-phased PIP was presented to the government of Mozambique that would reduce psychiatric morbidity and promote the child's developmental and adaptive capacities. *Phase I* provides the opportunity for immediate assessment of physical status, medical morbidity, coping and adapting styles, and an appraisal of the traumatic experience. An evaluation is made of the child's exposure to physical violence, the threats of injury and death, physical and psychological hardships, voluntary or forced participation in military activities upon others, and the child's definition and understanding of the traumatic experience. *Phase II* provides the opportunity to explore the child's psychiatric morbidity and psychosocial adaptation in a safe and organized residential milieu. Individual and group psychosocial interventions are provided, as well as realistic information as to what happened, to whom, and what will happen. The overall thrust is to extend and reinforce the child's support system, and to promote the child's adaptive capacities. *Phase III* is concerned with finding an extended solution and promoting the reintegration of the child into family and community.

There is evidence that many of these children can be rehabilitated when they are rightfully perceived as the victims of war and not as criminals or POWs. The psychosocial program serves as a parental surrogate providing a milieu in which the child will be safe and secure, where he can normalize his daily activities in community and school life in a way that will provide him therapeutic avenues for his distress. Lastly, the program promotes the reintegration of the child back to the larger community, family and village life, and hopefully, with restoration of his momentum to progress along his developmental and emerging psychosocial tasks.

References

Arroyo, W. & Eth, S. (1985). Children traumatized by Central American warfare. In S. Eth, & R. Pynoos, (eds.) *Posttraumatic stress disorders in children.* Washington, DC: American Psychiatric Press.

Carlin, J. E. (1979). Southeast Asian refugee children. In Noshpitz (ed.) *Basic Handbook of Child Psychiatry: Vol. 1. Development* New York: Basic Books, pp. 290–300.

Carlin, J. E. (1980). Boat and land refugees: mental health implications, for recent arrivals compared with earlier arrivals. Presented at the annual meeting of the American Psychiatric Association, San Francisco, CA.

Dodge, K., Bates, J. & Pettet, G (1991). Mechanisms in the cycle of violence. *Science,*

Duffy, B. (1989). An American doctor in the schools of hell. *US News and World Report*, January 16.

Dunsdon, M.I. (1941). A psychologist's contribution to air raid problems. *Mental Health*, **2**, 37–41.

Dyregrov, A., Raundalen, M., Lwanga, J. & Mugisha, C. (1987, October). Children and War. Paper presented to the Annual Meeting of the Society for Traumatic Stress Studies, Baltimore, MD.

Escalona, S. K. (1975). Children in a warring world. *American Journal of Orthopsychiatry*, **45**, 765–72.

Freud A. & Burlingham, D. T. (1943). War and children. *Medical War Books.* New York: Ernst Willard.

Gersony, R. (1988, September). Summary of Mozambican refugees' accounts of principally conflict-related experience in Mozambique. *Mozambique health assessment mission.* Division of Media and Publications: The Indiana State Board of Health.

Gillespie, R. D. (1942). *Psychological effects of war on citizen and soldier.* New York: W. W. Norton and Co.

Greenacre, P. (1943). Influence of infantile trauma on genetic patterns, *Emotional Growth*, **1**, 260–99.

Greenacre, P. (1952). *Trauma, growth and personality.* New York: W. W. Norton Co.

Horowitz, M. (1974). Stress Response Syndromes, *Archives of General Psychiatry*, **31**, 768–81.

Isaacman, A. (1987, June 28). An African war ensnarls the US ultra-right. *Los Angeles Times.*

Kinzie, J., Sack, W., Angell, R., Clarke, G. & Ben, R. (1989). A three year follow-up of Cambodian young people traumatized as children. Presented to the American Academy of Child and Adolescent Psychiatry. New York, New York, October 15.

Lin, K., Masuda, M. & Tazuma, L. (1984). Problems of eastern refugees and immigrants: adaptational problems of Vietnamese refugees Part IV. *Psychiatric J. Univ. Ottawa*, **9**, 79–84.

Milgram R. M., & Milgram, N. A. (1976). The effect of the Yom Kippur War on anxiety level in Israeli children. *Journal of Psychology*, **94**, 107–13.

Pynoos, R. S. & Nader, K. (1988). Psychological first aid and treatment approach to children exposed to community violence: research implications. *Journal of Traumatic Stress*, **1**, (4), 445–74.

Rofe,Y. & Lewin, I. (1982). The effects of war environment on dreams and sleep habits. In C. D. Spielberger, I. G. Sarason & N. A. Milgram (eds.) *Stress and Anxiety*, Vol. **8**. Washington, DC: Hemisphere Publishing Co.

Rosenblatt, R. (1983). *Children of War*. Garden City, New Jersey: Anchor Press/Doubleday.

Refugees from Mozambique, shattered land, fragile asylum, US Committee for Refugees. November 1986.

Sack, W. H., Angell, R. H. & Kinzie, J. D. (1986). The psychiatric effects of massive trauma on Cambodian children: II the family, the home, and the school, **25**, 377–83.

Shaw, J. (1987). Unmasking the illusion of safety: Psychiatric trauma in war. *Bulletin at the Menninger*, **51**, 49–63.

Terr, L. (1979). Children of Chowchilla: study of psychic trauma. *Psychoanalytic Study of the Child*, **34**, 547–623.

Terr, L. (1983). Chowchilla revisited: the effects of psychic trauma four years after a school bus kidnapping, *American Journal of Psychiatry*, **140** (12), 1543–50.

Terr, L. (1985). Children traumatized in small groups. In *Post-traumatic stress disorder in children*. E. Spencer & R. S. Pynoos (eds.) American Psychiatric Press, pp. 47–70.

Terr, L. (1991). Childhood traumas: an outline and overview. *American Journal of Psychiatry*, **148**, 10–20.

Ulman R., & Brothers, D. (1988). The shattered self. *Analytic Press,* Hillsdale, NJ.

Ziv, A. & Israeli, R. (1974). Effects of bombardment on the manifest anxiety levels of children living in the Kissutz. *Journal of Consultations in Clinical Psychiatry*, **40**, 287–91.

Zuckerman-Bareli, C. (1982). The effects of border tension on the adjustment of Kibbutzim and Moshavim on the northern border of Israel. In C. D. Spielberger, I. G. Sarason & N. Milgram (eds.) *Stress and anxiety*, Washington, DC.: vol. **8**, Hemisphere Publishing Co.

14

Stress and coping with the trauma of war in the Persian Gulf: the hospital ship USNS Comfort

MICHAEL P. DINNEEN, ROGER J. PENTZIEN and
JOHN M. MATECZUN

The trauma of war includes the preparation for war and the provisions of care to casualties. The crew of the USNS Comfort faced the prospect of a tragic, horrific war, for eight months from August 13, 1990 to April 15, 1991 in the Persian Gulf. The stress on the care givers in this war environment was substantial. As a wartime hospital ship, the Comfort was a unique trauma environment whose mission was the delivery of care to the victims of war.

The concept of a floating hospital is not new, nor is the provision of psychiatric services aboard a hospital ship. Spain employed a hospital ship during the Armada, and during the 17th century, the French provided one 100 bed hospital ship for every ten ships in the fleet. The first American hospital ship was the 'Red Rover' which carried volunteer Red Cross nurses and cared for union forces during the Civil War. (Mateczun, in press)

Psychiatrists have deployed with hospital ships for at least the last 50 years. A psychiatrist was aboard the hospital ship, USNS Solace in Pearl Harbor on December 7, 1941, and cared for both medical and psychiatric casualties. By the end of World War II, there were 12 hospital ships in the US Navy, and many of these had psychiatrists aboard. During the Viet Nam Conflict, two 500 bed hospital ships were kept busy providing care and respite for the forces ashore. These ships each had one psychiatrist and 48 dedicated psychiatric beds. Between 1973 and 1986, however, the Navy had no hospital ships. In 1986, funds were approved for two new hospital ships, the USNS Mercy and the USNS Comfort.

These identical ships began as San Clemente class tankers. Refitted as enormous floating hospital ships, the ships measure 894 feet long and displace nearly 70 000 tonnes. Each ship has 12 operating rooms and a capacity of 1000 beds, which include 80 for intensive care, 20 for recovery, 280 for intermediate care, 120 for light care and 500 for limited care. When

306

fully staffed, each ship has a crew of 1200 and functions as a small independent city. (Pentzien & Bonry, in press)

Once built, the USNS Comfort sat dormant for several years. She had never deployed and her capabilities had not been tested. On August 2, 1990, Saddam Hussein ordered the Iraqi army to invade Kuwait. Seven days later the crew of the Comfort was notified that they would be deploying in support of United Nations Forces. For many, this notification marked the beginning of an eight month odyssey. Given approximately five days' notice, men and women from disparate backgrounds were brought together, sent to sea, and faced a potentially imminent war.

The USNS Comfort crew consisted of 830 medical personnel, including 64 doctors, 3 dentists, 200 nurses, and 560 corpsmen. Mental health resources for the ship consisted of two psychiatrists, one psychologist, one social worker, approximately 18 psychiatric nurses, 20 psychiatric technicians, and three chaplains. During the Persian Gulf deployment, the USNS Comfort dedicated approximately 100 beds located on two contiguous wards to the care of psychiatric casualties.

Surprisingly little has been written about precombat stress and the effects on crew members of the rapid deployment that accompanies modern warfare. Accounts by psychiatrists from prior hospital ship deployments have described the number and diagnoses of psychiatric casualties, but have not commented on the adaptation of the crew members (Strange & Arthur, 1967). Doctor Morgan O'Connell, a British psychiatrist, served aboard the cruise liner Canberra during the Falklands war in 1982. Dr O'Connell spent nearly two years struggling to write about his experience during the Falklands War. He believed that, 'the delay may well be a reflection of my own problems', referring to the difficulties he experienced integrating his own traumatic experience and the trauma he had observed in others (O'Connell, 1986).

Much of the trauma that the crew of the Comfort faced has been referred to as 'the immediate precrisis period' (Mitchell, 1986). The anticipated stress of disaster and trauma may last for seconds, minutes, days, or even years for victims of traumas such as earthquakes, hurricanes, or hostage situations. When this stress is chronic, it is often overlooked by researchers, clinicians, and community leaders (see chapter by Davidson and Baum). During the anticipation phase, which can last from seconds to years, a person knows that there will be a disaster or trauma, yet does not know how serious it will be. The deployed forces of Operation Desert Shield faced 5 months of 'precrisis stress'. The atmosphere was characterized by tension, anxiety, boredom, heightened awareness, unpredictability, and radically altered personal and professional roles.

This chapter describes stress and coping aboard the hospital ship USNS Comfort during the Persian Gulf War. We describe one instance where members of the mental health team deployed to a nearby ship to provide onsite consultation and intervention after a disaster at sea.

Stressors

USNS Comfort crew members had little or no time to adjust to the idea of shipboard life and isolation from families and friends. Ninety percent of the crew had never deployed, and most never expected to go to sea. Despite being told repeatedly that the ship would be sailing, many believed that it would not actually occur. Some said, 'No way, they won't be able to get the engines running'. Precious last days with friends and families were lost as crew members rushed about purchasing sea bags, toiletries, laundry bags, uniforms, short wave radios, and stationery. For many, important family business remained undone. Many crew members had never been separated from their wives and children before.

The extreme time pressure and need for security resulted in people feeling out of control, disoriented, and fearful. Reliable information was scarce, physical stresses were plentiful, and the social milieu aboard ship was alien.

Before the cruise began, the ship's crew was assembled in a large auditorium and briefed on what to bring, and when to arrive at the busses, for departure to the ship. A legal representative instructed everyone concerning power of attorney and personal wills. Some people shed their first tears of the deployment as they sat down and decided who should inherit their money, and who should care for their children in the event they died. This was the first tangible blow to the crew's myth of safety and security; the threat of death seemed all too real.

Expectation of war

When the ship departed on August 13, war was imminent. The crew was told both that the ship would be protected and that allied warships would stay away from the Comfort in accord with the Geneva Convention. Everyone had a different fantasy of what this war would bring. These fantasies generated rumors that intensified the feelings of helplessness.

One rumor held that the Comfort was a primary target for Saddam Hussein, a despot who had destroyed hospitals in previous wars. The ship had huge red crosses painted on its sides that sat high in the water – seemingly an obvious target. When small boats approached, the crew were intensely observant. Plans were made for a defense of the ship. People wished for stinger missiles or a special forces team to provide security. The crew sought to decrease their anxiety and feelings of vulnerability by creating their plans for defense.

The threat of missile attack was a focal point for fear and anxiety. There was a general perception that the ship was extremely vulnerable to attack from exocet or silkworm missiles. People joked about sleeping inboard of the 'big red targets', i.e. the huge red crosses on the sides of the ship. Reassurance from the commanding officer that the ship was protected by unseen forces did little to quell the anxiety. People believed that, if attacked, the ship would sink like a stone.

In response to this fear, the leadership called together the crew for a briefing. The leaders informed the crew that the ship had a double hull and that most missiles would pierce only one layer of the ship's skin. In addition, the ship was compartmentalized to limit damage to one-fifth of the ship. Information spread that, since the Persian Gulf was only 60 feet deep, and the ship was over 100 feet tall, if it sank it would simply settle onto the floor of the Gulf and become a stationary hospital. This information was delivered in a calm, matter of fact manner, and questions were addressed.

After the briefing, the talk of missile attack diminished greatly. People wanted to believe that they were safe, and that those in charge would be able to provide protection. Despite the obviously unreasonable nature of the explanation of safety, people believed it, possibly because they were looking for some way to avoid thinking about the unthinkable.

During the height of the air war, there was an intelligence briefing given by a member of the medical intelligence group, an infectious disease specialist. He informed the crew that Saddam Hussein had an ample supply of anthrax spores that could easily be distributed using an agricultural sprayer. Such a sprayer could be mounted on a small boat and would be undetectable. Anthrax spores would float onto the ship and infect the entire crew. The early signs of infection would consist of flu-like symptoms but the illness would be 100% fatal and would make the ship 'uninhabitable' for decades. The briefer explained that there was a vaccine, but it was not yet available. Antibiotics could suppress an infection, but the supply of antibiotics was also limited and rationing would probably be necessary. Anthrax was a true weapon of terror.

Unpredictability

Shipboard life was structured. The day began at 0600 with reveille and, for most crew members, ended at 2200 with taps. Meals were uniform in timing and composition; muster was held everyday. Most other aspects of life were totally unpredictable. The mission was not clear to the crew. The ship's destination seemed to change daily. From the outset, the war was expected to generate anywhere between 300 and 30 000 allied casualties.

Even liberty ports were uncertain. The crew waited as long as 53 days for liberty on shore. People wanted to call their families, feel dry land under their feet, taste 'shore' food, or just have some privacy. On the day of liberty, excitement was always high. Inevitably, however, people would line up at 0700 for an 0800 liberty call – only to have liberty postponed for four hours, or cancelled altogether because of operational necessities or inclement weather and high seas. At first, crew members were enraged and complained bitterly about the lack of planning and poor leadership. However, once inconsistency became the norm, people became complacent or even apathetic, saying 'Why plan to go on liberty? Its not going to happen.'

While waiting for the war to start, people focused on special dates. The first and the fifteenth of each month took on special significance. The tension rose slowly then dropped precipitously after each date passed. Many acknowledged the irrationality of predicting the date the war would begin, but then participated in contests to predict the date of the first casualties, the outbreak of hostilities, etc. There was a sense of security on those days not identified as probable start dates.

Rumors of a rotation policy were ever present and provided much opportunity for disappointment, excitement, and conflict. It was very difficult to cope with being away for an unknowable amount of time. The Commanding Officer generated a rotation list that would allow the crew to return home in sections beginning in late December. This list was prepared in response to a message from the logistics command requesting such a list 'just in case'. Everyone wanted to be in the first section to go home and felt slighted if they were not chosen. Some crew members even wrote to their families telling them when they would be home.

Early in December, President Bush announced there would be no rotation policy. This announcement was passed over the ship's intercom by the Captain. The crew was informed that they should prepare to stay for a year. After this stark announcement there was increased anger and depression as well as complaints of headache, seasickness, muscle ache, and fatigue. Crew members joined in their rooms to cry. Others congregated in the halls to angrily decry the lack of leadership. There was a shared fantasy that the Commanding Officer could, and should, have prevailed on the ship's behalf. People feared that the ship was adrift and that no one cared.

For many, it was easier to cope with the unknown by not planning for return. Some physicians returned to the United States to take licensing examinations. The crew frequently voiced their fantasy that people would never return once they had 'escaped'. One physician wondered if he should go home to take his board exams. He was concerned that his son would be traumatized if he saw his father for two weeks and then had to say goodbye all over again. He didn't want to have to tell his son that he could not predict when he would be coming home. The father feared his own pain as much as that of his son.

Unpredictability is common on cruises but relatively unusual for deployments. Publications about deployment advise sailors that the first phase of deployment begins 6 weeks before deployment and that it is helpful to mark important dates, such as the halfway point in the deployment, with an appropriate celebration. Because they did not know how long their deployment would last, the crew of the Comfort could not plan for a reunion, nor prepare themselves for how long they must wait before being reunited with their families. This contributed to shared feelings of anger, helplessness, and lack of control.

Lack of information

The ship had very limited communication with the outside world. BBC broadcasts were sketchy and did not satisfy the crew's insatiable appetite for information. There was one telephone onboard ship and it was only available for true emergencies. Mail was the primary link with home but delivery was sporadic and unpredictable.

News was a precious commodity. Initially, news broadcasts were heard only via shortwave radios. The BBC broadcasts drew nightly huddle groups on the flight deck. Rumors, however, seemed to have more credibility than fact, filling the void left by the lack of information. The crew wanted overhead announcements by the Commanding Officer and opportunities to pose questions to the Captain. People believed that someone really knew what was going on, but was unwilling to share the information.

The public affairs officer began to publish a two-page daily summary of world events which was read with tremendous interest. After the war began, one crew member discovered that the ship could receive CNN using a simple antenna. Suddenly, the ship was able to receive news broadcasts 24 hours per day. After an initial period of euphoria, this thrill dissipated and the rumors started once again.

Contact with home was maintained through letters, videotapes, audiotapes, and brief phone calls. A weekly tape recorded message was sent to families by way of the Comfort Support Office in Bethesda, Maryland. The tape was made by the Commanding Officer and was available through a toll-free phone number. Family members used this resource regularly. The mail was a source of solace, excitement, sadness, anger, anxiety, and euphoria. Mail was unpredictable and came in waves. Often a large shipment of mail was announced, but only a small shipment would arrive, sometimes containing only a few large packages and no letters. Letters were sources of extreme pleasure and tremendous discouragement. One sailor tearfully went to the chaplain after he opened a letter, and his wife's gold wedding band rolled out onto the deck.

Mail served as a reminder that the people back home were real. It also reminded crew members that loved ones would not wait forever, that bills still needed payment, that family members died, and that civilian life went on. Some people coped with the situation by distancing themselves emotionally from their families and friends at home. In those instances, mail was avoided because it threatened to shatter this defense. People became frightened of losing their spouses and read between the lines for evidence of infidelity or lack of caring. In a study of adaptation to isolated environments, Earls (1969) noted that often submariners fantasized about their family's welfare, while they were away and unable to help. Earls hypothesized that it was '. . . as if he [the submariner] must create the image of a family problem which is as ominous as his impotence to deal with the problem. Some of these fears, including the conduct of his wife, may be well founded or they may be unrealistic and may approach a delusional intensity.'

Physical stress

The physical stresses of shipboard life were many. During the first several weeks, many of the crew members wore bandaids on their feet to protect blisters obtained from walking up and down the 20 flights of stairs on the ship. Most of the crew contracted a virus during the first month – affectionately termed 'The Comfort Crud'. Everyone was forced to adapt to a totally new diet which was bland, high in fat, and routine. Approximately 50 of the 1300 crew members visited sick call each day. Complaints were generally mild and included primarily seasickness, sprained joints, strained muscles, headaches, and viral syndromes.

Heat was a problem. Initially, the air conditioning system functioned so poorly that the sleeping spaces occasionally approached 95 °F. People often looked tired and acted irritable. The mess desk was located directly below the flight deck which, not uncommonly, registered 130 °F. As the heat permeated the mess deck, the embarrassment of dripping sweat into one's plate of food soon became the norm.

Noise was also inescapable, and only the quantity varied. During dinner conversations, crew members were forced to yell to be heard over the roar of the machinery. The need to constantly overcome background noise resulted in chronic fatigue. Conversely, successful adaptation to this somewhat hostile environment gave the crew members a much needed sense of mastery.

The social milieu

Adaptation to military shipboard life required a profound identity shift for many people. Those who had previously thought of themselves as civilians who occasionally wore a uniform, became acclimated to wearing a uniform 24 hours a day. Everyone had ideas about how the ship should be run. Few of the senior medical officers were comfortable with their loss of autonomy and the increased military structure which placed them squarely in a chain of command. Half of the crew felt that the ship should be a floating hospital and half wished that the Comfort could be a warship.

On this 900 foot ship with 1300 crew members, privacy was impossible. People who were accustomed to their own homes or apartments, their own rooms, and their own lives now shared space. The officers lived with five to seven others, while the enlisted crew lived with up to 126 roommates. This return to dormitory-type living frequently resulted in disagreements about issues such as when to turn out the lights, when and how many alarms to set, who gets the sink first, and who gets the top bunk. Yelling matches often ended in tears, and occasionally in fist fights.

Among the physicians, there was a general lack of purpose and activities. Several became compulsive about exercise, while others became excellent sleepers and spent what seemed like 20 hours per day in bed. The surgeon's motto became, 'Sleep till you're hungry, eat till you're tired.' People who were used to spending 12–14 hours per day working, now searched for ways to fill their time. Boredom was a major problem. Many crew members could not understand why they were not allowed to go home until they were needed. The concept that their job was to be available was alien and did not adequately support their sense of self-esteem.

On the other hand, there was excitement and freedom being in an environment where the rules had changed. The mundane grey tones of everyday existence were transformed into high intensity technicolor experiences at a moment's notice. For some, it did not matter that most days were spent cleaning, drilling, reading, or writing letters. This was where the action would be. The boredom was tempered by the promise of excitement.

People experienced guilt and confusion when they recognized that they enjoyed the freedom from home responsibilities. One crew member's wife was pregnant for the first time. The young man appeared anxious and struggled over requesting permission to leave the ship – despite his preference to remain at sea, free from the responsibilities at home. He wanted to be with his wife but did not want to miss the action at sea. When it became clear that a spouse's pregnancy was not a valid justification for leaving the ship, he relaxed. In a study of submariners, Mullin (1960) observed that, '. . . for a few men it was obvious that separation from home, wife, children, and family responsibilities meant subtraction of an element of stress in their personal adjustment.'

Describing his experience in Viet Nam, Dr Colbach wrote, 'How can I justify pleasure from horror? . . . This feeling was so improper that I fought against it [but] I was in the middle of a situation that highlighted the difference between life and death.' In times of war, expectations change and what seems bizarre can become the expectable. On Christmas Eve a group of people from the USNS Comfort dressed in their service dress blues and walked down the pier in Dubai to attend a midnight mass in the hanger deck of an amphibious warship. Chemical wands normally used by Marines during night operations were used in place of candles. The sights, sounds, and smells of war machinery surrounded the alter which was positioned directly below bomb shaped external fuel tanks. The congregation was squeezed in between Harrier Jets and Cobra attack helicopters. The contrast of peace and war was concrete, painful, and profound. There was a pervasive inescapable feeling that the coming war would extinguish the dim glow of the peace candles.

This setting was neither shocking nor alarming to the assembled congregation. Living with war machinery had become normal, it would have seemed abnormal to celebrate Christmas with family. A cultural shift had occurred, but this was not an easy transition.

After the cease fire, a peculiar phenomenon occurred. Several arguments erupted when a number of individuals admitted that they felt cheated because the ship had not received war casualties. When others heard this they became indignant, saying 'How can you wish that people had been injured or killed? You are a barbarian!' It was difficult for people to acknowledge their mixed feelings about having prepared for seven months only to return home. One surgeon said, 'I left a hero, and now I'm coming home a bum.'

Table 14.1. *Combat deployment stressors*

Separation
Terrorism
Biological and chemical warfare attack
Missile attack
Lack of information
Mail
Unpredictability
Physical stress
Boredom
Lack of privacy
Change in normal 'rules'

People were also reluctant to discuss their mixed feelings about leaving the steel cocoon that had provided their daily needs. Coming home was, for some, depressing because of the loss of this holding environment and the need to leave behind the dependent position (Table 14.1).

Coping and adaptation

Training and preparation often provided a sense of competence, activity, and mastery to replace boredom and fear. At the outset, staff devoted themselves to the task of setting up a hospital from scratch. Sixteen wards were opened and cleaned. When the cruise began, the entire ship had a thick coating of soot from being berthed next to a coalyard. The ship was cleaned at least three times on the way across the Atlantic. Simultaneously, Standard Operating Procedures (SOPs) were being written, watch, quarters and stations (abandon ship) lists were drawn up, and lifeboat drills were conducted. Although little medical care was being provided, everyone felt busy.

Gas mask drills were begun aboard ship almost immediately. During the drills the ship took on a surreal ambiance. Silent crew members walked slowly around the ship, avoiding exertion and the attendant shortness of breath. People looked anxious, but tried to appear calm – even jovial. Several individuals were unable to wear their masks, feeling trapped and claustrophobic. One said, 'I'd rather die from chemicals than feel trapped and in terror.' Group desensitization sessions were helpful for individuals frightened of their mask. (Becker et al., 1991).

The fear of biological and chemical attack was palpable. During the presentation on the potential anthrax attack, the crew sat in silence, appearing anxious and frightened. Many questions were raised, 'How would we ration the antibiotics?' 'If we could fill up our respirators in a matter of hours, then what?' The message was clear – there was no way to be protected. After the meeting, there was very little discussion of the threat, and people went back to discussing missile attacks and other matters. The concept of total vulnerability was not something that could be discussed or understood. It simply had to be ignored. The terrifying information was managed by avoidance, denial, and minimization to maintain a sense of safety, even though the safety was illusory.

Some people withdrew when fear was overwhelming in order to avoid being paralyzed. Others were more open about their fear. Often people would cry in their work spaces or on the decks. Expressions of fear were generally accepted but could become contagious. Later the expressions of fear were felt to be noxious; people turned away from those who appeared terrified. Many of the younger enlisted sailors denied any danger and ridiculed anyone who spoke of their fear.

Both writing and receiving mail were important avenues for maintaining contact with home and the feeling that one was not forgotten and still 'mattered'. Mail addressed to 'any serviceman' was received in enormous quantities. Crew members developed long distance friendships and spent many hours chronicling their experiences in letters. This process of putting thoughts and feelings into words to be read by interested but distant people provided solace and organized the experience. People with pens and pads scribbling fervently often populated the common areas of the ship. Many crew members raised in the video age rediscovered the written word.

A single telephone was available on the ship. The telephone cost $13.00 per minute and was often used, unfortunately, by junior enlisted personnel to attempt a reconciliation with a spouse or significant other. Inevitably, these calls resulted in frustration and enormous phone bills. Others received news of births, deaths, and illnesses. The telephone, located in the radio room, offered little privacy, and intimacies were often shared. The lack of privacy and limited support from the outside world resulted in closeness among crew members.

Shortly after the ship's departure from Norfolk, VA, five crew members began meeting each morning on the deck at 0530 to do calisthenics. Later, the small group began to meet at lunchtime. The group eventually grew to 50 individuals who devoted their lunch hour to strenuous activity. Officers, and enlisted males and females, met and sweated together. People took pride in the control they exerted over their waistlines, their weight, and their vitality. Jazzercise, aerobics, and on deck basketball also flourished. These organized activities fostered social support, decreased feelings of helplessness, improved self-esteem, and sublimated other desires.

Several physicians were addicted to their daily exercise. They found it extremely difficult to stop working out when injured. They would complain of rising tension, anxiety, and an increased depression. For many, improved strength, endurance, and physique resulted in an increased sense of mastery, control, and self-worth.

When injured, some were unable or unwilling to stop exercising and compounded their problems. One physician in particular arrived on the ship overweight, weak, and overworked. He began a strenuous exercise program, lost weight, and built muscles. He appeared driven and ultimately was injured and forced to cut back on his exercise program. He became sullen, tired, and forlorn. It was as if his replacement profession had been lost.

The flight deck was a hub of activity at the close of the working day. Runners circled the perimeter while the walking group took an inside track. The pace of the running often slowed as the conversations became more serious. After dinner, groups would huddle around short wave radios to ingest and then digest the tidbits of news available from the BBC. Smaller groups would then form and return to walking. Many became close friends and confidants as they tried to make sense of the situation, cope with the unknown, vent anger, and keep memories of home fresh. Friendships developed that would otherwise have been impossible. There was no escape. The crew ate meals, worked, worried, watched movies, wrote letters, and even showered together.

One person who had been content in a somewhat solitary existence found that she could develop close friendships. The closeness was situation specific, however, and did not last after she returned home. The shared experience of fear, loneliness, physical stress, lack of control, and sadness brought people together in profound ways, but faded quickly after the ship returned.

Saturday night parties in the officer's berthing spaces became a routine source of relief and a chance to unwind. Individuals brought their personal food from home to share. Slides were shown of recent ship activities. There were no couples and no alcohol. People mixed freely and developed warm relations. In some ways the deployment seemed similar to a summer camp experience. People were freed from their usual responsibilities but the resultant boredom took a toll.

Physical closeness and sexual intimacy were prohibited by edict. Those used to nightly intimacy found themselves cut-off and hungry. Rumors of sexual exploits were rampant. The command responded by setting clear limits '... no touching is allowed where body fluids could be exchanged.' Some, however, began to disregard even stern warnings about fraternization. They felt that so many pleasures had been removed that they deserved a little 'harmless' fun. Others rationalized their behavior saying that the war might expose them to atrocities, or might kill them, so why not do what was necessary to survive.

The horror of war and the very real threat of violence elicited some imaginative solutions. Movies served as an outlet or means to cope with thoughts or fears of violence. Movies also provided an escape to a world where happy endings were possible. Early in the deployment, the physicians began gathering in the operating room suite to view nightly movies. Later, these gatherings evolved into discussions of trauma management followed by a movie. The movies had primarily violent themes. The assembled group had an insatiable appetite for movies with names like 'Terminator', 'Predator', 'Lethal Weapon', 'Friday the 13th', and 'Rambo'. Movies that were played over the ship's closed circuit TV system had similar titles. At one point, a nine-hour Civil War Documentary arrived by mail. The segments were played nightly in the operating room and were viewed with intensity and fascination.

At the same time as the horror movies were being shown, another group in the officer's lounge viewed movies that elicited sadness. 'Beaches', a movie about a woman's death from cancer, was played numerous times. Many felt free to shed tears and display their loneliness and pain in the company of others sharing the experience. The officer's lounge group also viewed upbeat movies with happy endings. These movies provided an escape to a world that appeared to make sense. The operating room group never mixed thoroughly with the officer's lounge group (Table 14.2).

Prevention and consultation

'For me, the most frustrating part of the whole experience was trying to make people understand that I was not really interested in recounting the various types and numbers of psychiatric casualties that I saw, but, rather in emphasizing my discovery of the true role of the military psychiatrist – that of prevention. How do you quantify this aspect of your work' (O'Connell, 1986)? The role of the psychiatrist on a ship in a war zone is radically different than that of a colleague practising in an office in a peaceful setting. Primary prevention through consultation to community leaders and commanders, including education and early identification of at

Table 14.2. *Coping and adaptation*

Training/work
Denial/avoidance/withdrawal
Humor
Exercise
Social support and friendships
Contact with home:
   Letters to home
   Letters from home
   Audio/videotapes
   'Any serviceman' letters
Movies

---

risk individuals are critical functions of the psychiatrist at sea. Secondary prevention through crisis intervention and initial stabilization of patients are also critical functions for the psychiatrist. These concepts are the basis of care for patients and communities facing the stresses of war trauma (Glass, 1955).

Mental health care

The USNS Comfort deployed without a plan for the provision of mental health services. Almost immediately, the ship's psychiatrist, psychologist, and social worker combined forces with a psychiatric nurse and a chaplain to form a mental health team. Each member agreed to meet daily and share their activities and perceptions with the rest of the team. In this way, 'turf issues' and redundancy in the provision of services was minimized. Frequent meetings with open exchange of ideas promoted trust and camaraderie. The team members provided support to one another and developed a coherent and proactive mental health plan. Knowledge of the unique stressors on the USNS Comfort crew and other deployed forces allowed the mental health team to prioritize mental health services.

Education, command consultation, and group interventions were emphasized. The team agreed that if group function could be improved, individuals would withstand greater levels of stress. In parallel fashion, the mental health team fought off its own inclination to function as a set of individuals. Daily meetings were mandatory and provided a forum for both planning and team building.

The team agreed that it would be necessary to establish services for the ship's crew, servicemen in the theater of operations, and combat stress casualties during the war. If, however, the ship received large numbers of psychiatric casualties, mental health workers would be busy taking care of casualties, and the crew of the Comfort would need to be prepared to provide much of their own psychological support.

The mental health team identified its initial task as providing information and training to the crew as prophylaxis against combat stress. At the same time, development of traditional inpatient, outpatient, and consultation/liaison services were needed.

A ship's crew is a closed social system with a strong internal structure wherein each crew member relies on his shipmate for his survival. This system possesses extraordinary strength and resiliency when the group is strong, however, if this structure is weakened, group panic can occur. In a study of naval combat stress reactions, Weisaeth Gorm and van Overloop, (1986) proposed that group panic is bound to have more deleterious consequences on a ship as compared to a shore based facility. He stated that group panic '. . . is always a direct threat to the functioning of a naval ship as a whole'.

Nurses and corpsmen are at increased high risk for acute and chronic posttraumatic stress disorder (PTSD) (Norman, 1986). Several studies documented a high incidence of PTSD among Viet Nam era nurses (Baker, 1989; Norman, 1986). Navy nurses must possess superior clinical skills but they often serve primarily as supervisors, mentors, teachers, disciplinarians, and surrogate parents for young corpsmen (Shiffer, 1990). In a stirring account of her experiences in Viet Nam, RADM Frances Shea (1983) described how she was called upon to become a '. . . substitute mother, wife, lover, sister – the shoulder to cry on'. She went on to say, however, that nurses '. . . would not share [their own trauma] with anyone'. They simply 'toughed it out', and paid the consequences later.

An increase in patients' violent activity was noted by hospital ship psychiatrists during the Viet Nam conflict and was attributed to the situational approval of external aggression (Strange & Arthur, 1967). Training in the control of violent patients and the use of physical restraints is important to all corpsmen and nurses.

Many of the crew had young children at home. Conversations in lounges, at dinner, and before sleep often contained themes of loss, loneliness, and sadness. Several people asked for formal mental health consultations because they were dreaming that their children had died or that their families would be gone. A group was formed to cope with the separation. This tightknit group of parents transformed their sadness into creativity and activity. They devised systems for interactive long distance communication using videotapes, audiotapes, and mail. They organized a 'catalogue mail' for Christmas shopping for the entire crew. Mostly they grieved together the temporary loss of their children and their fear that they would be irrevocably estranged. For some, this loneliness and fear was overwhelming.

Case example In mid-January, the ship received 400 additional crew members, reservists who had been called up on several days notice. They were faced with adjusting to military duty, shipboard life, new jobs, new friends, and a war zone all at once. Screening was imperfect and added to the tension. One single mother was deployed as a corpsman six weeks after she had given birth to her fourth child. She had not complained to her reserve center because she felt powerless to change the situation and dutybound to serve her country. On the ship, her supervisor noted that she was listless, withdrawn, sad, and tired. During an initial evaluation, she spoke in a bland detached manner about her family and the stress of leaving her newborn child with an unproven caretaker. But when she was asked to describe her baby, tears flowed forth and she said 'I can't remember, I just can't remember what he looks like. I'm so bad.' Within days she returned home. Her departure caused a thoughtful yet heated discussion about the ethics of deploying mothers with young children, and the age when it would be acceptable for a mother to leave her child. There was no consensus except that perhaps the deployment was unhealthy but necessary.

The USNS Comfort did not have beds designated for psychiatric care prior to deployment. During the first week of the deployment, the mental health team met with the commanding officer and agreed that 10–20% of the beds on the hospital ship should be designated for psychiatric casualties. This estimate was based on the Viet Nam experience wherein the USNS Repose had 48 out of 500 total beds devoted to Psychiatry, and on projections that up to 30% of all casualties would be psychiatric.

The mental health inpatient service on the USNS Comfort was divided into two units. The first unit was a Combat Stress Center (CSC) with a 72 bed total capacity, and the second unit was a 60 bed combined psychiatry/medicine ward. The CSC was designed to apply lessons learned from recent conflicts and to use the principles of combat psychiatry: proximity, immediacy, and expectancy. Military personnel triaged to this unit were expected to return to duty within 48 to 72 hours. Combat stress casualties would remain in uniform, be addressed by their military rank, eat on the mess decks, and have daily work assignments. Treatment would consist of rest, replenishment, and psychological support combined with education on stress management and battle fatigue. Medications would be limited to sleeping aids except in very special cases. The unit would be run by corpsmen designated as 'squad leaders'. A military atmosphere would be preserved and access to the psychiatric ward would be severely limited. Servicemen assigned to the CSC would be referred to as soldiers, sailors, or marines – not as patients.

Case example The first crew member to be admitted to the psychiatry ward was a young female corpsman. Several days before the deployment she had become engaged and was transferred to a new work center with different people. She was having trouble sleeping and eating. She tried to tell friends, coworkers, and supervisors that she was not coping but 'no one would listen'. On the night of her hospitalization, she picked up one of the fire axes and carried it into her berthing area in a threatening manner. After the commotion subsided, she was escorted to the psychiatric ward. Her recovery was uneventful once she felt she was being heard and understood.

One measure of the crew's overall mental health was the rate of psychiatric hospitalization and subsequent departure from the ship. During the six and a half months of the deployment, 17 Comfort crew members accounted for 18 psychiatric admissions. Six of these patients were evacuated to await medical discharge from the Navy, and 11 were returned to duty. Of the 11 returned to duty, six were later returned to the United States because they were found unsuitable for further service on the basis of poor performance. The 12 crew members who left the ship after a psychiatric admission represented one percent of the ship's crew.

Disaster consultation and debriefing

On several occasions the mental health team deployed to provide consultation when accidents or disasters occurred. These consultations were important and tested the resolve of the team. One of the tenets of combat psychiatry is that mental health workers should be available for travel to the front lines to provide assistance and consultation. In practice this is difficult because it requires that mental health workers abandon the relatively protected hospital environment and travel to an unknown and potentially hostile environment. In addition, workers must serve as consultants, planners, teachers, and advocates. Verbal skills and one's power of persuasion become critically important and must be combined with a clear understanding of military mission priorities (Mateczun, in press).

One of the external consultations conducted by the mental health team took place aboard the USS Iwo Jima. The Iwo Jima is an amphibious assault ship that transports helicopters, marines, and equipment in support of amphibious operations. The ship had completed several demanding overseas deployments before being ordered to proceed to the Persian Gulf in support of Operation Desert Shield. On 30 October 1990, the USS Iwo Jima was steaming out of Bahrain after completing boiler repairs. The crew was somewhat anxious because the ship had recently experienced a series of mechanical failures. The boiler had been pressurized for the first time since repairs were completed, and the night crew had just been relieved.

A fresh crew had assumed duty in the boiler room when, suddenly, 600 pounds per square inch (psi) of steam began to escape from one of the main valves connecting the boiler to the turbine. One man was able to scamper up the ladder to safety, but within seconds the entire boiler room filled with superheated steam, scalding the remaining ten men. The ship went to general quarters, power was lost, and the medical and damage control teams went into action. Four men managed to climb the ladders out of the boiler room into the crew's mess deck screaming in agony. Their friends attempted to render aid. One sailor said later that he could not recognize one of the victims, a close friend, because the swelling and discoloration caused by the steam burns were so disfiguring. Several of the survivors were gasping for air as their wind pipes swelled shut. These men had to be intubated on the floor of the mess deck. Litter bearers pulled off large pieces of skin when they tried to move their friends. Six men died at the scene, but four were stabilized in the medical department and flown by helicopter to the USNS Comfort where they all eventually died despite heroic efforts on the part of the medical staff.

The Comfort received word of the disaster 30 minutes before the casualties arrived. Several members of the mental health team had served on Navy Special Psychiatric Rapid Intervention Teams (SPRINT), psychiatric consultation teams deployed for shipboard disasters. The Navy established SPRINT teams in 1977 following shipboard disasters aboard the USS Belknap and USS Kennedy in 1975, and the USS Guam and USS Trenton in 1977. These disasters resulted in long-term problems including increased psychiatric disability, poor work performance, marital discord, and psychiatric hospitalization (McCaughey, 1987). SPRINT teams used techniques developed by combat psychiatrists during World War I and World War II to provide aggressive psychological support to service members traumatized by disaster. The team's effectiveness was enhanced by its availability for immediate deployment and adaptability to a variety of situations. The team's goal was to provide crisis intervention, group debriefings, and command consultation which would catalyze the normal process of recovery from psychological trauma. The team was intended to temporarily augment and permanently strengthen existing support systems.

The commanding officer of the USNS Comfort, a psychiatrist, agreed that a psychological debriefing team should be sent to the USS Iwo Jima. This was not an easy decision because sending a team meant that a significant portion of the Comfort's mental health personnel would be temporarily lost at a time when war was potentially imminent.

Arrangements for transportation were quickly made and the ship's psychiatrist left by helicopter about four hours after the steam explosion. He arrived in Bahrain several hours later. The Iwo Jima was tied to the pier but had lost electrical power. The ship was quiet, hot, and filled with unpleasant odors. The psychiatrist was met by the ship's doctor and escorted to meet with the Commanding Officer of the Iwo Jima. The tragedy was discussed in detail and the commanding officer gave permission for a psychological debriefing.

During the initial meeting, the psychiatrist advised the Commanding officer not to immediately grant liberty for the crew, but to establish phone services for the crew, and to ensure frequent overhead announcements informing the crew of any developments. In addition, assuring proper rest and nutrition were emphasized as ways to limit stress reactions. After the meeting, the psychiatrist requested that a psychologist and two hospital corpsmen be sent from the Comfort to join the debriefing team.

The ship's executive officer conducted a tour of the boiler room. The entire room was shrouded in the white remains of the halon used in fire fighting, giving the dark space an eerie feel. Pieces of skin remained on walkways and ladders and one crew member's boot was lodged among some machinery. The executive officer described the accident and present status of the ship. He aided the consultation team in identifying sailors at risk for stress reactions. A schedule of debriefings was initiated.

The Comfort's psychiatrist met with the ship's chaplains, a psychiatric nurse, and other members of the ship's medical department. Practical suggestions concerning early interventions were traded for more information about the accident and about the ship. Finally, several hours were spent educating the ship's medical providers and chaplains about crisis debriefing and expectable responses to emotional trauma.

The initial intervention was guided by several principles (Table 14.3). First, the psychiatrist did not leave the USNS Comfort until he had received an invitation from the commanding officer of the USS Iwo Jima. This ensured that the psychiatrist arrived as an invited guest, not as a suspect

Table 14.3. *Disaster consultation*

Invitation to consult
Obtain comprehensive description before intervention
Identify high risk groups
Encourage rest and recuperation
Help must be practical and reasonable
Educate onsite care providers
Teach about normal responses to trauma
Provide debriefings
Encourage memorial services
Make follow-up plans

intruder. Secondly, a comprehensive picture of the trauma was reconstructed before group debriefings were conducted. The stance, 'I am your consultant, please educate me' was well received. Thirdly, the recipients of aid were assured that help would be practical and reasonable. Brief, concrete suggestions that prevented secondary trauma or exhaustion built credibility. Credibility and access were dependent on the crew of the Iwo Jima knowing that the SPRINT team was promoting a healthy response to trauma, not searching for weakness, sickness, or scapegoats.

The second day of the intervention began at 0700 with a briefing for the commanding officer and department heads. This provided an opportunity to explain to the ship's leaders the purpose of SPRINT interventions in general, and the specific plan for the Iwo Jima intervention. Immediately thereafter, all of the ship's officers were assembled for a lecture on responses to trauma and the likely sequelae of the disaster. At each session the message was clear. The crew of the Iwo Jima was a group of normal people who could be expected to have normal and predictable responses to a grossly abnormal event.

Formal debriefings for 20 to 30 individuals at a time began at 0900 (Table 14.4). The composition of the groups was based on the sailors normal working relationships within work spaces. Attendance was mandatory. The members at greatest risk were judged to be those who had been on firefighting teams, handled dead or dying sailors, or who had worked in the boiler spaces. The groups, which lasted about 90 minutes, were structured but allowed the open expression of thoughts and feelings about the disaster.

Group members were asked to describe their experiences during the steam explosion. This allowed the members to construct a coherent picture of the disaster. It was clear that, in the midst of confusion, heat, blackness, and terror, the sailors were unable to comprehend 'the big picture'. During

Table 14.4. *Debriefing*

Structured process
Encourage open expression of thoughts and feelings
Answer questions about stress reactions
Facilitate descriptions of personal experiences
Elicit thoughts/feelings/reactions
Construct the 'big picture'
Indicate the 'shared experience'
Advise about future reactions

this part of the debriefing, myths about what had happened were constructively shattered.

Next, people's thoughts and reactions concerning the tragedy were elicited. This naturally led to the expression of strong feelings. Many of the sailors clung to the belief that they could have prevented the tragedy, or saved one of their shipmates. Having said this out loud, however, they were able to see that it simply was not so. Crew members feeling the most anguish were comforted by their friends. Anger was frighteningly intense and was often directed at the group facilitators or other authority figures. Many of the men volunteered that they were not sleeping, or that they were avoiding sleep to prevent nightmares. One of the sleeping quarters had become a symbol of tragedy because several of the bunks were conspicuously empty.

The expression of thoughts, feelings, and reactions promoted an awakening to the fact of the shared experience. This was reinforced and given structure when group facilitators explained in detail that the crews' emotional, physical, cognitive, and behavioral symptoms were normal responses to the tragedy. Finally, crew members were advised to avoid alcohol, fist fights, and major life decisions until the impact of the immediate trauma had subsided.

The group debriefings were conducted over a period of 15 hours; more than 350 crew members were seen. Two teams of facilitators worked simultaneously and met with each other between groups to discuss progress and problems. After the last session, all of the debriefers met to discuss and digest the days events.

The following day, the team was asked to provide lectures on the crisis response to the 1500 Marines that were stationed on the ship. These lectures were delivered by a hospital corpsman on the flight deck. The team attended the memorial service for the deceased sailors, outbriefed the commanding officer, planned follow-up services with the ship's medical department, and then departed. The entire intervention lasted two days.

During the five months following the steam explosion, no crew member from the Iwo Jima was psychiatrically hospitalized for reasons related to the disaster. The ship was repaired and completed its mission in support of Operation Desert Storm. The ship's doctor reported that people continued to speak about their losses, anger, and fears of another accident, but they did their jobs and supported one another. Over time, the group's grief became less intense.

The Iwo Jima disaster had a profound effect on the crew of the Comfort. When word of the casualties was received, the burn unit on the Comfort was decorated for Halloween as a haunted house. Within hours, this room that had been prepared for a party, was converted back to an intensive care unit. Four Iwo Jima victims with burns over 90% of their bodies were treated. Many of the staff members in the ICU had never seen such catastrophic burns. Over the next 20 hours, the medical staff struggled to save the first burn victims to arrive on the Comfort. Tragically, they all died. There was sadness and a sense of demoralization even though the senior physicians repeatedly explained that burns of such severity were inevitably fatal.

Several of the crew members who had attended the critical incident stress debriefing seminar cofacillitated informal debriefing sessions for the ICU staff. Although people were reluctant to speak at first, they slowly revealed their sadness, anger, feelings of helplessness, and their fear that the Iwo Jima casualties were a harbinger of things to come. People felt unprepared for the horror of watching helplessly as young men died. The ICU staff debated whether to redecorate the unit as a haunted house and proceed with the Halloween party. After much discussion, the staff reached the conclusion that the party would go on. That evening the ICU became a fake house of horrors, and the crew relaxed. It was a most unusual memorial.

Several weeks later, eight soldiers were brought to the Comfort nearly comatose after they had accidently ingested methanol. The medical staff responded immediately, providing superior care. All of the patients recovered without any long-term sequelae. This successful experience restored the confidence of the medical unit.

Conclusions

In many ways, the Desert Shield/Storm deployment of the USNS Comfort was similar to other Naval deployments. Crew members were separated from their families, they lacked privacy, living was structured, and physical stress was plentiful. In other ways, the experience was unique. It was the first deployment for the ship, there was no time for the crew to prepare, the crew was unaccustomed to shipboard life, and the crew spent seven months preparing for mass casualties that never arrived. Operational necessities and the potential for war to begin any day contributed to the tension, anxiety, lack of reliable information, unpredictability, and radically altered personal and professional roles. The crew responded to this stressful environment by employing a variety of coping mechanisms that prevented disabling depression and despair.

Initial responses of the crew included denial and minimization of the stress. Over time, new or previously forgotten skills and strategies were used. Maintaining communication with each other and those back home, training, exercise, and the social network were important coping strategies. The mental health team focused its limited resources to catalyze these processes, 'inoculate' the crew, and provide command consultation, education, and identification of at-risk groups. Crew members were constantly encouraged to put their experience into words. Disaster at sea requires psychiatric consultation to minimize psychiatric morbidity and aid rapid return to function.

Care providers had to operate in a hostile environment under the chronic stress of impending war and the potential for overwhelming casualties. The role of salesman, educator, consultant, and cheerleader are a part of the mental health role in the treatment and prevention of war trauma psychiatric casualties.

References

Baker, R. R. (1989). The military nurse experience in Vietnam: stress and impact. *Journal of Clinical Psychology*, **45**, 736–44.

Becker, D. E. et al. (1991). *A gas mask desensitization program for sailors in a war zone*. Presented at the AMSUS Convention, New York.

Colbach, E. M. (1985). Ethical issues in combat psychiatry. *Military Medicine*, **150**, 256–65.

Earls, J. H. (1969). Human adjustment to an exotic environment: the nuclear submarine. *Archives of General Psychiatry*, **20**, 117–23.

Glass, A. J. (1955). Principles of combat psychiatry. *Military Medicine*, **117**, 27–33.

Mateczun, J. M. (in press). Navy-marine corps combat psychiatry, In F. D. Jones (ed.), *Textbook of Military Medicine*, Office of the Surgeon: Washington, DC, vol. 6.

McCaughey, B. G. (1987). US Navy special psychiatric rapid intervention team (SPRINT). *Military Medicine*, **152**, 133–5.

Mitchell, J. T. (1986). Assessing and managing the psychologic impact of terrorism, civil disorder, disasters, and mass casualties. *Emergency Care Quarterly*, **2**(1), 51–8.

Mullin, G. S. (1960). Some psychological aspects of isolated Antarctic living. *American Journal of Psychiatry*, **117**, 323–5.

Norman, E. M. (1986). A study of female military nurses in Vietnam during the war years 1965–73. *Journal of Nursing History*, **2**(1), 43–60.

O'Connell, M. R. (1986). Stress-induced stress in the psychiatrist: a naval psychiatrist's personal view of the Falklands' conflict. *Stress Medicine*, **2**, 307–14.

Pentzien, R. J. & Bonry, P. O. (in press). First to aid: USNS Mercy (T-AH19) and USNS Comfort (T-AH20) deploy to the Persian Gulf. *The Journal of the US Army Medical Department.*

Shea, F. T. (1983). Stress of caring for combat casualties. *US Navy Medicine*, **74**, 4–7.

Shiffer, S. W. (1990). Today's role of the Navy nurse. *Military Medicine*, **155**(5), 208–13.

Strange, R. E. & Arthur, R. J. (1967). Hospital ship psychiatry in a War zone. *American Journal of Psychiatry*, **124**(3), 281–6.

Weisaeth, L., Gorm, P. & van Overloop, M. (1986, September). *Naval combat stress-reactions.* Presented to NATO Conference on Disasters, Paris, France.

Weybrew, B. B. & Molish, H. B. (1979). Attitude changes during and after long submarine missions. Undersea Biomedical Research, Submarine Supplement.

15

Long-term sequelae of combat in World War II, Korea and Vietnam: a comparative study

ROBERT ROSENHECK and ALAN FONTANA

Introduction

In the years since the conclusion of the Vietnam conflict, mental health clinicians and social scientists have vigorously pursued the study of what was initially termed post-Vietnam stress syndrome. Pressed by urgent questions concerning the prevalence and etiology of psychological adjustment problems among Vietnam veterans, great strides have been made in the diagnosis, psychometric assessment, and treatment of the psychological sequelae of combat exposure in Vietnam.

A critical event in the study of war zone stress was the development of the diagnosis of Posttraumatic Stress Disorder (PTSD) for the third edition of the *American Psychiatric Association's Diagnostic and Statistical Manual* (American Psychiatric Association, 1980). Two features of this newly defined diagnostic entity were of particular importance. First, PTSD was conceptualized as a reaction to any type of extreme stress, not just to combat experience. Secondly, the cardinal features of the syndrome were identified in operational terms, encouraging empirical studies of the prevalence and presentation of the disorder in diverse populations.

The importance of comparative studies of PTSD

Although one of the distinctive features of the conceptualization of PTSD was its applicability to many types of traumatic experience, the preponderance of studies of PTSD among war veterans has focused on combat veterans of the Vietnam war. There have been a small number of clinical and empirical studies that have reported the existence of long-term sequelae of combat service among veterans of World War II (Archibald & Tuddenham, 1965; Brill & Beebe, 1955), and veterans of the Korean Conflict (Sutker, Thomason & Allain, 1989). There has been only one study, conducted on a medical ward in a Department of Veterans Affairs (VA) medical center, which compared the prevalence of combat stress among veterans of different wars (Blake et al., 1990).

In spite of the lack of empirical data, there is considerable speculation about differences in the experiences of veterans of different wars, particularly between veterans of World War II and the Vietnam Conflict. Some have suggested that both the guerilla nature of combat in Vietnam and the public controversy surrounding the war resulted in a degree of social alienation and psychological stress among Vietnam veterans that was relatively uncommon among veterans of World War II (Laufer, Gallops & Frey-Wouters, 1984). It is curious that there has been little discussion of the experiences of veterans of the Korean Conflict, even though, like Vietnam veterans, they fought in a war of containment that was undeclared, lacked sustained popular support, was fought on the Asian mainland, and ended in less than a military victory.

Comparative studies of different subgroups of veterans studied cross-sectionally are critical for an understanding of similarities and differences in the presentation of PTSD among veterans of different wars. While core symptoms may be similar, differences in 1) premilitary psychological and socioeconomic status, 2) combat experience, 3) quality of the postwar 'home-coming', and 4) the broad sociocultural milieu to which they returned are likely to have a significant influence on the nature of the readjustment problems experienced by veterans of different wars. Only through comparative empirical studies will it be possible to understand how the interaction of personal psychology, military experience, and changing societal circumstances shapes the long-term impact of combat.

The aging of World War II and Korean veterans lends a certain urgency to the conduct of cross-sectional comparative studies. In only a few years these veterans will be gone altogether, and comparative studies will be impossible. It seems appropriate and timely to apply knowledge and methods developed in the study of Vietnam veterans to the study of veterans of other wars.

Central issues in the study of PTSD among combat veterans

Studies conducted on Vietnam era veterans have typically focused on four questions: 1) Does PTSD exist among combat veterans years after the conclusion of their wartime service and, if so, what is its overall prevalence?, 2) How do combat veterans differ from noncombat veterans in their premilitary service characteristics (especially ethnicity, social class, and psychiatric illness)?, 3) What is the relative importance of premilitary risk factors versus war zone trauma in the emergence of chronic PTSD?, and 4) What relationships can be discerned between PTSD and other postwar psychiatric illnesses, problems in social adjustment, and patterns of service utilization (especially services from the Department of Veterans Affairs (VA), the federal agency whose primary mission is to heal the wounds of war)?

Studies have demonstrated the existence of postwar psychological problems among Vietnam (Kulka et al., 1988), Korean (Sutker et al., 1989), and World War II veterans (Archibald & Tuddenham, 1965). The National Vietnam Veterans Readjustment Study (NVVRS) convincingly demonstrated a 15.2% prevalence rate for PTSD among Vietnam theater veterans (Kulka et al., 1988). Numerous studies have shown that PTSD is significantly associated with combat exposure. Significant associations have been reported with premilitary psychological and sociodemographic characteristics (Boulanger & Kadushin, 1986; Kulka et al., 1988). Virtually every study addressing the issues has shown that PTSD is associated with serious concomitant psychopathology and social dysfunction (Laufer et al., 1981; Kulka et al., 1988).

Two studies of veterans of World War II, Korea and Vietnam

In an effort to extend the knowledge gained about Vietnam veterans to veterans of World War II and Korea, this chapter draws on two complementary sources of data: 1) the Third Survey of Veterans (SOV-III) (Department of Veterans Affairs, 1989), a national survey of veterans conducted by the United States Census Bureau in 1986–1987; and 2) a survey of 1900 war zone veterans who were assessed as part of the evaluation of a national VA clinical program in 1989–1990. The special strength of SOV-III is that it represents the total population of US military veterans. Its weakness is that data on premilitary and war zone experience, as well as current clinical status, are limited. In contrast, data from the clinical sample, while far richer in detail, are subject to the selection biases associated with a treatment seeking population.

Conclusions concerning the impact of combat on veterans of the three wars are complicated by the potentially confounding influences of current age and generational membership. Although the attribution of effects to either of these influences is largely a matter of interpretation, age effects such as increasing medical problems or widowhood are primarily biologically determined and could be expected to be essentially the same for all generations. In contrast, generational effects are likely to be determined by sociocultural factors. Divorce and drug abuse, for example, are more frequent among veterans who reached adulthood during the 1960s. Although these veterans are younger than their World War II counterparts, it is less their youth than the generation to which they belong that most likely accounts for these effects.

Using these two sources of data, we examine hypotheses concerning who went to war, what happened during their war zone service, and how their war zone experiences affected them after they came home. More specifically, we hypothesized that: 1) higher percentages of minority veterans and veterans of low socioeconomic status would be found among combat veterans than among noncombat veterans; 2) specific war zone experiences and traumas would differ among combat veterans of the three wars; 3) exposure to combat and other war zone stressors would be associated with increased psychiatric and social adjustment problems, and particularly with more severe symptoms of PTSD; 4) PTSD symptoms would be similar among veterans of all three wars; 5) social maladjustment problems would differ among veterans of the three wars, assuming that such problems are shaped as much by postwar sociocultural factors as by the psychological sequelae of combat; and 6) Vietnam veterans, as a result of their alienation from government agencies, would make less use of VA health care services and receive VA disability benefits less often than veterans of other wars.

The 1987 survey of veterans: methods

The 1987 Survey of Veterans (SOV-III) was designed by the Veterans Administration and was conducted by the United States Census Bureau to survey a representative national sample of noninstitutionalized veterans. Veterans were selected from citizens participating in the General Purpose Sample of the monthly Current Population Survey of April 1986 to January 1987 (for details of the sampling procedures see Department of Veterans Affairs, 1989). A total of 7058 wartime veterans were interviewed for SOV-III, and their responses were weighted on the basis of age, gender, and ethnicity to yield national population estimates.

Sociodemographic measures

Survey data of particular relevance to our study are age, ethnicity, marital status, military service history, highest educational level, current employment, income, and VA disability status. While data on premilitary socioeconomic status were not collected, educational level at the time of entry into the military was recorded, and will be used as a proxy for premilitary socioeconomic status.

Measures of general health and mental health status

Measures of current general health status in SOV-III include a five-point self-assessment of overall health status (excellent, very good, good, fair, and poor) and a self-assessment of health related limitations on ability to work.

While there are no measures of specific PTSD symptomatology in SOV-III, each veteran identified, from a list of 66 illnesses, those they had experienced in their lifetime. Three of these categories address lifetime experiences of mental illness: psychiatric problems, alcohol problems, and drug problems. Veterans reporting any one of these problems were considered to have had a mental health problem.

The overall reported prevalence of any mental illness in SOV-III was 4.8% for World War II veterans, 4.4% for Korean Conflict veterans, and 7.9% for Vietnam veterans. In general, these rates appear lower than one might expect and suggest a substantial underreporting of mental illness on a casual health survey of this nature. More precise lifetime rates of mental illness are available from the Epidemiological Catchment Area (ECA) Study, a collaborative research program conducted under the auspices of the NIMH during the early 1980s (Norquist et al., 1990). Although ECA lifetime rates of mental illness are up to 11 times greater than those recorded in SOV-III, there is a high correlation between the prevalence rates for specific psychiatric, alcohol, and drug disorders in the ECA study and the rates found in SOV-III ($r = .87$, $df = 7$, $p < .01$). This substantial correlation suggests that the rates of mental illness reported in SOV-III accurately reflect the *relative* rates of mental illness in the veteran population.

The sample

Analyses included all male veterans who reported military service during the official wartime eras of World War II (September 16, 1940–July 25, 1947), Korea (June 27, 1950–January 31, 1955), and Vietnam (August 5, 1964–May 7, 1975). Because of our interest in comparing characteristics of veterans from specific wartime eras, veterans who served in more than one era were excluded from the analyses. Data presented pertain to populations of 'single era' veterans: 8 553 416 male World War II era veterans (89% of the total), 3 766 357 male Korean era Veterans (73% of the total), and

7 157 674 male Vietnam era veterans (91% of the total). The lower proportion of Korean era veterans reflects the large number excluded because of dual service in World War II.

Analyses

Comparisons are presented between all veterans of each service era, within each service era, and between combat and noncombat veterans. Veterans who reported war zone service but no exposure to combat are classified with noncombat veterans.

For categorical data, standard errors of percentages and of differences between percentages were computed using the formulae presented in the statistical Appendix of SOV-III (Department of Veterans Affairs, 1989). These standard errors were used to evaluate the statistical significance of differences between pairs of percentages, reported as P values in Table 15.1. Differences in means were evaluated for significance by analyses of variance and multiple range tests.

Multivariate analyses of the relationship of combat experience to: 1) lifetime mental health problems, 2) current general health status, 3) divorce or separation, 4) current educational attainment, and 5) current income were performed for veterans of each war, controlling for premilitary service characteristics (ethnicity, premilitary level of education, and year of birth – entered as current age). Multivariate analyses were also performed on the utilization of VA health services by veterans of the three wars, controlling for combat experience, health status, current income, and ethnicity. VA is the federal agency directly responsible for healing 'the wounds of war'. Veterans' use of VA services is assumed by many to reflect their attitudes towards the society that sent them to war. Relationships for dichotomous dependent variables were obtained as adjusted odds ratios from simultaneous logistic regression analyses. Relationships for continuous dependent variables were determined by simultaneous ordinary least squares multiple regression procedures and were obtained as beta (standardized regression) coefficients.

The 1987 survey of veterans: results

Comparison of veterans of three wartime service eras

Data on age, ethnicity, and premilitary educational status are presented in Table 15.1. As expected, there is a wide discrepancy in mean age between veterans of the three wars. The percentage of minorities in the military has

Table 15.1. Demographic data, premilitary education and war zone service: health status and social adjustment, by combat exposure and military service era (single era veterans only) from the 1987 survey of veterans*

Population estimate	World War II		Korea		Vietnam	
	Combat 4434697	Non-combat 4118713	Combat 862901	Non-combat 2903457	Combat 2572085	Non-combat 4585589
Age (mean)	66.7	66.0[b]	55.7	55.2[a]	40.8	39.5[c]
Race (%)						
White	91.9	86.8[b]	86.3	88.7	83.2	84.4
Black	4.9	7.4[a]	9.8	6.5	9.1	8.4
Hispanic	2.7	3.6	3.7	3.4	6.0	5.1
Other	0.5	1.8	0.0	1.4[b]	1.7	2.0
Education at Service entry (%)						
< High school graduate	48.3	42.1[a]	50.5	31.0[c]	20.2	19.2
High school graduate	38.5	40.4	39.1	49.2[a]	55.7	51.2
Some college	13.3	17.5[a]	10.4	19.7[b]	24.0	29.6[a]
Health status score (mean) (1 = Excellent to 5 = Poor)	2.9	2.8[b]	2.6	2.3[b]	2.3	2.1[c]
Health related work limits (%)	25.6	22.1	11.9	7.1	6.5	2.9[c]
Lifetime mental health problems (%)						
Psychiatric problem	2.7	1.9	3.1	1.6	5.9	2.8[a]
Alcohol problem	3.6	2.2[a]	3.9	1.8	6.2	2.6[b]
Drug problem	0.0	0.0	0.0	0.9	2.1	1.3
Any mental health problem	5.5	3.9[a]	7.0	2.8[a]	12.0	5.6[c]

Marital status (%)						
Married	81.1	81.9	82.8	86.2[a]	80.8	77.1
Widowed	8.7	7.0	1.2	1.5	0.6	0.4
Separated/divorced	7.3	7.2	12.8	8.4	13.3	14.8
Never married	2.9	3.9	3.2	3.8	4.9	7.6[a]
Highest level of education (%)						
<High school graduate	36.4	32.0[a]	31.6	18.6[c]	5.0	6.0
High school graduate	35.0	32.6	38.3	37.5	38.7	35.5
Some college	28.6	35.3[b]	30.1	43.9[c]	56.4	58.5
Current employment (%)						
Employed	29.7	35.0[a]	79.3	81.9	88.5	93.2[a]
Retired/disabled	68.5	62.9[a]	17.3	14.3	4.6	2.1[a]
Unemployed/other	2.3	2.6	3.5	3.4	6.9	4.7
Personal income (mean)	$19749	$22905[c]	$27177	$31928[b]	$34519	$30617[c]
Ever used VA health Services (%)	30.2	21.5[c]	21.5	18.6	25.8	16.2[c]
VA disability (%)	12.1	5.8[c]	5.6	3.5	9.6	3.2[c]

Notes:
* Statistical comparison of combat and noncombat veterans by service era.

[a] $p < .05$.
[b] $p < .01$.
[c] $p < .001$.
Totals do not all add to 100% because of rounding.

increased steadily from one service era to another, as have educational levels at the time of entry into the service, mirroring developments among comparable age and gender cohorts in the general US population (US Bureau of the Census, 1989).

As expected, general health status (Table 15.1) is poorer among older veterans, and disabling health-related problems are more frequent. Mental health problems, in contrast, are significantly more frequent among Vietnam era veterans than among World War II and Korean era veterans. This is consistent with trends among matched age groups in the nonveteran population (Norquist et al., 1990).

Veterans of earlier war eras are also significantly more likely to be widowed, retired or disabled, and to have lower incomes. Vietnam veterans, overall, are more frequently divorced. These relationships follow trends in the general US population (US Bureau of the Census, 1989).

Contrary to our hypothesis that Vietnam veterans have been reluctant to use VA medical facilities, 19.7% of Vietnam era veterans report use of VA health care services, a significantly smaller percentage than for World War II veterans (26.0%) but about equal to the percentage of Korean era veterans (19.3%). The overall equivalence of VA service use among Vietnam and Korean era veterans is especially noteworthy, considering that Korean era veterans are a decade older and report poorer health status than Vietnam era veterans.

As with the use of VA health services, it is notable that the percentage of Vietnam era veterans receiving VA disability payments is greater than that of Korean era veterans, although smaller than the percentage of World War II veterans. These differences are not explained by differences in combat casualty rates (US Bureau of the Census, 1989).

Comparison of veterans by combat exposure

Ethnicity

Among World War II veterans, those who served in combat are less frequently black or Hispanic than those who did not see combat. Korean veterans show a reversal of this pattern, with a greater percentage of blacks among those who saw combat (Table 15.1). Among Vietnam veterans, in contrast, blacks and Hispanics are only slightly, and insignificantly, more frequently represented among combat veterans than among noncombat veterans. This finding also has been reported by others (Boulanger & Kadushin, 1986).

Premilitary educational levels

World War II combat veterans were somewhat less well educated at the time of entry into military service than those who did not serve in combat (Table 15.1). However, far greater differences in premilitary educational status exist among Korean veterans. Over half (50.5%) of Korean combat veterans had not completed high school as compared to only 31% of noncombat veterans. Among Vietnam era veterans 4.5% *more* combat veterans than noncombat veterans graduated from high school when they entered the military, while only 5.6% fewer attended college. These data seem to indicate that, contrary to popular belief, ethnicity and class differences between those who were exposed to combat and those who were not, were greatest in the Korean Conflict and smallest in the Vietnam Conflict.

Health status

Combat veterans in each era report poorer overall health, more frequent health related work limitations, and more frequent mental health problems than noncombat veterans (Table 15.1). While not offering direct evidence of the presence of PTSD among combat veterans, these data are suggestive of an adverse impact of combat experience on general health and mental health status.

Divorce

It has often been suggested that an especially high rate of divorce is characteristic of veterans suffering from PTSD. SOV-III data, however, suggest that the divorce rate is only higher among Korean combat veterans, although with only marginal statistical significance.

Educational achievement

Korean combat veterans also stand out when we examine levels of educational attainment. Although combat veterans of all eras are currently somewhat less well educated than those who were not in combat, these differences are greatest among the Korean veterans, largely reflecting differences that existed at the time of service entry.

Employment

Both World War II and Vietnam combat veterans, consistent with their poorer health status, are more likely to be retired/disabled than noncombat veterans. In view of the evidence of generally poorer adjustment of Korean combat veterans as compared to their noncombat peers, it is somewhat surprising that there is no significant difference in employment between Korean combat and noncombat veterans. This puzzling finding persists even when other factors (ethnicity, premilitary level of education, and current age) are statistically controlled.

Income

World War II and Korean combat veterans have lower incomes than their noncombat counterparts. In contrast, the mean income of Vietnam combat veterans is currently $3,902 *higher* than that of their noncombat counterparts.

VA health service use

Combat veterans of both World War II and Vietnam used VA services significantly more frequently than noncombat veterans (Table 15.1). VA service use is somewhat greater among Korean combat veterans than among noncombat veterans. This difference, however, is not statistically significant, a surprising finding in view of the fact that combat veterans reported significantly poorer health than noncombat veterans.

VA disability

Among both World War II and Vietnam veterans, the percentage of combat veterans receiving VA disability payments is more than twice that among noncombat veterans. However, among Korean veterans there is no significant difference in disability certification between combat and non-combat veterans. Furthermore, the percentage of Korean combat veterans receiving VA disability payment is only about half that of World War II and Vietnam combat veterans.

Multivariate models

When premilitary service factors (ethnicity, premilitary level of education, and year of birth – entered as current age) were statistically controlled, combat remained significantly associated with poor general health, work limitations, and mental health problems among veterans of all three eras. Combat veterans of World War II are 36% more likely to have a mental health problem than noncombat veterans (adjusted odds ratio = 1.36; 95% confidence interval 1.0 1.9). Combat veterans of Korea and Vietnam are more than two and a half times as likely to have a mental health problem as noncombat veterans. Adjusted odds ratio equals 2.6 (1.5–4.7) for Korean combat veterans, and equals 2.6 (1.9–3.5) for Vietnam combat veterans. The upper limit of the 95% confidence interval for World War II veterans is equal to the lower limit of the 95% confidence interval for Vietnam veterans. This suggests that the relationship between combat and mental health problems is significantly stronger among Vietnam veterans than among World War II veterans.

The results of the multivariate analyses were not as consistent for separation/divorce, educational attainment, and income. When premilitary characteristics are statistically controlled, combat is not significantly associated with current educational level for veterans of any era. Korean combat veterans are 1.6 times more likely than noncombat veterans to be divorced (adjusted odds ratio = 1.6; 95% confidence interval 1.2–2.0). Vietnam combat veterans have significantly higher incomes than noncombat veterans (beta = 0.27, p < .01).

Multivariate analysis of lifetime VA service use showed that when current health status, income, combat experience, and ethnicity are controlled, Vietnam era veterans were 23% *more* likely to use VA services than veterans of other eras (adjusted odds ratio = 1.2; 95% confidence interval 1.1–1.4).

Conclusions

Our examination of SOV-III results shows that trends in health status and social adjustment among veterans who served in different wartime eras follow age and generational trends in the general population. In addition, SOV-III data point to an increase in health care problems, particularly mental health problems, among combat veterans. Direct information concerning PTSD symptomatology is not available, however, these findings are indicative of an adverse effect of combat experience on general health and general mental health for veterans of all three wars.

Findings regarding the relative pre- and postmilitary circumstances of Korean and Vietnam combat veterans are quite unexpected. More than veterans of any other war, Korean combat veterans compared to noncombat veterans appear to be members of minority ethnic groups, from lower socioeconomic strata, currently divorced, reluctant to use VA health care services, and possibly were undercompensated for service related disabilities. In contrast, Vietnam combat veterans, compared to noncombat veterans of the same era, show the smallest differences in ethnicity and premilitary educational status, and have higher current incomes. It seems likely that while many Vietnam combat veterans have clearly suffered adverse health consequences of combat, other combat veterans have used their military service as a springboard toward their own socioeconomic improvement. These data indicate that Korean combat veterans, more than Vietnam combat veterans, are the forgotten warriors of today.

The VA clinical sample: methods

In 1988, the US Congress authorized and funded the establishment by VA of a national network of specialty clinics for the treatment of PTSD, the PTSD Clinical Teams (PCT) program. As part of a multiphase study of the implementation of this program, standardized assessment data were gathered on veterans who were evaluated for treatment during the first year of the program's operation. These teams operated in 24 cities (see acknowledgements) in every region of the country, and in small towns as well as large cities. It must be remembered, however, that veterans seen in this program were a help seeking sample and thus can not be taken as representative of the general population of combat veterans.

Measures

In addition to basic sociodemographic and military service data, detailed information was gathered on war zone experience, symptoms of PTSD, comorbid disorders, service utilization, and social adjustment.

Combat experience, combat trauma and postwar experience

A series of true–false items, incorporating the ten-item Revised Combat Scale of Laufer et al. (1981) were used to assess war zone military experiences. To determine the experiences that had been traumatic, or stressful in the postwar period for each veteran, clinicians were asked to make appropriate selections from a 18-item list.

PTSD

PTSD was assessed using the Structured Clinical Interview for Diagnosis (SCID) (Spitzer & Williams,1985). Subscores were determined for each of the three DSM-III-R PTSD symptom groups (intrusiveness, numbing, and hyperarousal) as well as for war-related guilt. As formulated in DSM-III-R, those veterans receiving criterial ratings for at least one intrusive, three numbing, and two hyperarousal symptoms were diagnosed positive for PTSD.

To assess the course of PTSD, veterans were asked to identify both: 1) the year of onset of PTSD symptoms and; 2) the year that they first became aware that these symptoms were related to their war zone experiences.

Additional clinical and social adjustment data

Clinical diagnoses of other psychiatric disorders were recorded, and a composite index of psychiatric distress was derived from items in the Addiction Severity Index (ASI) (McLellan et al., 1985). Alcohol problems were assessed using the CAGE screening items (Ewing, 1984), and drug problems were determined from a previously validated subgroup of items from the Diagnostic Interview Schedule (Vernez et al., 1988). Information regarding social adjustment, employment, and prior history of mental health service utilization was also obtained.

Sample characteristics

The data presented concern the first 1,900 veterans assessed in the PCT program. As in the analysis of SOV-III data, veterans who served in more than one wartime era were excluded. POWs were also excluded because they were far more frequent among World War II veterans, and we were concerned that their unique experiences might confound comparisons between combat veterans of the three eras. The sample for the present analyses, therefore, consists of 1731 veterans, the vast majority of whom were Vietnam veterans ($N = 1602$; 92.6%) followed by World War II veterans ($N = 75$; 4.3%) and Korean era veterans ($N = 54$; 3.1%).

Demographics

Comparison of the PCT sample with the sample of combat veterans in the general population as surveyed in SOV-III, showed the PCT veterans of each era to be older, more frequently divorced or unmarried, less likely to be employed, and far less well off financially than their counterparts in the general population (data available on request). Among Vietnam era veterans, greater percentages of blacks and Hispanics are present in the PCT sample than in the general population of veterans.

The VA clinical sample: results

Combat exposure

When the Revised Combat Scale was categorized into five levels, the majority of Veterans from all three eras had been exposed to the highest level of combat (Table 15.2), with significantly more Vietnam veterans (78%) scoring at that level. (In a nonhelp-seeking community sample, only 27% of Vietnam veterans reported equally high levels of combat exposure (Laufer et al., 1981).

To examine qualitative differences in combat experience, the frequency of positive responses to selected self-report items was compared across wars. Three patterns were discernible. For ten of the items, differences between veterans of the three wars were either not significant or were small ($p < .05$ for only one comparison) (Table 15.2). These ten items reflect the extremely high frequency, in this help seeking population, of harrowing encounters with danger and death. Only one item (participation in an amphibious invasion) was more frequent among veterans of World War II than among veterans of other wars. Three items were more frequent among veterans of Korea or Vietnam than among World War II veterans: receiving sniper or sapper fire, handling the dead away from the battlefield, and participation in atrocities. Most combat events were experienced with similar, and extremely high frequencies among veterans of all wars. Vietnam and Korean veterans, however, more often reported experiences that would be more common in the context of an unconventional war.

Traumatic experiences

Data concerning the experiences that clinicians judged to have been traumatic also revealed several different patterns. For seven of the fourteen trauma categories, once again, differences between veterans of different eras were absent or small (Table 15.2). These experiences included grief over the death of a buddy, experienced by over 80% of veterans, and four items involving guilt or feelings of failure.

World War II veterans, more than either Korean or Vietnam veterans, however, were judged to be suffering from sustained fears of being killed, perhaps related to their more prolonged duration of service (33 months, as compared to 19 in the Korean era and 23 during the Vietnam era)(US Bureau of the Census, 1989).

Both Korean and Vietnam veterans were judged to be suffering, more frequently than World War II veterans, from guilt over accidentally contributing to the death of another American. Vietnam veterans, more than veterans of the other two wars, were judged to be distressed from both witnessing and participating in atrocities. It is noteworthy, however, that more than one-fifth of Korean veterans were also troubled by witnessing and participating in atrocities.

Postwar experiences

Three items concerning feelings of alienation and bitterness towards their own country were also identified most frequently among Vietnam veterans, although they were also identified significantly more frequently among Korean veterans than among World War II veterans (Table 15.2).

Thus, while many of the basic experiences of conventional combat appear to be similar in all three wars, involvement in atrocities or abusive violence are more common among Vietnam veterans and to a lesser extent among Korean veterans than among World War II veterans. Postwar bitterness and alienation follow the same pattern.

PTSD diagnosis and symptoms

A total of 73.3% of veterans in the entire sample met DSM-III-R criteria for PTSD on the SCID, with a significantly greater percentage meeting criteria for PTSD among Vietnam veterans (Table 15.3). Vietnam veterans also more often met criteria for numbing, and manifested war related guilt more frequently than veterans of the other wars, although no differences emerged for intrusive symptomatology and hyperarousal. It appears that symptoms of numbing, as well as guilt, may diminish in intensity with the years, while intrusive symptoms and hyperarousal are more persistent.

Relationship between PTSD symptomatology and war zone stress

To determine the relationship of PTSD symptomatology to 1) combat exposure, 2) witnessing atrocities, and 3) participating in atrocities, multivariate analyses were conducted for veterans of each war. These analyses showed that PTSD symptomatology is associated, to some degree, with traumatic war zone experiences among veterans of all wars. As noted in the analysis of SOV-III data, these relationships appear weaker among older veterans. More detailed interpretation of these data, however, must await larger numbers of World War II and Korean Conflict veterans.

Table 15.2. *Combat experiences as reported by veterans and clinician assessment of traumatic experiences in PCT program clinical evaluations, by wartime era (single era veterans only)*

	World War II* (percent) N = 75	Korea + (percent) N = 54	Vietnam# (percent) N = 1602
High exposure to combat (combat scale)	68	67	78[a]
Combat experiences: veteran report			
Insignificant or small interwar differences			
Saw troops killed	95	96	96
Received incoming fire	95	93	98
Unit was in a firefight	76	78	86[a]
Stationed close to enemy lines	75	80	85[a]
Unit was ambushed or attacked	80	78	85
Encountered mines or booby traps	65	65	75
Sat with the dying	67	57	65
Veteran was wounded in combat	53[a]	35	46
Witnessed atrocities	29	23[a]	38
Member of an artillery unit	31	24	27
World War II > Korea > Vietnam			
Participated in an amphibious invasion	60[c]	30[a]	14[c]
Vietnam > Korea > World War II			
Unit received sniper or sapper fire	80	81[a]	92[b]
Handled dead away from the battlefield	37[b]	56	54[b]
Participated in atrocities	4[b]	21[a]	33[c]

Clinician assessment of traumatic experiences

Insignificant or small interwar differences			
Grief/anger death of a buddy	81	80	81
Horror at death & dismemberment	75	80	74
Guilt over surviving the war	46	51	60[a]
Guilt over killing others	42	49	53
Felt inadequate to save the wounded	33	38	36
Horror at the stream of human remains	30	31	35
Guilt over failing at responsibilities	15	24	26[a]
World War II > Korea = Vietnam			
Terror of being killed	70[b]	44	57[a]
Vietnam = Korea > World War II			
Guilt over accidentally contributing to the death of an American	6[c]	29	18[c]
Vietnam > Korea = World War II			
Horror over witnessing atrocities	25	24[c]	56[c]
Guilt over participating in atrocities	6	22[a]	34[c]
Vietnam > Korea > World War II			
Anger the country did not support their war	0[c]	18[c]	57[c]
Anger at being dehumanized by the military	3[c]	24[b]	42[c]
Anger at lack of public understanding	1[a]	9[c]	68[c]

Notes:
* Statistical comparison of World War II and Korean era veterans.
+ Statistical comparison of Korean era and Vietnam era veterans.
# Statistical comparison of Vietnam era and World War II veterans.

[a] = p < .05.
[b] = p < .01.
[c] = p < .001.

Table 15.3. *Mental health status and service use among PCT veterans by wartime service era (single era veterans only)*

	World War II* (percent) $N=75$	Korea + (percent) $N=54$	Vietnam# (percent) $N=1602$
PTSD (SCID)	55	65	75[c]
Intrusive symptoms	85	83	87
Numbing symptoms	63	70	82[c]
Hyperarousal	80	78	89
Guilt (2 of 2 items)	43	46[b]	62[b]
Other psychiatric disorders			
Anxiety disorder	19	15	19
Affective disorder	41	37	40
Schizophrenia	1	2	4
Anxiety disorder	19	15	19
Affective disorder	41	37	40
ASI psychiatric scale (mean)	0	1	1[a]
Suicide attempts			
Lifetime	8[c]	35	39[c]
Past 30 days	0	2	6[c]
Substance abuse disorders			
Alcohol abuse (Cage score = 3)	5	15[b]	28[c]
Drug abuse (3 of 3 DIS items)	0	0[b]	9[c]
Onset of PTSD symptoms			
Symptom onset during war era	89	83	91
Symptom onset after war era	11	17	9
Delay from onset to recognition			
None	51	55[b]	36[b]
1–2 years	21	21[a]	13[a]
3–10 years	6	6	24[c]
> 10 years	23	17[c]	27
Mental health service utilization			
Specialized PTSD program	11	19[b]	34[c]
Psychiatric hospitalization	36	50	50[a]
Psychiatric outpatient rx.	56	67	70[a]
Alcohol hospitalization	16	35	35[c]
Alcoholism outpatient rx.	16	31	36[c]
Drug abuse hospitalization	0[a]	4[c]	18[c]
Drug abuse outpatient rx.	0[a]	4[c]	14[c]
Any mental health hospitalization	47	65	66[c]
Any mental health outpatient rx.	63[a]	78	83[b]

Notes:
* Statistical comparison of World War II and Korean era veterans.
+ Statistical comparison of Korean era and Vietnam era veterans.
# Statistical comparison of Vietnam era and World War II veterans.
[a] $=p<.05$.
[b] $=p<.01$.
[c] $=p<.001$.

Comorbidity

Psychiatric comorbidity was assessed using a checklist of clinical diagnoses, completed by the clinician at the end of each veteran's evaluation (Table 15.3). Diagnostically, there were no differences among veterans of the three wars in the frequency of nonPTSD anxiety disorders, affective disorders, or schizophrenia. However, Vietnam veterans scored significantly higher than World War II veterans on the ASI psychiatric composite index, a measure of nonspecific psychiatric distress. Of particular note is the dramatic elevation in lifetime and recent suicide attempts among Vietnam compared to World War II veterans. Thus, while prevalence of comorbid psychiatric disorders does not differentiate veterans of the different eras, current psychiatric distress and suicidality do set Vietnam veterans apart from those of World War II.

As in SOV-III, both alcohol and drug abuse were most prevalent among Vietnam veterans, reflecting both their youth and generational affinity. However, a strikingly high percentage of Korean Conflict veterans were also diagnosed with alcohol abuse.

PTSD: course of illness

Over 85% of all veterans reported that symptoms of PTSD began during wartime; and, conversely, there were no significant differences between war eras in the percentages who reported delays in symptom onset (Table 15.3). Many more Vietnam veterans, however, identified a delay in *recognition* that their symptoms were related to their combat experience. Over a quarter of all help-seeking Vietnam veterans reported a lapse of over 10 years from symptom onset to the time they first identified their troubles as war related. These data suggest that the national attention focused on the problems of Vietnam veterans since 1980 may have had an important consciousness raising effect.

Social adjustment

As one would expect in a psychiatric patient population, the social and vocational status of PCT veterans (Table 15.4) is far below that of combat veterans in the general population (Table 15.1). As in SOV-III, however, clear differences in social adjustment status are apparent among these help seeking veterans of the three wars. Additionally, they seem to be influenced by both age and generational membership. Korean and Vietnam veterans in the PCT program, as in SOV-III, are considerably more likely than World War II veterans to be separated or divorced. Related to this is the finding that Vietnam veterans are far more socially isolated than others, with 47% reporting that they spend most of their free time alone, as compared to 35% of Korean veterans, and only 16% of World War II veterans.

Employment and income patterns also appear to be strongly influenced by age, with 73% of World War II veterans and 46% of Korean veterans reporting themselves as retired, while 68% of Vietnam veterans report either full- or part-time employment. Vietnam veterans, however, report far greater job instability than veterans of other wars, with 37.4% having quit or been fired from a job over 10 times in their lives. Both Korean and Vietnam veterans in this clinical sample have been incarcerated more frequently than World War II veterans.

Mental health service utilization

Vietnam veterans have used all types of mental health services more frequently than World War II veterans, and they have used PTSD and drug abuse treatment programs more often than Korean veterans (Table 15.3). These differences may well reflect 1) more frequent substance abuse among Vietnam veterans, 2) a reduction of the stigma attached to mental health service utilization in recent decades, 3) the development of specialized services for PTSD by VA during the past 10 years, and 4) the increase in public attention and acceptance of PTSD among Vietnam veterans in recent years.

Conclusions

The clinical data available from the PCT program support and extend the impressions gleaned from SOV-III. In many ways, war zone experiences and traumas are similar among help-seeking veterans of all three wars. The most notable differences concern the greater frequency of abusive violence reported by both Korean and Vietnam veterans, and the greater frequency of alienation and bitterness towards their own society among Vietnam, and to a lesser extent, Korean veterans.

Symptomatology of PTSD is similar among help-seeking veterans of all three wars. Numbing and guilt, along with general levels of psychiatric distress, appear to diminish with the passage of time. As expected, PTSD symptomatology was found to increase with increased war zone stress for veterans of all three wars.

Table 15.4. *Marital status, employment/income status, and social adjustment of PCT veterans by wartime era (single era veterans only)*

	World War II* (percent) N = 75	Korea + (percent) N = 54	Vietnam# (percent) N = 1602
Marital status			
Married	73	65^b	45^c
Widowed	7	2	1^a
Separated/divorced	15	28^a	44^c
Never married	5	6	10
How spend free time			
Family	68^a	48	37^c
Spouse/friends	16	17	15
Alone	16^a	35	48^c
Employment past 3 years			
Employed	21	37^c	69^c
Retired/disabled	73^b	46^c	14^c
Unemployed/other	5^a	17	17^c
Personal income (mean)	$12 600	$11 068	$13 217
Quit or fired from job			
Never	36	26^b	10^c
1–10 times	52	43	52
> 10 times	12^b	31	37^c
Ever incarcerated			
Never	77^c	46	40^c
Less than 2 weeks	20	33	32^a
Two weeks or more	3^b	20	28^c

Notes:
* Statistical comparison of World War II and Korean era veterans.
+ Statistical comparison of Korean era and Vietnam era veterans.
# Statistical comparison of Vietnam era and World War II veterans.
$^a = p < .05.$
$^b = p < .01.$
$^c = p < .001.$

Echoing findings from SOV-III, Vietnam veterans are more likely to have used mental health services than veterans of World War II, to have made suicide attempts, to have been involved in antisocial activities, and to be more frequently divorced, socially isolated, and vocationally unstable. Korean veterans fall in between Vietnam and World War II veterans on these measures, but it is not clear whether this reflects their intermediate age or the fact that the war in which they fought was in some ways like World War II, and in other ways like Vietnam.

Discussion

In this chapter, we have compared premilitary characteristics, war zone stressors, and postwar adjustment of veterans who served in World War II, Korea, and Vietnam. Using two complementary sources of data, a national community sample and a VA clinical sample, we identified characteristics of combat service and its aftermath that are similar among veterans of the three wars as well as those that are dissimilar. The principal findings of our examination of the Survey of Veterans and the VA clinical survey are listed in Table 15.5.

In our introduction, we presented six hypotheses which we shall now evaluate on the basis of these findings.

Hypothesis 1: Higher percentages of minority veterans and veterans of low socioeconomic status are found among combat veterans than among non-combat veterans.

Contrary to our original hypothesis, our data show that minorities and veterans with low premilitary educational attainment were not consistently overrepresented among combat veterans of the three eras. Racial and educational differences were modest during World War II, noteworthy during the Korean war, and negligible during the Vietnam War, a finding also reported by others (Martin, 1986). The Vietnam Conflict, in particular, was fought during a period of high public sensitivity to issues of social equality. The armed forces, early in the war, made a deliberate effort to balance exposure to combat danger among ethnic groups (Baskir & Strauss, 1978).

Hypothesis 2: Specific war zone experiences and traumas differ among combat veterans of the three wars.

By the available measures, veterans of the three wars were exposed to similar levels and types of conventional combat stress. Participation in abusive violence, however, was considerably more frequent among Vietnam and Korean veterans than among World War II veterans. These findings were based on data from a help seeking VA sample in which overall exposure to combat was especially high. We believe, however, these data accurately reflect the unconventional nature of these two wars, in which soldiers and civilians could often not be easily distinguished.

In addition to these differences in war zone stress, both Korean and

Table 15.5. *Summary of findings*

	WW II	Korea	Vietnam
Findings from the 1987 survey of veterans			
(National survey: representative of all US veterans)			
1. Is combat exposure associated with more frequent/more severe health and/or mental health problems?	Yes	Yes	Yes
2. Were socio-economic/ethnic differences apparent between combat veterans and noncombat veterans at time of service entry?	Yes	Yes	No
3. Is combat exposure associated with current health-related vocational dysfunction?	Yes	Yes	Yes
4. Are combat veterans more likely than others to use VA health-care services?	Yes	No	Yes
Findings from the PTSD clinical teams evaluation			
(Survey of help-seeking VA clinic users)			
1. Is there evidence, specifically, of current posttraumatic stress disorder among veterans exposed to combat and/or other war zone stressors?	Yes	Yes	Yes
2. Is the degree or type of war-zone exposure related to severity of current PTSD symptoms?	Yes	Yes	Yes
3. Is the presence of PTSD associated with evidence of other psychiatric, social or vocational dysfunction?	Yes	Yes	Yes
4. Are there major differences in combat exposure and clinical presentation from veterans of different wars?	Yes	Yes	Yes

Vietnam veterans, in contrast to World War II veterans, report bitterness about feeling exploited by the military and unsupported by the country on their return home. This combination of participation in atrocities overseas and rejection at home formed a disturbingly negative constellation for a sizable group of Korean and Vietnam veterans.

Hypothesis 3: Exposure to combat and other war zone stressors is associated with increased psychiatric and social adjustment problems, and particularly with more severe symptoms of PTSD.

In both the national survey and the VA clinical sample, the data we have reviewed indicate that exposure to war zone stress is associated with both physical and mental health problems. In and of themselves, each of these sources of data has notable limitations. In SOV-III, only general health problems are identified and their measurement is unidimensional. Although more elaborate and specific data on PTSD are available from the help-seeking PCT sample, they have limited generalizability. When considered together, however, the data lead us to believe that had more elaborate information been gathered in the national survey, the relationship of war zone stress and PTSD would have been clearly demonstrated in the general population.

Hypothesis 4: PTSD symptoms are similar among veterans of all three wars.

Although detailed data on symptoms of PTSD are only available for the clinical sample, they demonstrate that full-blown PTSD exists among some veterans of all three wars. The exceptionally high proportion of veterans with PTSD is due to the fact that these diagnostic data were collected from a clinical sample. The higher prevalence of PTSD among Vietnam veterans, relative to veterans of others wars, probably does reflect epidemiologic trends in the general veteran population. Two explanations for these trends are plausible. First, symptoms may attenuate with the passage of time or with ageing. World War II and Korean veterans may, in fact, experience less numbing 40 years after combat than Vietnam veterans do 20 years after combat. Moreover, older people may be less likely than others to report psychological symptoms as something out of the ordinary.

Secondly, some psychiatric epidemiologists believe that there has been a real increase in the prevalence of psychiatric disorder among more recent generations (Robins, Locke & Regier, 1991). While the explanation for this increase is unclear, increases in both substance abuse and family instability have played contributing roles. Regardless of the explanation, this trend is likely to have influenced the prevalence of PTSD among veterans of different war eras in the same way as it may have affected the prevalence of psychiatric disorder among other segments of the population. An explanation that does not seem plausible, however, is that differences in the prevalence of PTSD are due to differences in exposure to war zone stress.

Hypothesis 5: Social maladjustment problems differ among veterans of the three wars since these problems are shaped as much by postwar sociocultural factors as by the psychological sequelae of combat.

In contrast to the relative similarity of PTSD symptomatology among veterans of the three wars, substantial differences exist in social adjustment (e.g. marital status, vocational performance, and involvement with the criminal justice system). The typical clinical image of the combat veteran suffering from PTSD is of a divorced, vocationally unstable, substance abusing Vietnam veteran. As our review demonstrates, however, this contemporary stereotype of the traumatized veteran has less to do with specific problems associated with combat related PTSD than it does with the adaptive style of socially marginal men of the 1980s. The vast majority of World War II veterans with PTSD, for example, are married. These men, while deeply troubled and highly symptomatic, were members of a generation in which divorce was less acceptable and families more often stayed together through adversity.

In the VA sample, PTSD among Vietnam combat veterans has been significantly compounded by social marginality. The exceptionally high rate of social dysfunction reported in this group, in all probability, should be understood as reflecting selection biases that are inherent in surveys of VA clinical populations. In the VA, specific priority is given to serving those who are disabled and impoverished. As a result, the observed differences in social adjustment between veterans of different eras may not exist among those of higher socioeconomic status.

Hypothesis 6: Vietnam veterans, as a result of their alienation from government agencies, make less use of VA health care services and less frequently receive VA disability benefits than veterans of other wars.

In view of the evidence of adverse consequences of war zone stress, utilization of VA health services, i.e. services specifically offered to combat veterans by the federal government, is of particular importance. Surprisingly, Vietnam veterans have used VA health services more often than veterans of any other era. Korean veterans have used such services less often (after controlling for health status). Thus, in spite of evidence that many Vietnam veterans harbor bitter feelings towards the government and the VA, Vietnam era veterans as a group have not shown reluctance to use VA health care services. The public attention that was focused on the adjustment problems of Vietnam veterans during the 1980s may have led many of them to recognize the impact of the war on their lives and to seek assistance from the VA.

In contrast to Vietnam veterans, Korean veterans are less likely to have used VA health services or to be receiving VA disability payments. This relative underuse of VA services and benefits by veterans of the Korean Conflict is of particular interest. In contrast to the total victory achieved in World War II, the Korean Conflict ended in a negotiated stalemate (Stokesbury, 1988). There were no victory parades for the veterans who fought our first war of containment and, eight years after the Vietnam memorial was dedicated, there was still no national memorial to the 55 000 veterans who died in Korea. The abuse and neglect that Vietnam veterans were subject to on their return from Southeast Asia has been acknowledged and publicly rebuked. In contrast, few even remember the public controversies that surrounded Korean veterans after their return. In the mid-1950s, stimulated by reports that some Korean POWs had 'converted' to Communism (discredited by subsequent research), the conduct and valor of Korean veterans was publicly questioned. Their presumed poor performance in the war was touted as a harbinger of the deterioration of the American spirit (Severo & Milford, 1989). Vietnam veterans, who came of age during the 'activist' 1960s, were able to rally public attention and concern for their problems in the 1980s. In contrast, Korean veterans were part of a more politically passive generation that did not galvanize public interest or support on their behalf. Recent plans for construction of a national memorial to Korean veterans may signal a belated change in this situation.

Conclusions

This chapter has presented evidence of significant long-term consequences of combat experience on both the general health and the mental health of veterans of three wars, thus extending well-established findings from studies of Vietnam veterans to veterans of other American wars. Of perhaps greater importance is the observation that, while war zone experiences are closely associated with post war problems, public attitudes towards each war and contemporary sociocultural trends also have profound influences on the specific forms of postwar adjustment. The contemporary social envelope, along with the original traumatic experience, significantly influences the subsequent life course of young men who serve in war.

The substantial public support and concern for Vietnam veterans during the past decade appears to have generated increased use of VA services, while the relative public neglect of Korean veterans appears to have had the opposite effect. Although wars may continue in the minds of combatants long after the final gunshots have been fired, it is never too late for community helpers and health care providers to initiate the process of healing and social reintegration. Thus, in addition to attending to the needs of victims who identify themselves and seek treatment, special attention must be paid to fostering public understanding of the impact of combat (and, no doubt, other traumas as well) and of the availability of treatment. Such attention to public awareness and understanding may be as important, or even more important, in the overall healing process as direct professional care.

Acknowledgements

We would like to thank Louis Massari and Helen Spencer at NEPEC for their direct contributions to this study. We would also like to thank Paul Errera MD, Laurent Lehmann MD, Gay Koerber MA, and Robert Murphy of the Mental Health and Behavioral Sciences Service, VACO for their support of the PCT evaluation as well as the PCT staff who collected the data: Diane Castillo PhD, Raphael Chavas MSW, and Jo Anne Pennington (Albuquerque); Daniel Merlis MSW and Melvin Bond (Baltimore); Dharm Baines PhD and Karen Campbell (Battle Creek); Henry Parker ACSW, Hal Patterson PhD, and Leslie Steele (Boise); Robert Gerardi PhD and Peter Manale (Boston); Roger Lyman PhD and Betty Bowerman (Canandaigua); Angie Amick PhD and Charlene South-Gray (Charleston); Brenda Doherty RN and Alene Taylor (Chicago Westside); Reagan Andrews PhD and Cynthia Smith (Dallas); Charles Allen PhD and Florence Martin MA (Denver); Patricia Sohler PhD and Renee Hart (Gainesville); Edward Klama ACSW and Nanette Litturi (Hines); Judith Lyons PhD and Freda Triplett (Jackson); John Howell PhD and Launa Nuscis (Kansas City); Ebrahim Amanat MD and Rachel Stone (Los Angeles OPC); Harry Russell PhD and Barbara Peace (Minneapolis); Steven Giles PhD and Harriet Pipkin (Mountain Home); Karin Thompson PhD and Karen Roniger (New Orleans); Neal Daniels PhD, Frank Trotta PhD, and Helen Summers (Philadelphia); James Curran PhD, William Unger PhD, and Rochelle Fortin (Providence); Bruce Warren MD, Marvin Abney PhD, and Loren La Mora (San Antonio); Charles Marmar MD, Frank Schoenfeld MD, and Tony Allen (San Francisco); Ivonne Vicente MD (San Juan); and Miles McFall PhD and Chelle Holt (Seattle).

358   R. Rosenheck and A. Fontana

References

American Psychiatric Association (1980). *Diagnostic and Statistical Manual of Mental Disorders* (3rd ed.) Washington, DC, American Psychiatric Association.

Archibald H. C. & Tuddenham R. D. (1965). Persistent stress reaction after combat: a 20-year follow-up. *Archives in General Psychiatry* **12**: 475–81.

Baskir, L. M. & Straus, W. A. (1978). Chance and circumstance: the draft, the War and the Vietnam generation. New York: Knopf.

Blake D. D., Keane T. M., Wine P. R. et al. (1990). Prevalence of PTSD symptoms in combat veterans seeking medical treatment. *Journal of Traumatic Stress*, **3**, 15–27.

Boulanger G. & Kadushin C. (1986). *The Vietnam veteran redefined: fact and fiction*. Hillsdale, NJ: Lawrence Erlbaum Associates.

Brill N. Q. & Beebe G. (1955). *A follow-up study of War neurosis*, Washington, DC: US Government Printing Office.

Department of Veterans Affairs (1989). *1987 Survey of Veterans*. Washington, DC: Department of Veterans Affairs.

Ewing, J. A. (1984). Detecting alcoholism: The CAGE questionnaire. *Journal of the American Medical Association*, **252**, 1905–7.

Kulka, R. A., Schlenger, W. E., Fairbank, J. A. et al. (1988). *Contractual report of findings from the National Vietnam veterans readjustment study*. Research Triangle Park, North Carolina, Research Triangle Institute.

Laufer, R. S., Yager, T., Frey-Wouters, E. & Donnellan, J. (1981). *Legacies of Vietnam, Vol. III: Postwar trauma: social and psychological problems of Vietnam veterans and their peers*. Washington, DC, US Government Printing Office.

Laufer, R. S., Gallops, M. S. & Frey-Wouters, E. (1984). War stress and post-war trauma. *Journal of Health and Social Behavior*, **25**, 65–85.

Martin R (1986). Who went to War? in Boulanger and Kadushin (eds.) *The Vietnam veteran redefined: fact and fiction*. Hillsdale, NJ: Lawrence Erlbaum.

McLellan, A. T., Luborsky, L., Cacciola, J. et al. (1985). New data from the Addiction Severity Index: reliability and validity in three centers. *Journal of Nervous and Mental Disease*, **173**, 412–23.

Norquist G. S., Hough R. L., Golding J. M. & Escobar J. I. (1990). Psychiatric disorder in male veterans and nonveterans. *Journal of Nervous and Mental Disease*, **178**, 328–35.

Robins, L. N., Locke, B. Z. & Regier, D. A. (1991). An Overview of Psychiatric Disorders in America. In Robins, L. N. and Regier, D. A., (eds). *Psychiatric disorders in America*. New York: Free Press.

Severo R. & Milford L. (1989). *The wages of War: when American soldiers came home–from valley forge to Vietnam*. New York: Simon & Schuster.

Spitzer, R. L. & Williams, J. B. W. (1985). *Structured Clinical Interview for DSM-III-R*. New York: New York State Psychiatric State Institute.

Stokesbury J. L. (1988). *A short history of the Korean War*. New York, William Morrow.

Sutker P. B., Thomason B. T. & Allain A. N. (1989). Adjective self-descriptions of World War II and Korean prisoners of war and combat veterans. *Journal of Psychopathology and Behavior Assessment*, **11**, 185–92.

US Bureau of the Census (1989). *Statistical Abstract of the United States: 1989* (109th ed.) Washington, DC: US Government Printing Office.
Vernez, G., Burnam, M. A., McGlynn, E. A., Trude, S. & Mittman, B. S. (1988). *Review of California's Program for the homeless mentally disabled.* Santa Monica, CA: Rand Corporation.

16

Psychophysiological aspects of chronic stress following trauma

LAURA M. DAVIDSON and ANDREW BAUM

Exposure to traumatic events has been associated with a range of phenomena ranging from mild distress to more severe outcomes such as posttraumatic stress disorder (PTSD). At the heart of many of these outcomes is the stress process, which under acute conditions can be considered adaptive and essential for survival. To be sure, stress due to trauma is a normal response, despite the fact that emotional and psychophysiological processes may be at abnormal levels for a period of time. Disordered responses may follow an event which is outside the realm of normal human experience and which involves extreme threat or privation, including natural disasters, humanmade events such as war, fires, airplane crashes, chemical, nuclear, or toxic accidents, and more individual level traumas such as victimization by crime, rape, or automobile accidents. The vast majority of victims of these events experience only transient symptoms and recover readily. However, some victims appear to experience long-lasting stress following some kinds of trauma. Under some conditions, stress appears to persist and may form the basis of PTSD. In such cases, abnormal levels of response persist for abnormally long periods of time. Davidson and Baum (1986) suggested that situations which are not necessarily intense, but which pose lasting threats, may be associated with persistent symptoms of stress, and that these chronic stress reactions are very similar to posttraumatic stress disorder, and may differ only in the intensity of the symptoms. In this chapter we will describe the psychophysiological bases of traumatic stress, and discuss the parallels between chronic stress reactions and PTSD following exposure to trauma.

Symptoms of PTSD and chronic stress

Posttraumatic stress disorder and chronic stress reactions involve both psychological and biological changes. The three primary dimensions of

PTSD are persistent intrusive thoughts about the traumatic event, avoidance of stimuli which are associated with it, and persistent symptoms of hyperarousal (DSM-III R, American Psychiatric Association, 1987). Intrusive symptoms may include recurrent recollections, dreams, intense distress associated with reminders of the initial event, and feeling as if the event were occurring again. Avoiding reminders of the trauma may also be observed; avoidance of thoughts or settings associated with the trauma, decreased involvement with the outside world, and diminished interest in family, friends, and significant activities can also occur. Finally, individuals with PTSD exhibit symptoms of autonomic changes including difficulty sleeping, hyperalertness, difficulty concentrating, and memory impairment.

Stress is a central process in our adjustment to our environment. In the course of even the most routine events, we must adjust to changes in the environment, accommodate to situations and to other people's behavior, and manipulate settings so as to maximize desired outcomes. Under routine conditions, these adjustments are minor or automatic; many are so well learned or familiar that we may not even be aware of them. Sometimes, however, the changes or conditions to which we must adapt require a great deal of effort and involve hardship. When these adjustments require great effort or tax our ability to cope, they are stressful and cause us to experience unpleasant bodily and emotional states. This view of stress is consistent with earlier conceptualizations of it that suggest it is an adaptive process that is as inevitable as any natural phenomena (e.g. Seyle, 1976). Under most circumstances, the changes that characterize stress are transient and our discomfort brief. Under some conditions, however, the intensity or duration of stress can make it more unpleasant and dangerous.

Stress involves perceptions of environmental demands, be they threats, harm or loss, or challenge (Lazarus & Folkman, 1984). Some recognition or awareness of the presence of the need for adjustment appears necessary to initiate stress responding, though many aspects of the stress response are naturally occurring reactions that can be elicited by many nonstressful situations. Upon recognition that one's ability to cope is being taxed, sympathetic arousal occurs and the body gears up for effortful activity. This arousal supports cognitive and behavioral activity that is used in accommodating or manipulating the situation: If we seek to alter the situation and reduce the demand it is placing on us, this arousal typically facilitates these actions. Blood pressure, heart rate, and respiration increase and blood flow is altered to maximize nutrient rich blood supply to 'needed' areas such as the brain or skeletal muscles and minimize flow to less critical centers such as the digestive system. Catecholamines are released to extend and enhance these changes, and cortisol release and other hormonal changes alter metabolic rate and maximize glucose in the blood. These biological changes are only part of what occurs, but we need not describe the biological nature of this response further here. It is sufficient to note that physiological aspects of the stress response appear to form the basis for coping by maximizing our ability to act quickly and forcefully. This aspect of stress, then, leaves the organism in a state of readiness and hyperarousal.

At the same time, we experience emotional changes and our abilities appear to be affected as well. Emotional tone during stress is ordinarily negative: We feel anxious, upset, angry, uncomfortable, overwhelmed, or otherwise unhappy. Somatic distress is enhanced, symptom reporting increases, and our attention narrows as we approach and wrestle with stressful situations. We may become impatient or cut corners to cope with overload and we may therefore be less able to do certain kinds of things as well as when not challenged or stressed. Concentration, problem solving, frustration tolerance, processing of peripheral information, and creativity may all be affected.

The picture of an organism experiencing stress is one of a pumped-up, focused, active agent working to reduce threat or resolve situations requiring major adjustments. As was noted earlier, we are not the first to suggest that this is adaptive. Clearly, energizing an organism before action serves an important purpose and, since many stressors require very strong, very fast action, such readying may be needed for survival. However, under some conditions, this response may not be adaptive. There are at least two kinds of situations like this: when the most appropriate means of adjustment to a stressful situation is not one that is facilitated by arousal, and when the demand for adjustment persists beyond a relatively brief encounter.

What we have considered so far is a system for motivating and achieving strong responses when adjustments to physical or social environments are needed. This system is well designed for many of life's perils: if we found ourselves in the path of a speeding truck or being chased by a mugger, the kind of adjustments needed to achieve desired outcomes (escape) are facilitated by arousal. However, many of the stressors that one encounters are not ones for which direct action or manipulation of the situation will be effective. There are situations in which the best way to proceed is accommodation – learning to live with unresolved demand for adjustment by changing one's relationship with it or by managing emotional responses. Learning that a good friend has AIDS, or being in a stressful situation from which there is no escape, clearly require adjustment, but the arousal described earlier may not facilitate intrapsychic or palliative coping and may interfere with it, particularly when the most effective adjustment is to inhibit responses.

It is also evident that long-term adjustments require a different context: the heightened arousal that is so conducive to coping with acute demand is not practical over a long period of time. The enhanced sympathetic tone, if maintained for a long time, may have important physiological costs: prolonged elevations in blood pressure may contribute to hypertension or heart disease, as may chronic elevations or enhanced responses of a variety of hormones. Immune system changes, as well as long-term changes in mood, and metabolism, and behavior may also be associated with unde-sired outcomes. Management of these long-term patterns when stress persists is a critical aspect of efforts to reduce the contribution stress makes to illness.

The point is simple, but the implications are complex. The stress response is not always adaptive and may produce important negative 'side effects'. For studies of traumatic stress, this suggests that the sources of chronic stress must be better understood. Most traumatic events are acute events (Baum, O'Keeffe & Davidson, 1990). The mechanisms underlying the long-term effects of these brief events should provide information about response management and about possible health effects. This is particularly true for PTSD, given that the disorder marks a clear minority of trauma victims who, for whatever reason, are not able to deal with the trauma in its immediate aftermath and for whom long-term stress responding is neither pleasant nor conducive to coping.

Posttraumatic stress

Recognition of a psychological syndrome following trauma has been in the works for centuries but it is only in the past 50 years or so that the causes and sequelae of the syndrome have been clearly established. Early theories of the etiology of posttrauma pathology were largely biological, focusing on the possibility of CNS damage as a cause (Trimble, 1985). At one time, railway trauma syndromes were referred to as 'Railway Spine', and Erichsen (1882) argued that symptoms of the disorder were a result of changes in the molecular structure of the cord. Not all early theorists conceptualized the disorder in this way. Page (1885) argued that some cases of traumatic stress were organic in origin whereas others were due primarily to psychological factors. The development of psychoanalytic theory also had an impact on conceptualizations of posttrauma pathology. Janet

Table 16.1. *Factors believed to be involved in etiology of PTSD*

Organic causes (microlesions, compression of spine)
Unconscious motivation
Psychological factors
Premorbid emotional disturbances
Memory and social context
Situational and personal variables
Abnormal adrenergic function
Endogenous opioid peptide function
Stress

(1893) introduced the concept of unconscious motivation in the development of these symptoms, and several early twentieth century writers suggested that symptoms were a function of repressed memories of the traumatic event. Kardiner and Spiegel, (1941) in a study of World War I veterans, concluded that the long-term consequences of trauma are discontinuous, persistent, and of very long duration. Symptoms of this syndrome included abnormal dreams, irritability, exaggerated startle responses, withdrawal, and aggressive behavior.

During, and after, World War II, researchers gained a clearer picture of the trauma syndrome. Kardiner and Spiegel updated the work Kardiner had done earlier, and Archibald and Tuddenham (1965) reported persistence of symptoms up to 20 years after combat. Dobbs and Wilson (1960) compared brain waves, pulse and respiration of combat veterans and university students when exposed to combat sounds. Combat veterans showed increases in pulse and respiration and a decrease in alpha wave production during the combat stimuli while control subjects did not.

Today, theories can be grouped in a similar way, some emphasize psychological factors and others are more biological (see Table 16.1). Haas and Hendin (1983) emphasized the importance of premorbid factors in the development of posttrauma problems. They suggested that pretrauma and trauma factors interact to give meaning to specific trauma experiences. Holloway and Ursano (1984) took a similar approach to understanding the development of the disorder emphasizing the importance of memory, social context and metaphor. Memories are modified by subsequent experiences, and what is remembered about what actually happened during a traumatic event will be influenced by available information, the surrounding community, reactions at home, and the development of each individual. War experiences might later be used to represent current troubling life experiences and traumatic events may be reexperienced as a function of current difficulties.

Green, Wilson, and Lindy (1985) also focused on psychosocial processes in describing reactions to trauma. They developed a conceptual model to take into account the characteristics of the individual and the characteristics of the environment. Whether a person is able to recover following exposure to a trauma is dependent on the way the individual perceives, understands, and deals with the event. These individual characteristics also interact with the social environment. Some environments may be more conducive to recovery than others.

Recently, there has been an increase in theories of PTSD that involve physiological processes and both peripheral and central nervous system mechanisms. Unlike early theories, they do not focus on physical damage or CNS lesion caused by the trauma. Instead, they consider processes that follow from the psychological appraisal and processing of trauma. The cause of distress in most of these theories is the continuing distress associated with persistent stress. The biological changes seen as supporting abnormal responses and PTSD are associated with this stress response.

Psychophysiology of posttraumatic stress

At least two major theories of posttrauma pathology are primarily concerned with biological changes. Kolb, Burris & Griffiths (1984) suggested that many of the symptoms of PTSD may be related to abnormalities of the central adrenergic system 'either as a result of excessive secretion or enduring hypersensitivity at receptors consequent to a resetting of discharge potential' (p. 101.). During trauma, information overloads the cortical neuronal barrier. Stimulation may initially lead to sensitization of neuronal synapses, but, if trauma continues or is repeated over time, depression of synaptic processes may occur which may then lead to increased receptor sensitivity. Kolb (1987) hypothesized that the affected structures are in the temporal–amygdaloid complex. Because of changes in these structures, hypersensitivity develops and a variety of stimuli can then cause arousal. In addition, with excessive and repeated stimulation, cortical control over the lower brainstem structures such as the medial hypothalamic nuclei and the locus ceruleus is diminished leading to aggression and alterations in the sleep–wake cycle.

Van der Kolk et al. (1985) also proposed a physiological explanation for the disorder. They suggested that the symptoms of PTSD can be explained by alterations in the nonadrenergic and the endogenous opioid systems.

Comparing trauma in humans to inescapable shock and stress induced analgesia in animals, they posed the possibility that inescapable shock leads to catecholamine release and eventual depletion and activation of the endogenous opioid system. In humans reexposure to trauma may cause activation of the opioid system which may induce paradoxical feelings of control, but subsequent opioid withdrawal may lead to anxiety, hyperreactivity, and aggression. Hyperreactivity was seen as a product of vulnerability to respond to situations with excessive autonomic reactivity due to alterations in locus coeruleus activity and many of the psychological symptoms of PTSD caused by hyperreactivity of sympathetic and opioid systems (Pitman et al., 1990).

These two theories offer biological explanations for the etiology of PTSD and representative symptoms. Each focuses on activity of the sympathetic nervous system, and studies have tested the central role of sympathetic arousal in generation of PTSD symptoms. Kolb et al. (1984) treated patients with two sympathetic blocking agents, propranolol and clonidine. Clonidine acts centrally in the brain, and propranolol acts centrally and peripherally at beta receptors. Preliminary work suggested that some of the symptoms of PTSD improved with each of these drugs, providing partial support for the hypothesized relationship between sympathetic arousal and symptom formation in PTSD. Other drug protocols have been tested and have provided patients some relief, but long-term drug treatment for PTSD seems unlikely at this time (Davidson et al., 1990; Reist et al., 1989).

Research has documented peripheral physiological differences between people with PTSD and control populations, and these studies have also provided some information about biological bases of response to trauma. Blanchard et al. (1982) exposed a group of Vietnam veterans with PTSD and a group of nonveteran controls to evocative combat sounds and several mental arithmetic tasks. They found that heart rates, systolic blood pressure, and EMG changed for both groups during the mental arithmetic task but that changes for combat sounds were observed only in the PTSD group. Thus, PTSD patients appeared to exhibit peripheral sympathetic hyperresponsiveness to stimuli reminiscent of the traumatic events they experienced, and these stimuli may have assumed special meaning for them. Other studies that have found no evidence of such response to combat stimuli among combat veterans who do not have PTSD suggest that the salience of these evocative cues is increased as part of the disorder (Davidson & Baum, 1989).

Malloy, Fairbank and Keane (1983) also compared the physiological responses of veterans with PTSD to the responses of veterans without the disorder and a group of veterans with psychiatric diagnosis other than PTSD who had never been assigned to combat. Again, indices of arousal, heart rate, and skin conductance were elevated during exposure to combat scenes only among those veterans with PTSD. In a more recent study, Pitman et al. (1987) examined psychophysiological responses (heart rate, skin conductance, and frontalis EMG) to imagery of traumatic experiences in a group of combat veterans with PTSD and a group of combat veterans without the disorder. They found greater skin conductance and EMG changes and a similar trend for heart rate for the PTSD group only when they were read scripts which described their traumatic experiences. Similar findings were also reported when an anxiety disorder control group was included. Again, PTSD subjects were more responsive to trauma relevant imagery (Pitman, Orr & Steketel, 1989). Veterans with PTSD have exhibited elevated heart rate, blood pressure, epinephrine secretion, and self-reported distress following viewing of a combat film compared to nonPTSD controls (McFall et al., 1990), and combat veterans with PTSD have exhibited a naloxone reversible increase in pain tolerance after watching the last 15 minutes of the movie *Platoon* (Van der Kolk et al., 1989; Pitman et al., 1990).

Among the most important research programs on stress during the second half of this century has been the work of Mason and his colleagues. Recently, this effort has included studies of posttraumatic stress disorder. Kosten et al. (1987) measured catecholamine levels in a group of PTSD inpatients, comparing mean levels of norepinephrine and epinephrine in hospitalized patients with PTSD, major depressive disorder, mania, paranoid schizophrenia, and undifferentiated schizophrenia. Results indicated that norepinephrine and epinephrine were significantly elevated in the PTSD group relative to the others, though there were no differences between the PTSD and manic patient groups in the first sample immediately after hospital admission. The relative elevations among PTSD patients were sustained throughout the course of hospitalization, and characterized response long after the initiating trauma. They also appeared to occur in the absence of any specific eliciting stimuli.

In a similar study, mean levels of cortisol were found to be significantly lower among PTSD patients than in groups of depressed, manic, and undifferentiated schizophrenic patient groups (Mason et al., 1986). There were no differences between the PTSD group and paranoid schizophrenics. This finding was not consistent with those for catecholamine levels: stress ordinarily is associated with elevations in both catecholamines, reflecting sympathetic response and activation of the adrenal medulla, and in corticosteroids, reflecting activation of the pituitary–adrenocortical axis. Because of the apparent dissociation of these two neuroendocrine systems in PTSD patients relative to others, Mason et al. (1986) examined the relationship between norepinephrine and cortisol levels in another sample of inpatients. They found that the ratio of norepinephrine to cortisol was significantly elevated in the PTSD group relative to depressed, manic, and undifferentiated schizophrenia patients. This ratio provided a diagnostic sensitivity of 78% and specificity of 94% for correct classification of PTSD. To extend these findings, a group of PTSD outpatients were also studied. Again, mean cortisol levels in the PTSD group were lower (Yehuda et al., 1990). However, Pitman and Orr (1990) did not find comparable differences in a study of 13 combat veterans and 10 healthy controls.

Other studies have also found evidence of altered sympathetic response in PTSD patients. As a marker of beta-adrenergic receptor function, Lerer et al. (1987) measured cAMP signal transduction in intact lymphocytes and in platelet membranes in 10 Israeli PTSD patients and compared their results to those from 10 healthy controls. They found a lowered cAMP signal transduction in PTSD patients compared to controls. These data suggested a functional deficit rather than an alteration in receptor number. Perry, Giller, and Southwick (1987) studied CNS adrenergic receptor dysregulation in Vietnam Veterans with PTSD and age matched controls by examining binding parameters of platelet $alpha_2$ adrenergic receptors. They found fewer total $alpha_2$ receptor binding sites in the PTSD group and an altered ratio of receptor affinity states. These findings suggest a down regulation of receptors.

Other researchers have found a relationship between PTSD and platelet monoamine oxidase (MAO) which is involved in the synthesis of serotonin and in the degradation and reuptake of catecholamines (Davidson et al., 1985). Lower MAO activity was detected in the PTSD group when compared to age-matched controls (Davidson et al., 1985). However, when the PTSD group was divided into those with a history of alcoholism and those without such a history, only the alcohol group showed altered MAO levels. It may be that the alcoholism and PTSD develop independently, or that PTSD might lead to alcohol abuse and, consequently, lower MAO activity.

Given clear similarities between simple stress responding and psycho-physiological characteristics of more profound response to trauma, such as PTSD, how may these syndromes be best integrated? Are PTSD and other long-term disordered response patterns simply an exaggerated stress response? If so, what makes them so persistent?

One answer suggested by several different research groups, attempts to explain how exposure to traumatic events may be translated into long-term psychological and biological changes. Trauma victims may experience a conditioned response; that is, they may come to respond to once neutral stimuli that have come to be linked with stressful events (Davidson & Baum, 1986; Kilpatrick, Veronon & Best, 1985; Keane et al., 1985). Stimuli that are reminiscent of the initial trauma or stressor may also evoke responses similar to those elicited in the original situation. The range of responses that are possible include all the responses that may occur following exposure to an acute stressor (affective changes, behavioral changes, organ system changes, and physiological changes).

The logic of conditioned responding to trauma is derived from classical conditioning theory that can be traced back to Pavlov's work with dogs. A stimulus such as food was presented because it evoked an observable response, salivation. The food was an unconditioned stimulus (UCS) and the salivation was an unconditioned response (UCR). When a neutral stimulus such as a tone was paired with the UCS, it came to elicit the same kind of response as the UCS. This new response was called the conditioned response. In responding to a traumatic stressor the sequence of events are similar. Traumatic events are paired with neutral stimuli that come to elicit psychophysiological symptoms of stress. Through higher order conditioning an ever widening array of routine stimuli may come to evoke a stress response, leading victims to experience stress in more prolonged and often out-of-context fashion.

This notion has two important corollaries (Davidson & Baum, 1986). The first is that traumatic responding is an exaggerated stress response and may be understood and studied in light of the extensive literature on stress. This is not to say that there are not some differences in responding based on the nature of the stressor. In fact, there is literature documenting patterns of endocrine responses to different stressors based on extent of threat, perceived ability to cope and so on. Secondly, there are probably individual differences which may help explain why traumatic responding becomes long lasting for some people and not for others. Why some people are immune to the long-term effects of stressors is a relatively unexplored area. To better understand these individual differences it becomes important to evaluate all aspects of stress responding.

Measuring the effects of trauma

There are four primary ways to measure stress: they include self-report measures, performance assessments, psychophysiological measurements

Table 16.2. *Levels of measurement of chronic stress*

Self-report measures
ratings of distress
symptom experience
irritability
previous mood and behavior
ratings of events

Behavioral measures
performance (stress-sensitive tasks)
coping
motivation and tolerance for frustration
indirect effects (e.g. reduced exercise, drug use)

Physiological measures
sympathetic arousal
reactivity
parasympathetic arousal

Biochemical measures
sympathetic arousal (catecholamines)
pituitary–adrenal axis arousal (cortisol)
endogenous opioid peptide activity

---

and biochemical measures (see Table 16.2). Baum, Grunberg, and Singer (1982) argued that a simultaneous assessment of self-report, performance, and biologically based responses constitutes an optimal measurement strategy that potentially provides clearer and more broad understanding of stress. Self-report measures assess somatic experiences, emotional changes and ratings of events surrounding the initiating stressor. Affective and somatic components of stress may be measured using scales like the Beck and Zung Depression Inventories, and the Symptom Checklist-90 (Derogatis, 1977). Scales have also been developed which assess characteristics of stressors or symptoms of PTSD like the Horowitz Impact of Events Scale (Horowitz, Wilner & Alvarez, 1979), the Mississippi Scale for Combat-related PTSD (Keane, Caddell & Taylor, 1988), and the MMPI subscale for PTSD (Keane & Fairbank, 1983).

Performance measures are based on the notion that stress will affect persistence, motivation, or concentration, or other factors which may influence performance during or after stressor exposure (Glass & Singer, 1972). Although a variety of tasks have been identified which distinguish stressed from nonstressed subjects, performance on proofreading tasks has proven to most reliable. Subjects are asked to read a seven-page passage and circle any errors that they find. Errors have been systematically inserted and they include punctuation errors, spelling errors, grammatical errors and so on. Subjects are typically given five minutes to work on this task.

Psychophysiological measures assess activation of the sympathetic nervous system. Changes which result from sympathetic activation include increased heart rate, elevations in systolic and diastolic blood pressure, and increased skin conductance. In the laboratory these are fairly easy to assess. In the field, telemetric devices may also be worn for extended periods of time allowing more complete assessment of daily variations in systolic and diastolic blood pressure.

Finally, many biochemical changes occur throughout the body during periods of stress. These changes can be assessed in the blood and in some instances in the urine. Perhaps the most widely studied endocrine glands are the adrenal cortex and the adrenal medulla. The primary hormones secreted by the adrenal cortex are aldosterone and cortisol, and epinephrine and norepinephrine are secreted by the adrenal medulla. Other hormones which have been studied include testosterone, prolactin, insulin, growth hormone, and glucagon.

The utility of this multimethod assessment strategy has been documented in various settings. We have used this approach over a ten-year study assessing stress among residents living near the damaged Three Mile Island (TMI) power station. Using behavioral measures and biological measures in conjunction with self-report measures has proven useful for several reasons. Since subjects may try to answer questions 'correctly', self-report measures are prone to sources of error. Behavioral and biological indicators of stress may be subject to fewer deliberate sources of error. Also, although these parameters typically vary in parallel, this is not always the case. For example, through 1984 we found that TMI residents as a whole reported more symptoms, performed more poorly on behavioral tasks, and exhibited more symptoms of stress related arousal than did control subjects (Baum, 1990; Baum, Gatchel & Schaeffer, 1983; Davidson & Baum, 1986; McKinnon et al., 1989). However, following the restart of the undamaged reactor in 1985, there was some decoupling in these measures (Davidson et al., in press). The Three Mile Island group no longer reported more distress than did subjects in a control group. However, they still exhibited the same behavioral deficits, and they showed evidence of biological arousal.

The exact implication of these findings remains to be explored. However, these data are important for several reasons. They highlight the significance of measuring stress in several different ways. If we had merely assessed stress using self-report measures, we may have concluded that the residents had finally adapted, and discontinued our study. However, we know from our other measures that this is not completely true. Why different aspects of response change at different rates and some indices of stress continued to be elevated is yet to be explored. It may be that complete behavioral and biological adaptation to the stress lags behind or that these changes are permanent. Either of these alternatives would have implications for posttraumatic stress.

In studying combat related PTSD, Malloy et al. (1983) suggest using a similar approach. They assessed symptoms of PTSD while veterans viewed combat relevant visual and auditory stimuli. As a behavioral measure of PTSD, they counted the number of aversive stimuli that the subject voluntarily viewed, their biological indicators were tonic heart rate and magnitude of electrodermal response, and they assessed patient's ratings of subjective distress. The authors reported that, by using this multimeasure assessment procedure, they were able to correctly identify 100% of PTSD patients. No control patients were incorrectly classified.

Susceptibility vs. immunity

This research suggests that traumatic events may have a number of different long-term consequences, most of which are consistent with chronic stress. However, it does not provide direct information about why some people are more susceptible to the effects of these events while others are more resistant. The figures vary across situations and types of traumas, but it is clear that, at most, only a substantial minority of trauma victims develop serious difficulties or are diagnosed with substantial emotional disorders. Most victims appear to be capable of handling even the most severe stressors moderately well. Why do some develop long-term distress and disability?

As noted earlier, some believe that premorbid problems or comorbid disorders define those most vulnerable to exhibit long-term distress following traumatic events. While the amount of variance accounted for by these factors is unknown, it is clear that they contribute to ultimate outcomes. It is also possible that perceptual or cognitive factors that predispose certain kinds of information storage or retrieval could be involved. Traumatic events are often acute; that is they are usually brief events that dissipate rapidly once they conclude. However, some aspects of these events, some as brief as a few minutes, appear to become chronic stressors and support the persistence of stresslike responding. Recollections or memories of the event and how accessible they are could be involved in this. We know that recurrent images, particularly intrusive images and thoughts about an event, are characteristic of PTSD. These images appear in dreams, intrude on making consciousness and daydreams, and, in serious form, can lead to dissociation. At the same time, individuals experiencing a good deal of intrusive thought may also be reliving the original trauma often, thereby experiencing stress over a very long period of time. Thus the frequency of intrusive images and thoughts may not be a consequence of PTSD and chronic stress, but rather a cause or facilitating agent of chronic stress.

Using a multimethod assessment strategy, we have found that TMI area residents have been differentially affected by the trauma, and that some have experienced more stress than have others. Some TMI area residents have consistently shown elevations on criteria intended to measure stress, and also had higher blood pressure and more medical complications and prescriptions than did others (Baum et al., 1986). Using the Impact of Events Scale (Horowitz et al., 1979) we found that area residents who reported the greatest frequency of intrusive thought exhibited the most symptoms of stress. Further, this relationship was developmental: three years after the accident, intrusive thoughts were not related to stress: TMI area residents exhibited stress regardless of whether they reported experiencing intrusive imagery. However, six years after the accident, only those subjects experiencing intrusive images exhibited stress. Intrusive thinking was assessed with items measuring unwanted thoughts, recollections, dreams, images and so on. Although intrusive thinking was assessed with items measuring unwanted thoughts, other reminders of the accident are prominent at TMI too. For example, the reactor's large cooling stacks dominate the landscape, and since the plant is an important part of the local economy, it is frequently in the news. Following other traumatic events, continuing sources of threat are less tangible. We were interested in investigating whether intrusive recollections were related to chronic stress in the absence of obvious external clues. To do this, we studied a group of Vietnam Veterans who had experienced combat at least 14 years earlier. None of the subjects was experiencing PTSD at the time of the study. Combat veterans were compared to noncombat military and nonmilitary control groups of similar age and background. We assessed stress using questionnaires, performance on a stress sensitive task, levels of urinary catecholamines, and blood pressure and heart rate. Intrusive thinking was measured using the IES. Level of stress exposure was assessed using a combat intensity scale.

We found that, irrespective of combat exposure, subjects who reported more intrusive symptoms were more likely to experience symptoms of chronic stress 14 years later. In fact, combat experience alone was not a good predictor of stress. These data, together with our data from subjects living near TMI suggest that intrusive thinking may be an important individual difference variable which could help predict long-term responding to traumatic events. There may also be individual differences that make intrusive thinking more or less likely. People may differ in the way that they initially process incoming stimuli. The way that images are stored, processed, or recalled may later influence intrusive thinking. If the initial processing of an event is vivid, images may be recalled more often and may be more bothersome when they are remembered. In addition, these vivid images may be more readily conditioned thereby increasing the range of evocative stressors.

Conclusions

Posttraumatic stress may be viewed as a special case of stress in any form: traumatic events, usually acute in duration, are generally extraordinary events that stretch the envelope of one's adaptive skills and require a great deal of effort for satisfactory resolution and integration. Because these events have the potential to be relived, reexperienced, or otherwise made to last longer than the physical occurrence, they appear to cause chronic stress for many victims. In doing so, they may also cause changes in fundamental psychophysiological response systems that can lead to long-term changes and a variety of negative outcomes. If we are to effectively understand and avoid these consequences, multiple measurement strategies that consider the entire organism and that focus on the psychological relevance of both situational contexts and bodily responses must be adopted. By better characterizing the events that initiate these long-term difficulties, the means by which some are able to cope in healthy fashion while others do not, and the nature and duration of affective, cognitive, and biological changes that ensue, we may be able to better treat and prevent a range of posttrauma syndromes.

Acknowledgements

This work was supported by the Uniformed Services University of the Health Sciences Protocols C07205 and R07265. The opinions or assertions contained herein are the private ones of the author(s) and are not to be construed as official or reflecting the views of the Department of Defense or the Uniformed Services University of the Health Sciences.

References

American Psychiatric Association (1987). *Diagnostic and Statistical Manual of Mental Disorders* (DSM-IIIR). Washington, DC: American Psychiatric Press.

Archibald, H. C. & Tuddenham, R. D. (1965) Persistent stress reaction after combat: a twenty-year follow-up. *Archives of General Psychiatry*, **12**, 475–81.

Baum, A. (1990). Stress, intrusive imagery, and chronic distress. *Health Psychology*, **9**(6), 653–75.

Baum, A., Gatchel, R. J. & Schaeffer, M. A. (1983). Emotional, behavioral and physiological effects of chronic stress at Three Mile Island. *Journal of Consulting and Clinical Psychology*, **51**(4), 565–72.

Baum, A., Grunberg, N. E. & Singer, J. E. (1982). The use of psychological and neuroendocrinological measurements in the study of stress. *Health Psychology*, **1**, 217–36.

Baum, A., O'Keefe, M. K. & Davidson, L. M. (1990). Acute stressors and chronic response: the case of traumatic stress. *Journal of Applied Social Psychology*, **20**(20), 1643–54.

Baum, A., Schaeffer, M. A., Lake, C. R., Fleming, R. & Collins, D. L. (1986). Psychological and endocrinological correlates of chronic stress at Three Mile Island. In R. Williams (ed.), *Perspectives in Behavioral Medicine*. NY: Academic Press, pp. 201–217.

Blanchard, E. B., Kolb, L. C., Pallmeyer, T. P. & Gerandi, R. J. (1982). Psychophysiological study of post-traumatic stress disorders in Vietnam veterans. *Psychiatric Quarterly*, **54**, 220–7.

Davidson, J., Kudler, H., Smith, R. et al. (1990). Treatment of posttraumatic stress disorder with amitriptyline and placebo. *Archives of General Psychiatry*, **47**(3), 259–66.

Davidson, J., Lipper, S., Kilts, C. D., Mahorney, S. & Hammett, E. (1985). Platelet MAO activity in posttraumatic stress disorder. *American Journal of Psychiatry*, **142**, 1341–3.

Davidson, L. M. & Baum, A. (1986). Chronic stress and posttraumatic stress disorders. *Journal of Consulting and Clinical Psychology*, **54**(3), 303–8.

Davidson, L. M. & Baum, A. (1989, August). Chronic stress and combat exposure. Paper at the meeting of the American Psychological Association, New Orleans.

Davidson, L. M., Weiss, L., O'Keeffe, M. K. & Baum, A. (in press). Acute stressors and chronic stress at Three Mile Island. *Journal of Traumatic Stress*.

Derogatis, L. R. (1977). *The SCL-90 Manual I: Scoring, administration, and procedures for the SCL-90*. Baltimore: Johns Hopkins University School of Medicine, Clinical Psychometrics Unit.

Dobbs, D. & Wilson, W. P. (1960). Observations on persistence of war neurosis. *Diseases of the Nervous System*, **210**, 686–91.

Erichsen, J. E. (1882). *On concussion of the spine: nervous system in their clinical and medicolegal aspects*. London: Longmans, Green.

Glass, D. C. & Singer, J. E. (1972). *Urban stress: experiments on noise and social stressors*. New York: Academic Press.

Green, B. L., Wilson, J. P. & Lindy, J. D. (1985). Conceptualizing post-traumatic stress disorder: a psychosocial framework. In C. R. Figley (ed.) *Trauma and its wake: the study and treatment of post-traumatic stress disorder.* New York: Brunner/Mazel, pp. 53–69.

Haas, A. P. & Hendin, H. (1983). Suicide among older people: Projections for the future. *Suicide and Life Threatening Behavior*, **13**(3), 147–54.

Holloway, H. D. & Ursano, R. J. (1984). The Viet Nam veteran: memory, social context and metaphor. *Psychiatry*, **47**, 103–8.

Horowitz, M., Wilner, N. & Alvarez, W. (1979). Impact of events scale: a measure of subjective stress. *Psychosomatic Medicine*, **41**(3), 209–18.

Janet, P. (1893). *Etat mental des mysteriques: les stigmates mentaux*. Paris: Reuff and Cie.

Kardiner, A. (1932). The bio-analysis of the epileptic. *Psychoanalytic Quarterly I*, **3–4**, 375–83.

Kardiner, A. & Spiegel, H. (1941). *War stress and neurotic illness*. London: Hoeber.

Keane, T. M., Caddell, J. M. & Taylor, K. L. (1988). Mississippi scale for combat-related posttraumatic stress disorder: three studies in reliability and validity. *Journal of Consulting and Clinical Psychology*, **56**, 85–90.

Keane, T. M. & Fairbank, J. A. (1983). Survey analysis of combat-related stress disorders in Viet Nam veterans. *American Journal of Psychiatry*, **140**(3), 348–50.

Keane, T. M., Fairbank, J. A., Caddell, J. M., Zimering, R. T. & Bender, M. E. (1985). A behavioral approach to assessing and treating posttraumatic stress disorder in Vietnam veterans. In C. R. Figley (ed.) Trauma and its wake. New York: Brunner/Mazel, pp. 257–94.

Kilpatrick, D., Veronen, L. & Best, C. (1985). Factors predicting psychological distress among rape victims. In C. R. Figley (ed.) *Trauma and its wake: traumatic stress theory, research, and intervention*. New York: Brunner/Mazel, pp. 113–41.

Kolb, L. C. (1987). A neuropsychological hypothesis explaining posttraumatic stress disorders. *American Journal of Psychiatry*, **144**, 989–95.

Kolb, L. C., Burris, B. C. & Griffiths, S. (1984). Propranolol and clonidine in treatment of posttraumatic stress disorders. *Psychiatry Annals*, X.

Kosten, T. R., Mason, J. W., Giller, E. L., Ostroff, R. B. & Harkness, L. (1987). Sustained urinary norepinephrine and epinephrine elevation in posttraumatic stress disorder. *Psychoneuroendocrinology*, **12**, 13–20.

Lazarus, R. S. & Folkman, S. (1984). *Stress, appraisal and coping*. New York: Springer.

Lerer, B., Ebstein, R. P., Shestatsky, M., Shemesh, Z. & Greenberg, D. (1987). Cyclic AMP signal transduction in posttraumatic stress disorder. *American Journal of Psychiatry*, **144**, 1324–7.

Malloy, P. E., Fairbank, J. A. & Keane, T. M. (1983). Validation of a multimethod assessment of post-traumatic stress disorder in Vietnam veterans. *Journal of Consulting and Clinical Psychology*, **4**, 488–94.

Mason, J. W., Giller, E. L., Kosten, T. R., Ostroff, P. B. & Podd, L. (1986). Urinary free cortisol levels in post-traumatic stress disorder patients. *Journal of Nervous and Mental Disease*, **174**, 145–9.

McFall, M. E., Murburg, M. M., Ko, G. N. & Veith, R. C. (1990). Autonomic responses to stress in Vietnam combat veterans with posttraumatic stress disorder. *Biological Psychiatry*, **27**(10), 1165–75.

McKinnon, W., Weisse, C. S., Reynolds, C. P., Bowles, C. A. & Baum, A. (1989). Chronic stress, leukocyte subpopulations, and humoral response to latent viruses, *Health Psychology*, **8**(4), 389–402.

Page, H. D. (1885). *Injuries of the spine and spinal cord without apparent mechanical lesions.* London: J. and A. Churchill.

Perry, B. D., Giller, E. L. & Southwick, S. M. (1987). Altered platelet 2-adrenergic binding sites in psottraumatic stress disorder. *American Journal of Psychiatry*, **144**, 1511–12.

Pitman, R. K. & Orr, S. P. (1990). Twenty-four hour urinary cortisol and catecholamine excretion in combat-related posttraumatic stress disorder. *Biology and Psychiatry*, **27**(2), 245–7.

Pitman, R. K., Orr, S. P., Forgue, D. F., deJong, J. B. & Claiborn, J. M. (1987). Psychophysiologic assessment of posttraumatic stress disorder imagery in Vietnam combat veterans. *Archives of General Psychiatry*, **44**, 970–5.

Pitman, R. K., Orr, S. P. & Steketel, G. S. (1989). Psychophysiological investigations of posttraumatic stress disorder imagery. *Psychopharmacology Bulletin*, **25**(3), 426–31.

Pitman, R. K., van der Kolk, B. A., Orr, S. P. & Greenberg, M. S. (1990). Naloxone-reversible analgesic response to combat-related stimuli in posttraumatic stress disorder: a pilot study. *Archives of General Psychiatry*, **47**, 541–4.

Reist, C., Kauffmann, C. D., Haier, R. J., Sangdahl, C., DeMet, E. M., Chicz-DeMet, A. & Nelson, J. N. (1989). A controlled trial of desipranine in 18 men with posttraumatic stress disorder. *American Journal of Psychiatry*, **146**(4), 513–16.

Seyle, H. (1976). *The stress of life.* New York: McGraw-Hill.

Trimble, M. R. (1985). Post-traumatic stress disorder: history of a concept. In C. R. Figley (ed.) *Trauma and its wake.* New York: Brunner/Mazel, pp. 5–14.

van der Kolk, B., Greenberg, M., Boyd, H. & Krystal, J. H. (1985). Inescapable shock, neurotransmitters, and addiction to trauma: toward a psychobiology of posttraumatic stress. *Biological Psychiatry*, **20**, 314–25.

van der Kolk, B. A., Greenberg, M. S., Orr, S. P. & Pitman, R. K. (1989). Endogenous opioids, stress-induced analgesia and posttraumatic stress disorder. *Psychopharmacology Bulletin*, **25**(3), 417–21.

Yehuda, R., Southwick, S., Nussbaum, G., Wahby, V., Giller, E. & Mason, J. (1990). Low urinary cortisol excretion in patients with posttraumatic stress disorder. *Journal of Nervous and Mental Disorders.*

17

Individual and community reactions to the Kentucky floods: findings from a longitudinal study of older adults

FRAN H. NORRIS, JAMES F. PHIFER and KRZYSZTOF KANIASTY

In June 1981, south-eastern Kentucky experienced serious and widespread flooding. Losses amounted to over nine million dollars and, despite the sparse population of the area, over 500 families were left homeless for varying periods of time. In May 1984, a storm system brought tornadoes, strong winds, and severe, extensive flooding to this same area. More than 6000 homes were damaged and over 5000 persons were forced out of their homes by the flooding. The losses, totalling over 20 million dollars, prompted a presidential disaster declaration.

What impact did these two floods have upon their rural Appalachian victims? Were these individuals able to take these events 'in stride' or did they present a serious challenge to their ability to cope? Did these floods leave a lasting impact upon the mental and physical wellbeing of these individuals or did they only result in relatively minor and short-lived emotional upset? Were some people more affected than others? What was the impact on the community as a whole? Were these communities able to 'rally around' their members or were they shattered and split apart? Did daily life in the community 'bounce back' to normal in a few weeks or was the sense of community irreparably altered? These questions and others were the focus of our study of the psychosocial impact of the Kentucky floods.

A considerable body of scientific literature has examined the impact of such disasters on the mental and physical health of victims. Results of previous studies of disasters have run the gamut from revealing a high incidence of severe, chronic psychiatric problems among victims (e.g. Gleser, Green & Winget, 1981) to concluding that the psychological impact is minimal and that many victims even perceive the experience as a positive one (e.g. Taylor, Ross & Quarantelli, 1976). Thus, despite the proliferation of studies addressing this issue, much remains unknown about the nature and severity of the health consequences of natural disasters.

Study design

The study described in this chapter had three features that held particular promise for increasing what we know about the effects of disaster. The first is the study's prospective and longitudinal design. This feature allowed us to overcome many of the methodological problems that have plagued this area of research, problems that have made it difficult to establish whether disasters do, in fact, affect the wellbeing of victims. The major problem arises because, almost by definition, it is not known where or when a disaster will strike. Thus it is usually not possible to obtain information about a group of people *before* a disaster strikes. Without some knowledge of the victims' level of functioning before the disaster, it is difficult to establish whether the disaster was responsible for the symptoms observed. For instance, if 20% of victims are depressed after a disaster, this figure must be compared with the percentage of depressed persons in that area *before* the disaster to determine if this represents an increase, a decrease, or no change in the rate of depression.

Occasionally, predisaster information is available because it had been collected for another reason. Such information was available for the St Louis studies, for example, because that city had been included in a large epidemiological study conducted about a year before the flooding there occurred (Smith et al., 1986). The study we will describe was all the more unusual because the Kentucky floods occurred during the course of an ongoing panel study of older adult mental and physical health. A statewide sample of older adults, including many people who resided in the flooded area, was interviewed within three months before the 1981 flood. They were interviewed a second time about three months after that flood, and many were also interviewed three to four additional times after that. Because these floods occurred during the course of the panel study, predisaster assessments were available to provide a point of comparison to the assessments made after the floods. The design is illustrated in Fig. 17.1.

The second unusual feature of the present study was its consideration of both individual and collective aspects of disaster exposure. Our sample was drawn from ten different afflicted counties, some of which had heavy and severe losses in the floods and some of which experienced relatively little destruction. We also included a few adjacent counties that had been spared by the floods. With the help of data provided by the Kentucky Division of Disaster and Emergency Services, we were able to measure and take into account these county level losses when examining the impact of the incidents on the people involved. It has generally been assumed that, as the proportion of victims to nonvictims within a community increases, the

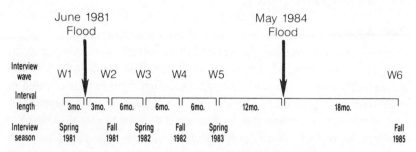

Fig. 17.1. Time frame of interview waves and flood occurrences.

mental health impact of the disaster also increases (Green, 1982). As this proportion increases, victims are more likely to be displaced from their communities, and it becomes more difficult for them to avoid being exposed to physical destruction (and even death following the more severe catastrophes). In studies of the Buffalo Creek dam collapse, these aspects of exposure were found to combine with victims' more personal losses in predicting long-term symptom consequences (Green & Gleser, 1983). Erikson (1976) proposed that the trauma experienced by survivors at Buffalo Creek had two facets, 'individual trauma', and 'collective trauma', the impairment of the prevailing sense of communality. In most human disasters, 'the two traumas occur simultaneously, and are experienced as two halves of a continuous whole' (p. 154).

Our study was thus unusual in its consideration and assessment of *both* types of impact: the experience of personal losses and exposure to community destruction. Following Bolin (1985), we will sometimes refer to two broad categories of victims when describing our findings: 'primary victims' were those who directly experienced physical, material, or personal losses; 'secondary victims' were those who lived in the affected area, but sustained no personal injuries or damages. Conceptually, this distinction is important because disasters are community level events with the potential to precipitate change and stress even for those who experience no direct losses. That is, secondary victims are also subjected to the 'collective trauma'. We thought that they might also have mental health consequences from their experiences.

The third feature of the study that we feel is important is its focus on older people. The statewide panel study that preceded the disaster study was concerned with the reaction of older adults to various potentially stressful life events such as bereavement, medical illness, and financial difficulties. All respondents were aged 55 or older. Friedsam (1960, 1962) suggested that older persons constitute a special risk group in times of disaster in that they may be less likely to receive warning, more reluctant to evacuate, and more disturbed by altered patterns of life. Kilijanek and Drabek (1979) concluded from their review of the literature that, relative to younger persons, elderly disaster victims are at greater risk to experience substantial financial losses and injured family members. Older persons may sustain a disproportionate share of personal losses and physical injuries because they are more likely to live in flood plains or in dwellings more susceptible to damage from natural disasters.

Given the relatively greater impact of disasters on older adults, and their fewer social and economic resources, researchers have generally expected older adults to exhibit high rates of emotional difficulties following disaster. However, the findings have been contradictory. A number of prior studies have observed detrimental mental health effects in older persons (e.g. Krause, 1987; Logue, Melick & Struening, 1981; Miller, Turner & Kimball, 1981; Ollendick & Hoffman, 1982). Yet, other studies have suggested that older persons either are not seriously affected by disasters (Cohen & Poulshock, 1977; Kilijanek & Drabek, 1979), or are affected less than younger victims (Bell, Kara & Batterson, 1978; Bolin & Klenow, 1982–83; Huerta & Horton, 1978). Thus, it is not known whether older adults cope better or worse than younger persons with the stress of disaster.

In sum, our primary goal was to examine the impact of the Kentucky floods on mental, physical, and social functioning, using a methodologically conservative prospective design. Two somewhat broader purposes overlapped with this goal. One was to learn something about who may be rightly considered the 'victims' of disaster, i.e. are only those who sustain personal losses affected or are others in the community affected as well? The second was to learn how the elderly, in particular, may be affected by natural disaster.

The setting and sample

The setting for the study was a rural and mountainous area in southeastern Kentucky. Of most concern was the general ability of this region to cope with the needs of its citizens following disasters and emergencies. Southeastern Kentucky is an impoverished area characterized by disproportionate numbers of persons under the poverty level, high unemployment (estimated as up to 20% at the time of the 1981 flood), and inferior housing. Educational levels of its citizens are among the lowest in the country. According to a statewide needs assessment conducted only a few years before the floods (Schulte & Murrell, 1980), this area provided fewer local health, mental health, and social services than did any other area of the state. These conditions might be expected to have exacerbated the impact of disaster.

The study encompassed a total of 15 south-eastern Kentucky counties that varied in 'impact ratio', i.e the number of homes that were damaged or destroyed relative to the population size of that county. For the 1981 flood, values ranged from 0 (for nonvictims residing in adjacent, nonflooded counties) to 13.1 homes damaged per 1000 population. For the 1984 flood, these values ranged from 0 to 15.6 homes damaged per 1000 population. There was considerable redundancy in exposure to the two incidents; most of the counties flooded in 1981 were flooded again in 1984. In addition, because the later flood was more widespread, it also struck many of the adjacent counties that had not been flooded in 1981.

All participants in the study were aged 55 or older, averaging 67. All had participated in a statewide panel study beginning in the spring of 1981 and all were interviewed a final time in the fall of 1985 (see Fig. 17.1). The interviews took place in the respondents' own homes, and were usually conducted by indigenous interviewers. Other than its advanced age, the most notable feature of the sample was its limited education (an average of 8 years). Of the 222 older adults interviewed, primary victims numbered 37 in 1981 and 44 in 1984, secondary victims numbered 106 in 1981 and 135 in 1984, and nonvictims numbered 79 in 1981 and 43 in 1984.

The findings

Throughout this chapter, we will focus on the effects of two variables. The first, *personal loss*, was scored on a 5-point scale based on primary victims' perceptions of their losses (from minimal to total). Secondary victims and nonvictims received scores of 0. The second, *community destruction*, was the impact ratio, described above. Based on archival data, it was independent of the respondent's psychological state. It applied to primary and secondary victims alike; nonvictims received scores of 0. In the analyses (primarily hierarchical regression), the effects of personal loss were statistically controlled when assessing the effects of community destruction; thus the latter's effects may reasonably be interpreted as being over and above those accounted for by personal loss. Except where otherwise noted, the effects described in this chapter were those of the 1981 flood. As shown in Fig. 17.1, it is for this incident that our data are more complete.

Effects on mental health

One purpose of the study was to examine the impact of the floods on the emotional wellbeing of older adults over the two years following each flood. (For detail on these findings, see Phifer & Norris, 1989.) Previous studies have provided little information about the natural course of observed psychological reactions. Many crucial questions have thus remained unresolved: do psychological reactions occur immediately after the disaster or do they develop at a later point in time? How long do these changes in emotional wellbeing continue? Do symptoms remain at the same level or do they fluctuate over time?

Because most of our participants had been interviewed four times after the 1981 flood, we were able to provide some answers to many of these elusive questions. The questionnaire included three measures of psychological symptoms: the 20-item Center for Epidemiologic Studies Depression Scale (Radloff, 1977), the trait half of the State-Trait Anxiety Scale (also 20 items; Spielberger, Gorusch & Lushene, 1970), and the 18-item General Well-Being Scale (Ware et al., 1979). These scales, which correlate highly with one another, have all been found to be acceptable to, and reliable for, older adults (Himmelfarb & Murrell, 1983).

There was clear evidence from these standardized measures that disasters adversely affect mental health. With predisaster symptoms and sociodemographic characteristics controlled, each symptom scale was affected by one or both of the disaster measures for at least some interval of time. This was true both for the 1981 flood and for the 1984 flood. With regard to the severity of these symptoms, flood exposure appeared to produce mild to moderate levels of emotional distress, but these reactions did not appear to be severe enough to be considered psychiatric disorders. The severity of these reactions was similar to that experienced following other types of stressful life events such as bereavement, medical illness, or loss of a job.

Initially, however, the findings were not terribly informative concerning the nature and duration of symptoms, because the pattern of significant effects across the three symptom measures, two exposure measures (personal loss and community destruction), and five postflood waves was complex (perhaps even unclear). For this reason, we conducted a factor analysis of the three scales to yield more conceptually distinct outcome measures. Four distinct factors emerged: negative affect (e.g. sad mood, crying spells, feeling hopeless; alpha = .90), cognitive symptoms (e.g. indecisiveness, preoccupation, lacking self-confidence; alpha = .76),

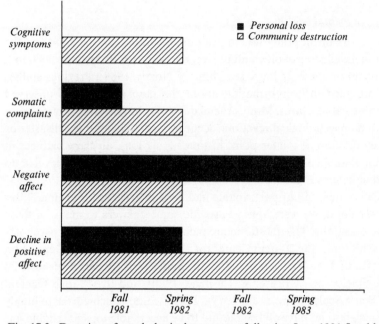

Fig. 17.2. Duration of psychological symptoms following June 1981 flood by dimension and aspect of exposure.

psychosomatic complaints (e.g. feeling fatigued, lacking energy, having sleep or appetite problems; alpha = .92), and declines in positive affect (e.g. feeling less happy or cheerful, being less interested in or satisfied with life; alpha = .88).

The results of regression analyses using these factors are summarized in Fig. 17.2. It shows the duration of symptoms attributable to the 1981 flood for the four dimensions of mental health and the two aspects of flood exposure. The 'bar' ends at the last wave where a statistically significant effect was observed, with predisaster symptoms again controlled. For example, exposure to community destruction was still associated with an increase in 'cognitive symptoms' (indecisiveness, preoccupation, lack of self-confidence) at the second postflood interview (Spring 1982, one year after the flood) but these effects had dissipated by the following Fall.

The two aspects of flood exposure had somewhat different consequences. Experiencing personal losses was associated most strongly with increases in negative affect, that is, sadness, anxiety, discouragement, worry, and agitation. For many, these emotional reactions were still apparent after two years. In contrast, exposure to high levels of community destruction was associated most strongly with declines in positive affect, reflecting a community-wide tendency for people to feel less positive about their surroundings, less enthusiasm, less energy, and less enjoyment of life. Again, these effects could still be observed two years after the flood.

Not apparent in Fig. 17.2, because of the way those data are presented, was a tendency for the observed effects to be stronger at 'Spring' interviews than at the 'Fall' interviews. These stronger emotional reactions appeared to coincide with the 'anniversary' of the flood, the time of year when the threat of flooding is at its peak. This finding is consistent with Bolin's (1982) specific observation that tornado victims experienced renewed stress with the onset of tornado season, as well as with the general idea that posttraumatic stress may be triggered by environmental events that serve as reminders of the original stressor (Green, Lindy & Grace, 1985).

Other findings lent further support to the idea that symptoms may fluctuate according to the time or season of the year. In the final interview, we included one scale (4 items; alpha = .76) that measured the level of anxiety experienced in situations of mildly threatening weather (situations reminiscent of the flood). Levels of anxiety during periods of threatening weather were considerably higher among persons exposed to the floods (either 1984 or 1981) than among other older adults. Moreover, these levels were also higher than could be accounted for by victims' own general tendencies to be anxious in other situations. This appeared to be one symptom outcome where personal losses usually did not matter. Secondary victims showed as much heightened sensitivity to threatening weather as did primary victims. (For more details on these findings, see Norris & Murrell, 1988.)

Effects on physical health

In addition to mental health, the study also was concerned with the potential impact of disaster on the physical health of these older victims. (For more detail on these findings, especially as they relate to the 1984 flood, see Phifer, Kaniasty & Norris, 1988.) The basic assumption of this research was that prolonged stress could lead to 'wear and tear' on various bodily systems, resulting in an increase in various physical symptoms. Our measure of health was a revised version of the General Health Scale (Belloc, Breslow & Hochstim, 1971; alpha = .89). A factor analysis of this 20-item measure yielded three distinct subscales: physical symptoms (e.g. headaches, trouble breathing, pain in the joints; alpha = .80), fatigue (e.g. lack of energy, general malaise; alpha = .80), and functional impairment (e.g.

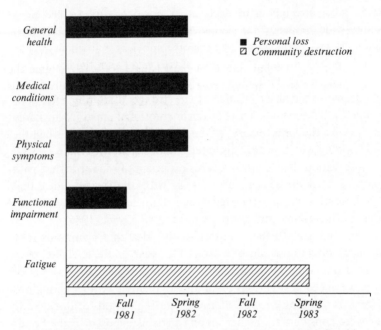

Fig. 17.3. Duration of physical symptoms following June 1981 flood by dimension and aspect of exposure.

trouble getting around; alpha = .77). These scales were supplemented with a 10-item index of medical conditions, such as high blood pressure, ulcers, and diabetes.

Statistically significant findings for the 1981 flood are illustrated in Fig. 17.3. (Effects of predisaster symptoms and sociodemographic characteristics were again controlled.) Exposure to the floods was related to a decline in general health functioning, with victims reporting increased difficulties performing day-to-day activities, more general physical complaints, greater fatigue and more medical conditions.

In general, however, the floods' effects on different aspects of physical health were less strong and less lasting than they were on mental health. Most physical complaints peaked at Wave 3, about one year following the flood. Only fatigue showed more lasting increases, with these symptoms still elevated two years later. These symptoms were associated with exposure to community destruction rather than personal loss, indicating a community-wide tendency toward feeling greater fatigue than felt before the flood. This finding is quite consistent with that shown for positive affect in Fig. 17.2, and it is reasonable for elevations in fatigue to co-occur with declines in positive affect.

In a manner actually more pronounced than for mental health, the impact of the flood on physical health exhibited some seasonal variations, with the level of medical symptoms peaking in the first spring after the incident, decreasing by that fall, then increasing to a lesser degree the following spring. A trend analysis (see Phifer et al., 1988) confirmed this impression. This seasonal trend was found only for those people who had experienced both high personal losses and high community destruction in the floods and, thus, was not the general pattern among this sample of older adults. As discussed previously, in this particular setting, Spring inevitably brings the threat of flooding. It may be that this threat of future incidents 'stirs up' feelings of anxiety, tension, and nervousness, leading to associated physical symptoms, such as muscle tension, fatigue, loss of appetite, and sleep problems.

Effects on social relations and support

In our study, we also examined some areas of functioning that have been examined less frequently in previous research than have mental and physical health. One such area concerned social functioning. This included both the adequacy of support exchanged during the crisis, and subsequent social functioning, i.e. quality of social relationships, extensiveness of social networks, and the perceptions people maintain about the support that would be available to them if needed. (For more detail on these findings, see Kaniasty, Norris & Murrell, 1990; Kanisty & Norris, 1993.)

In the floods themselves (1981 and 1984 data combined), help of some form was received by 61% of primary victims. Victims were aided most by their immediate families and relatives (41%), followed by neighbors and friends (34%). Only 7% obtained some form of assistance from governmental, agricultural, or charity organizations.

Our ability to examine the adequacy of assistance received was aided by the inclusion in the original panel study of the 13-item Louisville Social Support Scale, a scale modified from the earlier scales of Phillips (1967) and Andrews et al. (1978). For the present purposes, the scale was divided into three subscales: social participation (size and closeness of one's network; alpha = .62), kin support (expectations of help from family members; alpha = .75), and nonkin support (expectations of help from friends, neighbors, and churches; alpha = .62). Thus, in the interview preceding the flood, all respondents had been asked a series of questions concerning how much help they could expect to receive in a *hypothetical* emergency. It is interesting to compare these predisaster expectations with the help received in the actual emergency from various sources.

Flood victims (primary victims only but combined across incidents) received much less help than they had expected to receive when asked about a hypothetical emergency prior to the floods. Looking at both kin support and nonkin support, we found that victims' expectations of how much help they would receive in a crisis were about three times higher than the amount of help actually received in the emergency. For example, only 22% actually received a 'fair' or 'great' amount of help from their neighbors, compared with 73 percent who had expected to receive this much help in a hypothetical emergency. Similarly, 24% received a fair or great amount of help from relatives outside the home, compared with 73% who had expected to receive this much help. Only 6% received a fair or great amount of help from churches in the area, compared with 60% who thought they would receive help from this source.

Why didn't these flood victims receive more help? One possibility is their advanced age. Previous research (Kilijanek & Drabek, 1979; Poulshock & Cohen, 1975) has shown that the elderly may have a 'pattern of neglect' in that they receive less help than younger victims. In fact, we since have found that age was a strong predictor of the social support received by victims of Hurricane Hugo in Charleston, SC. It may be that the elderly are overlooked by sources of aid or that they are less likely to request assistance from family, friends, or organizations.

It is also quite possible that these findings generalize past the older population. The likelihood is high that potential support providers, such as victims' families, neighbors, and friends, were victims themselves. Consequently, the need for support by victims simply exceeded its availability. Those who were supposed to help in times of emergency might have been affected themselves by the crisis, thus rendering them temporarily unable to provide extensive aid to others.

In addition to examining social support *during* the floods, we looked at whether the flood affected its victims' later expectations for social support (again in a hypothetical emergency). Given the overall low levels of helping observed, it is not terribly surprising that perceptions of support declined from preflood levels. These findings are illustrated in Fig. 17.4. Initially, the effects of the 1981 flood were more profound for primary victims than for the community as a whole. These victims reevaluated both their kin and nonkin networks. However, concerning kin, these declines were relatively short-lived, lasting only 3 to 6 months. That is, people soon regained their optimistic assessments that their relatives would be available to help them in spite of past experiences that failed to support these expectations.

In contrast, both primary and secondary victims appeared to have

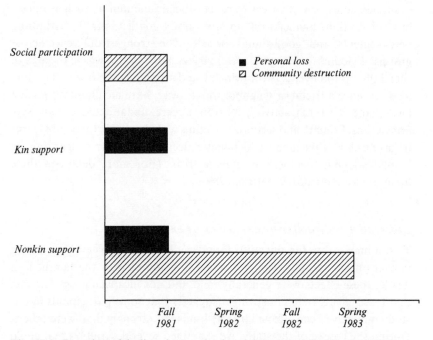

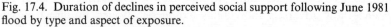

Fig. 17.4. Duration of declines in perceived social support following June 1981 flood by type and aspect of exposure.

lowered expectations concerning the helpfulness of their *nonkin* networks (friends, neighbors, and churches). This decline was still observable two years postflood. Of the two aspects of flood exposure studied, it was exposure to community destruction that had the most lasting effects on expected nonkin support. This is an excellent reminder that natural disasters impact upon whole communities, not just selected individuals.

This observation is further corroborated by the finding that community destruction was also associated with decreased participation in social activities with relatives, friends, and community organizations. Primary and secondary victims alike reported decreased social participation. Destruction of the physical environment may have altered usual patterns of social interactions – disrupting daily activities such as visiting, shopping, recreation, church-going, etc. This finding, as well as that for nonkin support, is consistent with the previous findings of Drabek and Key (1976).

Additional evidence of impaired social functioning emerged when we examined the life events experienced by disaster victims over the next 18 months after the 1984 flood. Life change in the postdisaster period was examined across several areas of psychosocial functioning, such as household disruption, financial disruption, family conflict, health disruption, bereavements, and 'good things for self'. The strongest difference across groups of victims (primary vs. secondary vs. nonvictims) was in the area of social disruption events, with primary and secondary victims being more likely to have a friend or neighbor move away, have a child move farther away, stop a church activity, or stop a recreational activity than were nonvictims. Primary and secondary victims were *less* likely than nonvictims to have a child leave home, which may reflect cultural norms regarding the family 'sticking together' through a crisis. (For more detail on these findings, see Hutchins & Norris, 1989.)

Differential vulnerability by age and experience

To summarize thus far, this study found evidence that disasters have lasting impact on mental, physical, and social functioning. For the sample as a whole, these effects were generally mild and not incapacitating. The fact that these effects were not stronger suggests that some participants in our study may have been affected by the floods less strongly than were others. During the course of the study, we examined several variables that could influence how adversely individuals would be affected by disaster (See Phifer, 1990 for details.) In this chapter, however, we have limited ourselves to considering the influences of age and past experience.

It should be noted that a sizeable proportion (45%) of our sample was under 65, i.e. comprised persons who would be better characterized as 'middle aged' than as old. These middle-aged victims (55 to 64) had the most difficulty coping. As shown in Fig. 17.5, it was in this age group that losses in the 1984 flood were most strongly associated with increases in depressive symptoms. Adults aged 65 to 74 were affected relatively little. Very old adults (75 +) were intermediate – affected more than those 65–74 (perhaps due to poorer health) but affected less than middle-aged victims.

That older adults were found to be less at-risk than middle-aged adults could be due to several different factors. The elderly tend to experience less change in other aspects of their lives than do younger persons (e.g. Hughes, Blazer & George, 1988; Masuda & Holmes, 1978), which may prevent them from becoming overwhelmed by the stress of the flood. The 55 to 64 year-old group may also have had more of an emotional reaction to the flood because they were approaching retirement age. The disruption and material losses associated with the flood may have threatened various goals they had for retirement. For instance, a couple whose home was severely damaged in

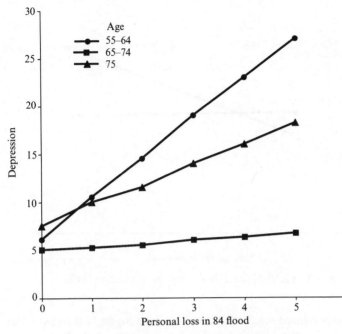

Fig. 17.5. Personal loss in 1984 flood by depression and age.

the flood may have worried that they must abandon various 'dreams' they had for retirement, such as buying a vacation home.

Of the potential explanations, the one of most interest to our research team was the role of prior experience. Relative to younger adults, older people bring a rich history of experience to bear on any crisis. Bell et al. (1978) proposed that it was this experience with crisis – and the resulting ability to accept loss and suffering – that accounted for the resilience of older adults following the 1975 Omaha tornado. More generally, Eysenck (1983) proposed an 'inoculation hypothesis', which states that exposure to stress *increases* resistance to subsequent stress. Eysenck's hypothesis appeared to us to be strikingly relevant for both our setting (a flood prone area in Appalachia) and population (older adults).

Thus, having lived through many crises in the past, the elderly may have already possessed the wealth of coping strategies needed to adapt success-fully to the Kentucky floods. Floods are not uncommon in south eastern Kentucky, but those that occurred in 1981 and 1984 were more severe and widespread than most previous ones had been. As a result, our sample included both 'newly exposed' and 'formerly exposed' subsamples of disaster victims at a ratio of about 2:1. In addition, roughly one-third of the

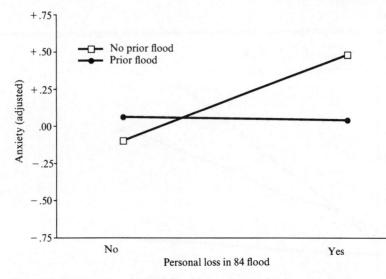

Fig. 17.6. Personal loss in 1984 flood by anxiety and prior experience.

sample had experienced some other event over the course of their lives that could be considered traumatic such as a serious accident, physical assault, or fire. We therefore could study how these past experiences (before 1981) interacted with recent exposure (either 1981 or 1984) in predicting postdisaster mental health. (See Norris & Murrell, 1988.)

As illustrated in Fig. 17.6, for personal loss and the 1984 flood, our results supported the advantages of prior experience quite strongly. More experienced older adults took their losses in stride, showing no increase in psychological symptoms. Less experienced older adults were affected more strongly. The study provided stronger evidence of 'direct tolerance' (the inoculating properties of experience with the same type of stressor, i.e. prior floods) than of 'cross tolerance' (the inoculating properties of experience with different but related stressors, e.g. prior fire, assault, or accident). Both sets of findings, however, were generally consistent with the inoculation view.

Conclusions

Compared to most disaster impact studies, this study had a number of advantages: it used a community sample of older adults who reported diverse psychological and physical symptoms; it provided comprehensive measurement with psychometrically sound measures; and perhaps most importantly, it provided a prospective design with preflood measures. With this more defensible design, our study focused on whether older disaster victims – both primary and secondary – experience declines in their mental health, physical health, and social functioning following disaster.

The results of this research project suggested that these floods did influence the mental and physical health of their victims. The findings suggest it is common for people who experience losses or damage to feel blue, down in the dumps, worried, anxious, and fearful, and to be more easily upset. However, victims did not develop psychiatric illnesses in response to the floods. They also experienced physical symptoms of fatigue, feeling worn out, having trouble sleeping, and having more aches and pains, but they did not develop major illnesses. It was not surprising to find emotional distress following these floods. What was surprising was that these reactions continued for many months, and even years, after the floods. Although similar in magnitude to the reactions to other types of stressful events, the duration of these reactions was not similar. The emotional reactions of older adults to life events have generally been limited to about six months (Murrell & Himmelfarb, 1989; Norris & Murrell, 1987). In contrast, their reactions to the floods persisted for up to two years. In our work, the only other event that we have found to engender such enduring effects is death of one's spouse (Norris & Murrell, 1990).

The disruption of social relations and support may be one of the most difficult aspects of the flood experience with which to cope – particularly given the violation of expectations this reality represents. In an individual level event such as bereavement, friends and family rally around and support the bereaved individual. In a community level event, such as disaster, these people may be attending to their own problems, leaving other victims to feel lonely, isolated and abandoned. The people typically counted on for support in times of crisis may be victims themselves and unable to offer help. Thus, in a sense, when they are needed the most they are not able to be there.

Thus, our study suggests that disasters result in emotional problems through two different 'paths' (Kanski & Norris, 1993). One path is a direct impact related to the immediate loss and trauma of the disaster. Disasters precipitate a constellation of losses including physical injury, damage to one's home and possessions, and symbolic losses of photographs or keepsakes. The emotional trauma of disaster may come through exposure to death (horror), extreme physical force (terror), and life threatening situations. Disasters may shatter the myth of personal invulnerability and threaten the sense of control over one's environment. All of these facets may precipitate emotional distress. The second path is indirect: disasters disrupt the social network of the community and daily social routines, which, in turn, results in emotional distress. Without the presence of emotional support and material aid from family and friends, disaster victims may face the full emotional brunt of the disaster on their own.

As we noted at the outset of this chapter, two somewhat broader purposes overlapped with our goal of examining the impact of the Kentucky floods on mental, physical, and social functioning. One was to learn something about who may be rightly considered the 'victims' of disaster, i.e. are only those with personal losses affected or are others in the community affected as well? The second was to learn whether the elderly, in particular, are affected by natural disaster.

The answer to the first question was quite clear: the emotional impact could not be understood without reference to both the individual and collective impact of the disasters. There were mental and physical health effects even for those who, in the absence of personal loss, were exposed to community destruction only. Following these disasters, the community at large (i.e. both primary and secondary victims) felt less positive and less satisfied with their lives. They got less enjoyment from day-to-day activities. They shared a heightened perception of danger (weather related distress) and unceasing fatigue. Their confidence in the helpfulness of their communities was never quite the same. No one would suggest that such 'symptoms' constitute psychopathology. Nonetheless, for the community as a whole, these disasters did impair the quality of life for quite some time. In this field, there perhaps has been an undue emphasis on uncovering disorder. We also need to understand the broader implications of disaster for community life.

Our findings concerning secondary victims have methodological as well as substantive implications. In many studies, 'nonvictim' controls would be described better as secondary victims; often, they are those persons who live in the same area as primary victims, but had no personal loss or property damage. Studies of the 1974 Brisbane floods are a good example here because the authors themselves (Abrahams et al., 1976) raised this point as an issue for their study. This approach does improve the comparability of victims and controls. Conceptually, however, it is problematic because it is no longer clear what a finding of 'no difference' means. Were primary victims unaffected or were secondary victims affected also?

Finally, our study should increase what we know about how the elderly, in particular, cope with disaster. Although our sample as a whole experienced mild to moderate levels of distress, older persons (65+) as a group were more resilient to the emotional impact of these floods than were mid-aged persons (55–64). Certainly, like others in the community, older adults should be told that the feelings of sadness, fear, anger, and worry they experience following a disaster are normal and to be expected, and that they are not alone in having these feelings. And, those older adults who experience distress should be encouraged to seek help from formal or informal sources, in order to prevent more severe problems from developing. Furthermore, it is important to remember that older adults constitute an extremely heterogenous population, in which some persons, such as those of lower socioeconomic status, have greater postdisaster needs than others (Phifer, 1990), yet may receive less help (Kaniasty et al., 1990). Nonetheless, it is equally important to remember that many (and perhaps most) older people in disaster stricken communities are coping quite successfully, perhaps even better than their young and mid-aged neighbors.

Implications for crisis intervention

Our results and a large body of literature on the stress process suggest that there is typically an immediate, shortlived psychological reaction to stressful events such as disasters. Under certain situational and psychological conditions, this transient stress reaction may develop into more severe or chronic emotional problems (Dohrenwend, 1978). Numerous authors have advocated the use of crisis intervention services following disasters to prevent the development of psychopathology (e.g. Bailey et al., 1985; Cohen, 1985; Farberow, 1978; Frederick, 1981; Hartsough, Zarle & Ottinger, 1976). Crisis intervention is particularly suited as an intervention method for natural disasters, in which case the group to be targeted for intervention is relatively easy to identify.

However, it is important to remember that people who need help may not seek it. The elderly in particular tend to rely upon informal support structures such as family, friends, and religious organizations (Bell et al, 1978; Poulshock & Cohen, 1975). This reluctance to use formal assistance may reflect a generational emphasis on independence and 'carrying one's own weight' and the stigma of 'public welfare'.

Given that older adults are generally reluctant to request assistance and do not seek outpatient mental health services, a traditional 'office' approach in which the clients are self-referred is not effective (Farberow, 1978; Michael et al., 1985). Crisis intervention must assume a proactive posture rather than a reactive one in identifying those older adults in need of services. This involves active casefinding and outreach services in the community (Okura, 1975; Richard, 1974). These outreach efforts are most effective if they take the form of assisting older victims with the variety of practical problems arising during the impact period, such as needs for housing, medical care, material aid and social services. Older adults are more likely to accept help for such 'problems in living' than to accept help for 'mental health problems' (Farberow, 1978; Seroka et al., 1986).

A few more specific recommendations for crisis intervention may be drawn from these findings. First, we believe that it is important to recognize the limits of formal service programs. Professionals and outsiders are important sources of assistance when the level of need is high, but they must not and cannot supplant natural helping networks. We would encourage crisis teams to experiment with ways of mobilizing people to help one another. This task is neither as simple nor as simplistic as it sounds. People should be encouraged (or at least reminded) to check on and assist their neighbors, friends, and relatives. The direct result should be a maintenance of perceptions of social support. The indirect result should be better mental health.

Secondly, crisis teams should encourage people *not* to abandon their social activities, as they so often do when crisis strikes. Such activities keep people informed about the relative needs of network members. And, these are undoubtedly the best forums for the sharing of experiences and feelings that is believed to be so important for disaster victims. One of the basic tenets of crisis counseling is that people need to recognize that some distress is a normal reaction to an abnormal event. What better way to recognize this than through the social comparisons provided by routine social interactions? Most importantly, such activities may serve to preserve both a sense of social embeddedness and the quality of community life.

Thirdly, our results suggest that crisis teams might target older persons to serve as indigenous community workers. Older people are seldom enlisted for the physical work of rescue and recovery, but surely there are other roles in relief efforts that they could perform quite well. Through sharing their experiences and coping strategies, many older adults living in disaster prone communities might constitute a useful resource in preparing or conducting pre-event interventions and in helping others to cope during the aftermath of a natural disaster. Overall, this study suggests that there is much we could learn from 'experienced' victims about how to cope with stressful situations. Presumably, this knowledge can be applied to developing crisis interventions for other, less experienced, victims.

It is always difficult to know to what extent one should attempt to generalize findings from a given research study. This issue is particularly problematic for disaster research because we must study these events as they occur naturally and cannot assign subjects to experience specific agents in specific socioeconomic contexts. It is for this reason that integrative review articles (e.g. Bolin, 1985; Green, 1982; Lystad, 1985) play such an important role in this field. For example, the present study may be judged as relevant to understanding the Buffalo Creek (e.g. Gleser et al., 1981) and Wyoming Valley (Logue et al, 1981) disasters because of certain similarities in their settings. On the other hand, the intensities of these crises differed dramatically. They also may be judged as relevant to understanding disasters such as the Mt. St. Helens eruption (Murphy, 1984) because both involve the continuing presence of an environmental threat. Here, however, the settings are quite different. The clearest applicability of these findings is to areas that face both depressed economies and recurring disasters. While they may or may not generalize to other settings, such high risk settings would seem important to study in their own right.

Acknowledgements

This chapter summarizes the major findings from a four-year research project, 'Flood Exposure and Older Adult Mental Health' (NIMH Grant No. MH40411, Fran H. Norris, Principal Investigator). The work was performed while the authors were employed at the University of Louisville's Urban Studies Center. Appreciation is extended to Center staff for their assistance in all phases of the project and especially to Gerald Hutchins (now at Transylvania University) for his computer expertise. The authors also wish to thank Bonnie Green and Susan Solomon for their invaluable consultation and advice throughout the project. Finally, the authors are indebted to Stanley A. Murrell, Department of Psychology, University of Louisville, who was principal investigator of the original panel study (NIMH Grant No. MH33063) and mentor to us all.

References

Abrahams, M., Price, J., Whitlock, F. & Williams, G. (1976). The Brisbane floods, January, 1974: their impact on health. *Medical Journal of Australia*, **2**, 936–9.

Andrews, G., Tennant, C., Hewson, D. & Schonell, M. (1978). The relation of social factors to physical and psychiatric illness. *American Journal of Epidemiology*, **108**, 27–35.

Bailey, B. E., Halliman, M. M., Contreras, R. J. & Hernandez, A.G. (1985). Disaster response: The need for community mental health center (CMHC) preparedness. *Journal of Mental Health Administration*, **12**, 42–6.

Bell, B., Kara, G. & Batterson, C. (1978). Service utilization and adjustment patterns of elderly tornado victims in an American disaster. *Mass Emergencies*, **3**, 71–81.

Belloc, N., Breslow, L. & Hochstim, J. (1971). Measurement of physical health in general population surveys. *American Journal of Epidemiology*, **91**, 105–11.

Bolin, R. C. (1982). *Long-term family recovery from disaster*. Boulder, CO: Institute of Behavioral Science, University of Colorado.

Bolin, R. C. (1985). Disaster characteristics and psychosocial impacts. In B. T. Sowder (ed.) *Disasters and mental health: selected contemporary perspectives*. Rockville, MD: National Institute of Mental Health, pp. 3–28.

Bolin, R. & Klenow, D. J. (1982–1983). Response of the elderly to disaster: an age-stratified analysis. *International Journal of Aging and Human Development*, **16**, 283–96.

Cohen, R. (1985). Crisis counseling principles and services to disaster victims. In M. Lystad (ed.) *Innovations in mental health services to disaster victims*. Rockville, MD: NIMH, pp. 8–17.

Cohen, E. S. & Poulshock, S. W. (1977). Societal response to mass relocation of the elderly: implications for area agencies on aging. *The Gerontologist*, **17**, 262–8.

Dohrenwend, B. S. (1978). Social stress and community psychology. *American Journal of Community Psychology*, **6**, 1–14.

Drabek, T. E. & Key, W. M. (1976). The impact of disaster on primary group linkages. *Mass Emergencies*, **1**, 89–105.

Erikson, K. T. (1976). *Everything in its path*. New York: Simon & Schuster.

Eysenck, H. (1983). Stress, disease, and personality: the 'inoculation' effect. In C. J. Cooper (ed.) *Stress research*. New York: Wiley, pp. 121–46.

Farberow, N. L. (1978). *Training manual for human service workers in major disasters*. Washington, DC: US Government Printing Office, DHEW Publication No. (ADM) 79–538.

Frederick, C. J. (ed.). (1981). *Aircraft accidents: Emergency mental health problems*. Rockville, MD: National Institute of Mental Health.

Friedsam, H. J. (1960). Older persons as disaster casualties. *Journal of Health and Human Behavior*, **1**, 269–73.

Friedsam, H. J. (1962). Older persons in disaster. In G. W. Baker & D. W. Chapman (eds.) *Man and society in disaster*. New York: Basic Books, pp. 151–82.

Gleser, G. C., Green, B. L. & Winget, C. N. (1981). *Prolonged psychosocial effects of disaster: a study of Buffalo Creek*. New York: Academic Press.

Green, B. L. (1982). Assessing levels of psychological impairment following disaster: Consideration of actual and methodological dimensions. *Journal of Nervous and Mental Disease*, **170**, 544–52.

Green, B. L. & Gleser, G. C. (1983). Stress and long-term psychopathology in survivors of the Buffalo Creek disaster. In D. Ricks and B. S. Dohrenwend (eds.) *Origins of psychopathology: problems in research and public policy*. Cambridge, MA: University Press, pp. 73–90.

Green, B. L., Lindy, J. D. & Grace, M. C. (1985). Posttraumatic stress disorder: toward DSM IV. *Journal of Nervous and Mental Disease*, **173**, 406–411.

Hartsough, D. M., Zarle, T. H. & Ottinger, D. R. (1976). Rapid response to disaster: the Monticello tornado. In I. Parad, H. J. Resnik & H. L. P. Parad (eds.) *Emergency and disaster management: a mental health sourcebook*. Bowie, MD: Charles Press, pp. 363–74.

Himmelfarb, S. & Murrell, S. A. (1983). Reliability and validity of five mental health scales in older persons. *Journal of Gerontology*, **38**, 333–9.

Huerta, F. & Horton, R. (1978). Coping behavior of elderly flood victims. *The Gerontologist*, **18**, 541–6.

Hughes, D. C., Blazer, D. G. & George, L. K. (1988). Age differences in life events: a multivariate controlled analysis. *International Journal of Aging and Human Development*, **27**, 207–20.

Hutchins, G. L. & Norris, F. H. (1989). Life change in the disaster recovery period. *Environment and Behavior*, **21**, 33–56.

Kaniasty, K. & Norris, F. H. (1993). A test of the social support deterioration model in the context of natural disaster. *Journal of Personality and Social Psychology*, **64**, 395–408.

Kaniasty, K., Norris, F. H. & Murrell, S. A. (1990). Received and perceived social support following natural disaster. *Journal of Applied Social Psychology*, **20**, 85–114.

Kilijanek, T. S. & Drabek, T. E. (1979). Assessing long-term impacts of a natural disaster: a focus on the elderly. *The Gerontologist*, **19**, 555–66.

Krause, N. (1987). Exploring the impact of a natural disaster on the health and psychological well-being of older adults. *Journal of Human Stress*, **13**, 61–9.

Logue, J. N., Melick, M. E. & Struening, E. (1981). A study of health and mental health status following a major natural disaster. In R. G. Simmons (ed.) *Research in community and mental health*. Greenwich, CT: JAI Press, vol 2., pp. 217–74.

Lystad, M. H. (1985). Human responses to mass emergencies: A review of mental health research. *Emotional First Aid: A Journal of Crisis Intervention*, **2**, 5–18.

Masuda, M. & Holmes, T. (1978). Life events: perceptions and frequencies. *Psychosomatic Medicine*, **40**, 236–61.

Michael, S., Lurie, E., Russell, N. & Unger, L. (1985). Rapid response mutual aid groups: a new response to social crises and natural disasters. *Social Work*, **30**, 245–52.

Miller, J. A., Turner, J. G. & Kimball, E. (1981). Big Thompson flood victims: one year later. *Family Relations*, **30**, 111–16.

Murphy, S. (1984). Stress levels and health status of victims of a natural disaster. *Research in Nursing and Health*, **7**, 205–15.

Murrell, S. A. & Himmelfarb, S. (1989). Effects of attachment bereavement and preevent conditions on subsequent depressive symptoms in older adults. *Psychology and Aging*, **4**, 166–72.

Norris, F. H. & Murrell, S. A. (1990). Social support, life events, and stress as modifiers of adjustment to bereavement in older adults. *Psychology and Aging*, **5**, 429–36.

Norris, F. H. & Murrell, S. A. (1988). Prior experience as a moderator of disaster impact on anxiety symptoms in older adults. *American Journal of Community Psychology*, **16**, 665–83.

Norris, F. H. & Murrell, S. A. (1987). Transitory impact of life-event stress on psychological symptoms in older adults. *Journal of Health and Social Behavior*, **28**, 197–211.

Ollendick, D. & Hoffman, M. (1982). Assessment of psychological reactions in disaster victims. *Journal of Community Psychology*, **10**, 157–67.

Okura, K. P. (1975). Mobilizing in response to a major disaster. *Community Mental Health Journal*, **11**, 136–44.

Phifer, J. F. (1990). Psychological and physical sequelae of natural disaster: differential vulnerability among older adults. *Psychology and Aging*, **5**, 412–20.

Phifer, J. F., Kaniasty, K. Z. & Norris, F. H. (1988). The impact of natural disaster on the health of older adults: a multiwave prospective study. *Journal* of Health and Social Behavior, **29**, 65–78.

Phifer, J. F. & Norris, F. H. (1989). Psychological symptoms in older adults following natural disaster: nature, timing, duration, and course. *Journal of Gerontology*, **44**, 207–17.

Phillips, D. L. (1967). Mental health status, social participation, and happiness. *Journal of Health and Social Behavior*, **8**, 285–91.

Poulshock, S. W. & Cohen, E. S. (1975). The elderly in the aftermath of a disaster. *The Gerontologist*, **15**, 357–61.

Radloff, L. (1977). The CES-D scale: a self-report depression scale for research in the general population. *Applied Psychological Measurement*, **1**, 385–406.

Richard, W. (1974). Crisis intervention services following a natural disaster: the Pennsylvania Recovery Project. *Journal of Community Psychology*, **2**, 211–19.

Schulte, P. S. & Murrell, S. A. (1980). *Kentucky's social service needs assessment: the telephone survey*. Louisville, KY: Urban Studies Center, University of Louisville.

Seroka, C. M., Knapp, C., Knight, S., Siemon, C. R. & Starbuck, S. (1986). A comprehensive program for postdisaster counseling. *Social Casework: The Journal of Contemporary Social Work*, **67**, 37–44.

Smith, E. M., Robins, L. N., Przybeck, T. R., Goldring, E. & Solomon, S. D. (1986). Psychological consequences of a disaster. In J. H. Shore (ed.) *Disaster stress studies: New methods and findings*. Washington, DC: American Psychiatric Press, pp. 50–76.

Spielberger, C., Gorusch, R. & Lushene, R. (1970). *STAI manual for the state-trait anxiety inventory*. Palo Alto, CA: Counseling Psychologists, Inc.

Taylor, V., Ross, G. & Quarantelli, E. (1976). *Delivery of mental health services in disasters: the Xenia tornado and some implications* (Disaster Research Center Book and Monograph Series 11). Columbus, OH: The Ohio State University.

Ware, J. E., Johnson, S. A., Davies-Avery, A. & Brook, R. H. (1979). *Conceptualization and measurement of health for adults in the health insurance study vol. III, Mental health* (R-1987/3-HEW). Santa Monica, CA: Rand Corporation.

Part V
Conclusions

18

The structure of human chaos

ROBERT J. URSANO, BRIAN G. McCAUGHEY and
CAROL S. FULLERTON

Even in the midst of the human chaos that results from traumatic events, the excellent contributors to this volume have identified elements of structure. The structure of trauma – predictable responses of individuals and communities – can be either helpful or harmful to health, family, and community. The complex web of human trauma is a challenge to clinicians, researchers, community leaders and, of course, the victims of trauma. Trauma and disasters come in many forms. The victims of these events are widespread and include not only those directly experiencing the disaster but, also, family, friends, disaster workers, and others who may be a part of the 'community of meaning' of the traumatic event. The structure described in the contributions to this volume brings us back to the basic questions addressed in the model presented in the opening chapter. What is the nature of trauma? Who are the victims of traumas and why are they at risk? How does the recovery environment affect outcome?

The stress of trauma

Trauma and disasters are primarily defined by their risk to life, however, this only begins the definition. It is the interaction of the nature of the stressor and its mediators that results in the individual's experience of traumatic stress (Table 18.1). Some groups are exposed to the threat of a traumatic event long before its occurrence. The anticipation of a trauma or a disaster is an infrequently looked at chronic stressor for some populations. Disaster workers, rescue workers, police, fire fighters, and communities in which natural disasters (earthquakes and floods) or manmade disasters (violence, war, and contamination) are common and frequent create a climate of anticipatory stress prior to any traumatic event. Contamination disasters produce long-term anticipatory stress of the possible, the probable and the imagined risks to health and family.

Table 18.1. *Nature of traumatic stress*

Stressors
Risk to life
Exposure to death and the dead
Physical injury
Duration
Loss
Degree of terror
Mediators
Anticipation
Assessment of the threat
Natural versus man-made
Control
Stigmatization
Role constraint
Prior disaster experience

Individuals vary in their assessment of the threat of a traumatic event, even when the risk is dramatic and clearly evident. The interaction between the actual risk and the threat assessment greatly influences behaviors which can be relevant to health and disaster/trauma preparedness. From the decision to walk late at night in an unlit park, to the decision to buy a home near an earthquake fault, the interaction of risk and threat assessment is an ongoing process which affects chronic stress and the identification of high risk individuals and communities.

The distinction between natural, manmade, and technological disasters is, at times, difficult to maintain. Although some disasters can be clearly defined along this continuum (war as manmade and hurricanes as natural), other disasters such as earthquakes are clearly an interaction between natural risk and man's propensity to disregard known risk and create buildings and cities which can become weapons of destruction rained upon individuals during a natural earthquake.

Individual and community responses to disaster vary based on the degree to which they are seen as preventable. Generally, natural disasters are felt to be outside of human control, however, technological disasters – increasingly common in the modern day world – are 'preventable'. The perceived 'preventability' of a disaster is an important area for study in relation to the degree of stress experienced by individuals and communities after a traumatic event. Prior disaster experience is an important moderating variable which can provide some protection from the experiences of traumatic events and certainly affects acute disaster behaviors.

Some aspects of traumatic events, such as exposure to death and the dead, contain no actual risk to life but clearly evoke high anxiety, thoughts of death, dismemberment, and imagined risk. Identification and emotional involvement play an important role in the experience of disaster workers, rescue workers, and families of victims. This mechanism is an important avenue through which the trauma of disaster is propagated to wider and wider circles. Our understanding of this mechanism is in its infancy.

Physical injury is a prominent part of the psychological experience of trauma and disasters. Response to physical injury varies greatly among individuals but it is often a powerful psychological event. Physical injury can increase the risk of psychiatric disease and inevitably leads to a rethinking of one's life goals and perspectives, at least in short run. Understanding acute and long-term responses to physical injury, including organic brain syndromes, is important to managing the psychiatric responses to trauma and disasters. Nearly all studies which have examined the question have shown higher rates of psychiatric disorders among victims of traumatic events who have been injured. Injury adds an additional stressor to the threat and risk experience. Injury brings home the experience of individual vulnerability; creates loss or potential loss of family, friends, and work; and can be a long and enduring reminder of the traumatic event. Each of these aspects of injury contributes to the psychological experience of trauma.

Generally, events which endure the longest have the greatest psychological impact. Thus, the psychological experience of a traumatic event is greatly influenced by the loss of family, friends, income, and community as well as physical injury. These experiences can endure for days, months, and years, affecting behavior, health, and the ability to create a life plan.

All traumatic events create terror. Terror includes the feelings of extreme vulnerability, helplessness, loss of control, uncertainty, and threat to life which are part of the psychological experience of trauma. Human induced trauma may create the highest levels of terror because of the rupture of the expectation of safety and trust in one's environment. Terror is a common experience throughout one's life, however, the intensity and duration of terror in a traumatic event is overwhelming.

A frequently overlooked aspect of trauma is the stigmatization of victims. As individuals, families or communities, we frequently wish to avoid the victims of trauma or disasters. These victims remind us of our own profound vulnerability to unexpected and unplanned for events. Such stigmatization increases the isolation of the victims and frequently their experience of self-blame. Often the stigmatization of the victim is the result

Table 18.2. *Victims of*
trauma and disaster

Children – Elderly
Rescue and disaster workers
Hospital personnel
Community leaders
'The hero'
Single parent
Community of shared meaning

of the expectation and wish of others that the individual 'be all better now'. The length of time required for recovery is difficult for the surrounding community to accept and, at times, endure. Recovery requires the expenditure of resources – time, energy, and money – by the victims' family, friends and community. This burden of the trauma spreads the stresss of the traumatic event to the wider community.

The stereotypic roles of victims and helpers following traumatic events can limit the possible behaviors of victims, rescuers, family members and community leaders. Such role constraints require identification in order to facilitate a return to a more flexible social setting in which the wide range of human experiences – vulnerabilities, strengths, and resources – can be experienced by all members of the disaster community. The experience of 'hero' in particular can be burdensome and disruptive to ongoing family and work environments. At times, the experience of being a hero is felt to be so desirable that it is difficult to give up and return to one's everyday life.

Victims of trauma and disaster

The victims of traumatic events span the entire life cycle, from the young to the elderly. The disaster community and its victims are much more widespread than in the past (Table 18.2). Disasters and traumas may be more common in the modern urbanized world; certainly, the impact of natural disasters on highly developed areas is immense. Disaster victims include those who were not even at the disaster site and who frequently go unrecognized.

Rescue workers, disaster workers (including medical personnel) and community leaders experience intense stress during traumas and disasters. Their exposure to the destruction of the disaster, the primary victims and the pressure under which they work to relieve the distress of others, makes them high risk groups. Denial, humor, and communication with the 'outside' nondisaster world can all be important coping strategies during, and after, the exposure to trauma. Community leaders experience the intense stress of the modern day mass media. Communications can both aid the recovery of a community and can end the career of a community leader. From military commanders to mayors, from company presidents to prime ministers, the management of trauma and disasters is extremely complex and stressful.

Trauma and disasters change individuals' lives. The effects are acute, long term and chronic and may endure for years. The chronic stress of trauma also has a physiologic cost. For most, recovery from the effects of a traumatic event is the norm. For some, the impact of trauma also includes the development of psychiatric disease.

Children are frequently the most disturbing victims of trauma. Child victims stir our feelings of the protection of the innocent and the irrationality of disasters. Child victims of war highlight the way in which trauma robs children of their childhood. Children are swept up into the maelstrom of war through their direct exposure and through the loss of involvement of their family members in their lives. There is now considerable evidence that posttraumatic effects in children can be serious and enduring. The disruption of a child's family and community has profound effects on the child's ongoing development. The children of trauma live in an out of control world of 'big people'.

Elderly people may not necessarily do worse in times of disaster or trauma. Older people bring with them previous experiences and well established community links. The nature of the trauma and the extent of recovery of the community and its resources can be very important to the impact of a disaster on the elderly.

An individual's social and familial role may decrease or increase the risk of psychological distress. Individuals working with the dead of a disaster report taking comfort in recognizing their role in contributing to the families' recoveries. The role of 'hero' in a community may carry increased risk. Family roles and perceived support are also important to the degree of stress. Single parents may be a high risk group because of the demands upon them to provide care to their children and their relatively low level of available supports.

Recovery environment

The contribution of the recovery environment to individual and community responses to traumatic events cannot be overemphasized. Community leaders and families can critically influence the speed and direction of

Table 18.3. *Recovery environment*

Rest
Respite
Safety
Social organization
Outreach programs
Self-help groups
'Talk'
Media director
Housing and work

recovery by first constructing an environment of rest, respite and safety (Table 18.3).

Social supports are an important element in both instrumental and emotional reconstitution; however, high levels of social support may bring their own burden, particularly for women. Individuals reporting high levels of social support may also be asked to provide high levels of social support to others. This additional stress can affect individual psychological recovery.

Communities cannot be assured that those who need help will seek assistance. The elderly, in particular, may both experience more need for independence and have less available means for seeking support. Outreach programs are important in order to reach the wide array of victims. Relying upon victims to reach resources disregards the experience of stigmatization, lack of transportation, and difficulties of communication which characterize disaster communities.

Mobilizing self-help groups can be important to maximizing the use of resources as well as increasing access for those individuals who might not seek formal assistance. The development of indigenous community workers in disaster struck communities can be an important resource. Community leaders can make use of previously existing community structures such as churches, schools, employers and community service organizations to establish outreach programs with which to extend services and support.

The importance of maintaining or reestablishing formal and informal social structures is underlined by the growing literature on debriefing as an important intervention in the recovery process. A known social structure decreases apprehension and distrust and encourages emotional and informational sharing among disaster victims. Empirical studies in this area are lacking. However, clinical observations support the importance of 'talking' among victims to the development of a coherent, cognitive understanding of the trauma events; the sharing of emotional perspectives; and the development of new social networks for ongoing contact. The role of debriefing requires further study. The use of debriefing requires recognition of the phases of a disaster. Rest, respite, and safety are the most important elements in the initial response to the traumatized victim. In the long run, countering the experience of stigmatization and reestablishing normal social ties and activities facilitates the return to normalcy.

Inevitably the return to normalcy takes longer than expected. Community leaders frequently hope to declare recovery accomplished long before the event has transpired. Community leaders can more accurately gauge the return to 'normal' by when their 'in box' no longer contains bills, memos, and complaints related to the disaster.

Respite for community leaders should include respite from the mass media. In large communities with established communication patterns this is frequently not a problem. However, in small communities it can be important to appoint a media director. One of the primary tasks of the media director is to serve as liaison between the community leader and the media, relieving the community leader of day-to-day exposure and fear which the media can engender.

The family is an important unit of study and intervention following a disaster. The development of new housing and business opportunities are important psychological as well as community interventions to reestablish normalcy. Community losses must be recognized and achievements in heroism identified. Community wide events can be important markers of community recovery and serve themselves to reestablish individual and community life.

Directions

Understanding psychological responses of individuals and communities to traumatic events is an important part of recognizing the world in which we live. The variables that influence outcome following a traumatic event are many. The chaos that appears to those in, and outside of, a traumatic event overlays an emergent structure, a structure which is just now becoming evident through research, clinical work, and community concern. The development of community disaster plans, of medical intervention and prevention plans to address the psychological responses to trauma, and the training of leaders in the stresses and resources of traumatic events can greatly help individuals and their communities. The principle of traumatic stress care for individuals and organizations is taking on a form which had been unseen only a few years before. Education about the nature of psychological trauma is needed to increase the knowledge base for intervention and the resources for furthering our understanding. Consultation and mutually helpful relationships among clinicians, researchers, and community leaders are essential to these efforts. These collaborations are potentially mutually enriching, and can serve the best interests of the many yet unidentified victims of future traumas and disasters.

Index

hostage victims (*cont.*)
  feeling of guilt, 38–9
  recovery from trauma, 40–2; awareness
    of pre-existing psychiatric disturbances
    or life events, 41; opportunity to regain
    self-esteem, 41–2
human chaos, structure, 403–10
  see also Stress of trauma
hurricanes, *see* Relocation stress following
  natural disasters
hypomanic behavior after accident, 111

identification of dead bodies, stress, 56–7
Impact of Event Scale, 50, 127
  for Fernald, Ohio, disaster enquiry, 163
indecisiveness after floods, older adults,
  383–4
industrial density, and magnitude of
  disaster, 83
industrialization and increased disaster
  threat, 84
informed of Radioactive Contamination
  Syndrome, 174
injury, denial, 107–8
Injury Severity Score, definition, 105

Kentucky floods, reactions of older adults,
  378–400
  see also Floods
Korean war, long-term sequelae, studies,
  331–8
  see also war sequelae

*Late Effect of Accidental Injury
  Questionnaire*, 127
learned helplessness, posttraumatic stress
  disorder, 12
legal aspects of physical injury, 127–9
literature, terror experiences, 34–7
  voluntary, 34
Loma Prieta earthquake, 1989, natural
  disaster, 137–8, 146–50
  local government problems, 146–7
  mechanical problems, 148
  mental health problems, 150
  news media, 148
  rescue work, 146–7
  residents reactions, 144–5, 149
  resource and support, 146
  rumors, 150

major depression, posttraumatic stress
  disorder, 12
manic behavior after accident, 111
manmade disasters, statistics, 179–80
manmade/natural disasters
  aspects of responsibility, 75

classification, 137–40
global climatic changes, 75
Marina District after Loma Prieta
  earthquake, 148–9
marital state and response to disaster,
  189–90
Marshall's debriefing method, 204–9
media, respite from in small communities,
  409
  see also news media
Memorial Service, Gander military air
  disaster, 276
mental disorders, organic, following
  accident, 125
mental health
  care, on hospital ship, 319–20, 321–2
  effects of floods, older adults, 383–5
  services, intervention and relocation,
    237–42
  team, on hospital ship, 321
mining disaster, Messina, 1908, 79–80
  psychiatric studies, 79–80
Mississippi riverboat disasters, 79
Mitchell's method of debriefing, 209–11
The Monkey's Paw, terror evoked by, 34–5
mood and dioxin exposure, *see* St Louis
  disasters
mortality, 1960s–1970s, 3–4
  trauma, 1987, 4
  violence, 1987, 4
mothers on combat duty, 321
Mount St Helen's volcanic eruption,
  psychological effects, 7
Mozambique war, child victims, 287–305
  background, 287–90
  see also child victims of terrorism,
    Mozambique

natural disasters
  relocation stress, 200–47; *see also*
    relocation stress following natural
    disasters
  statistics, 179–80
natural/manmade disasters, classification,
  137–40
negative response to disaster, 191–2
news media
  Loma Prieta earthquake, 148
  in postearthquake period, 145
  respite from in small communities, 409
Night of the Living Dead, terror evoked by,
  36
Norway
  avalanche disaster, 1986, 254–64; *see also*
    avalanche disaster
  effect of Chernobyl on population, 94–5,
    96–7